OXFORD MEDICAL PUBLICATIONS

Endocrinology
Key questions answered

Endocrinology
Key questions answered

John Laycock
Senior Lecturer, Department of Neuroendocrinology,
Division of Neuroscience and Psychological Medicine,
Imperial College School of Medicine, London

and

Peter Wise
Honorary Consultant Endocrinologist, Department of Endocrinology,
Charing Cross Hospital, London

OXFORD   NEW YORK   TOKYO

OXFORD UNIVERSITY PRESS

1997

Oxford University Press, Great Clarendon Street, Oxford OX2 6DP

Oxford   New York

Athens   Auckland   Bangkok   Bogota   Bombay   Buenos Aires
Calcutta   Cape Town   Dar es Salaam   Delhi   Florence   Hong Kong
Istanbul   Karachi   Kuala Lumpur   Madras   Melbourne
Mexico City   Nairobi   Paris   Singapore   Taipei   Tokyo   Toronto, Warsaw
and associated companies in Berlin   Ibadan

Oxford is a trade mark of Oxford University Press

Published in the United States
by Oxford University Press Inc., New York

ISBN 0 19 2628461

Typeset by
Footnote Graphics, Warminster, Wilts.

Printed in Great Britain by
Biddles Ltd, Guildford & King's Lynn

How to use this book

Readers will have their own approaches to the process of self-assessment. Although the structure of this book is not unique, a few comments may prove useful. Physiology and clinical questions are identified by 'P' and 'C' respectively, and within each section follow a sequence. In physiology, this sequence is merely a systematic coverage of factual material within each domain: we have attempted to provide a probe of knowledge which is equally applicable to the undergraduate and early postgraduate with matching answers and explanations in the subsequent answer section.

In the clinical questions, there is a natural progression from aetiology/pathology to diagnosis and then treatment for most disorders. As in the physiology sections, the sequence of disorders within each chapter generally mirrors the content of *Essential Endocrinology*. However, material which we assess as being beyond the undergraduate syllabus is marked by a double asterisk. We do not wish in any way to dissuade the undergraduate from exploring more advanced concepts and less common disorders: our cutoff point was necessarily arbitrary.

In the more common endocrinopathies, we have provided certain question sequences. Our purpose was to simulate clinical situations, and the logical progression which takes place both in diagnosis and treatment in clinical endocrine practice. These sequences are not marked. Such groups of questions should ideally be identified in advanced and dealt with in one 'sitting'.

Although short answer questions are more appropriate to certain areas of physiology and medicine, their marking system may create problems. We recommend that in the self-marking process, reproducing a catalogued item should attract a positive point, and omitted items a minus point. Items recorded over and above what is listed in the catalogued answer should attract a further point, if it can be shown to be a valid response either by cross-reference to *Essential Endocrinology* or an alternative text.

As in all branches of clinical science, correctness of a catalogued answer may be questioned. Where 'correct' responses appear to challenge previously-held views, we can only urge readers to access the relevant bibliography for a broader discussion than can be provided in the relatively short answer items.

Preface and Acknowledgements

The concept of self evaluation is certainly not new. Yet it was only during our recent preparation of the text for *Essential Endocrinology* (3rd edition) that we conceived the idea of a companion self-assessment volume dedicated to endocrinology. As with *Essential Endocrinology*, the target population is the medical undergraduate and early postgraduate. As in our textbook, the physiological and clinical aspects are dealt with separately within each endocrine domain. The assessment concept embraces both multiple choice and short answer questions. These are not always formulated exactly as might be encountered in examinations, but are structured to systematically and comprehensively probe knowledge and decision-making skills from within a data-bank of almost 400 questions and answers. Some items are indeed factual (as in most of the physiology section); others involve practical choices based on a series of clinical and laboratory variables. Great care has been taken to avoid ambiguities, and all work has been peer reviewed by one or two further endocrinologists or physiologists to ensure accuracy. In this respect we are very grateful to Ann-Marie Cowell, Mary Seed, Saffron Whitehead, Donal O'Shea, and Baldev Singh.

We have not been content just to provide 'yes' or 'no' question responses at the end of each chapter as a simple self-marking exercise. Answers are provided in such a way that correct or incorrect choices are fully clarified and explained, with links (if applicable) to other domains of endocrinology (the endocrine 'web' is surely not a new concept!). As we proceeded in our task, we realised that in providing detailed responses we were actually treading new ground that was not contained in the parent text. This largely resulted from the more practical approaches which formulated themselves in the clinical sections. Accordingly, we identified that not only did this work complement *Essential Endocrinology* but actually supplemented it. From our limited experience, we feel that this concept of supplementation will also apply when the book is partnered with other endocrine textbooks.

We have provided up-to-date references to stimulate further reading, minimizing the number to reduce confusion, but at the same time covering all domains evenly. The bibliography at the end of each chapter contains references to work which is mostly in the nature of a 'review', and is located in the more readily accessible journals. The chosen papers and chapters are written by opinion leaders, and yet avoid bias as much as possible. We have exercised the right to provide or substitute simplified 'topic' titles which clearly identify the area covered by the reference. Many journal articles have confusing or daunting titles which appear 'specialized': yet their discussion sections are often intelligent, informative, and in turn well-referenced. The reader searching for additional information is unlikely to be disappointed.

We are grateful for the confidence with which OUP has approached our concept. If our self-assessment formula is successful, we hope to create updated versions at regular intervals, to keep pace with interesting and important developments in the science and practice of endocrinology.

London   J. L.
June 1997   P. W.

Contents

1 Hormone synthesis, storage, release, and transport (Physiology)

Multiple Choice Questions

P.1 Hormones

a are molecules released by endocrine gland cells into the extracellular fluid to act on specific target cells
b are either proteins, polypeptides, or steroids
c are released from specific nerve endings in the hypothalamus
d can act on target cells near to their point of release, in which case they have a paracrine function
e include energy substrates such as glucose

P.2 Biologically active protein and polypeptide hormones

a are normally synthesized following specific gene transcription in the endocrine cells
b are often derived from larger precursor molecules called pre-prohormones
c when first translated on the ribosomes may contain a signal peptide as part of the amino acid chain
d often exist initially as larger precursor prohormones
e can be produced in their final form within secretory granules

P.3 Steroid hormone synthesis

a necessitates initial gene activation
b generally starts with acetate as the precursor molecule in the endocrine cells
c produces hormones which share a common basic structure
d consists of a series of enzyme-regulated molecular conversions
e requires a minimum time of 20 minutes

P.4 Storage of protein and polypeptide hormones

a within the endocrine cells of origin is rare
b in the endocrine cells is generally by containment in secretory granules
c as free protein in the endocrine cell cytoplasm is common
d is unnecessary because of the rapidity of the synthesis process
e is a function of the liver

P.5   Storage of steroid hormones

a   in large quantities in their endocrine cells is common
b   can occur in the form of fat-soluble esters within the endocrine cell
c   occurs mainly in adipose tissue (in the adipocytes)
d   is represented by the hormone fraction which is bound to plasma-binding proteins
e   is in the form of colloidal gel within the endocrine cells

P.6   The release of specific protein/polypeptide hormones

a   occurs by exocytosis of granule contents
b   is dependent on the endocrine cell membrane potential remaining in the resting state
c   is by simple diffusion across the phospholipid component of the membrane
d   often requires the presence of calcium ions in the extracellular fluid
e   can be elicited in vitro by increasing the potassium ion concentration in the extracellular medium

P.7   Steroid hormones

a   are lipophilic molecules
b   are released as soon as they are synthesized
c   enter the circulation by exocytosis from the endocrine cells
d   fail to be released if the microtubular network in the endocrine cells is disrupted
e   are released in response to specific hypothalamic releasing factors

P.8   In the circulation, specific protein/polypeptide hormones

a   are usually transported entirely as 'free' (i.e. bioactive) molecules in the plasma
b   may be transported within cellular components of the blood
c   are synthesized from circulating precursors by the actions of specific enzymes
d   are transported within the secretory granules
e   are inactivated by very efficient plasma enzymes

P.9   The transport of steroid hormones

a   is partly in association with plasma proteins
b   in the circulation is by linkage to cholesterol molecules
c   is mostly within the lymphatic circulation
d   is mostly as free unbound molecules
e   is a function of the platelets

Short Answer Questions

P.10

Briefly describe the principal features of protein/polypeptide hormone synthesis, storage, and release.

P.11

Briefly explain the role of plasma proteins in the transport of hormones in the circulation

P.12

List *three* ways in which hormones can be transported in the circulation, giving specific examples in each case.

P.13

Briefly identify the general principals of steroid hormone synthesis, storage, and transport.

MCQ Answers

P.1 a **True**. This could be the essence of a definition for hormones.

  b **False**. This statement implies that there is no scope for other types of molecule also being hormones. Examples of other molecular structures having an endocrine (i.e. hormonal) role are quite plentiful, however, including the iodothyronines from the thyroid and the catecholamines from the adrenal medulla which are all amino acid derivatives. Prostaglandins and related compounds are also candidates, as is the latest newcomer to the family nitric oxide.

  c **True**. The hypothalamic releasing and inhibitory factors which act primarily on specific cells of the adenohypophysis (anterior pituitary) are all neurosecretions which are clearly hormones. Other examples are the neurohypophysial (posterior pituitary) hormones which are also synthesized in cell bodies in the hypothalamus.

  d **True**. Paracrine (and autocrine—i.e. acting on their own cells of production) systems all have similarities and overlap with the endocrine system. Definitions become very confusing!

  e **False**. Energy substrates are generally excluded from the strict definition of hormones since they are required by, and influence, all cells of the body.

P.2 a **True**. Most protein and polypeptide hormones are normally synthesized following specific gene activation in the nuclei of their endocrine cells of origin. *However*, certain hormones may be derived from precursors elsewhere (e.g. angiotensin II formed from angiotensin I in the blood).

   b **True**. Protein/polypeptide hormones are initially synthesized as larger precursor molecules (pre-prohormones) with a signal peptide at the amino end of the amino acid chain.

   c **True**. This signal peptide is probably necessary to enable the molecule to enter the endoplasmic reticulum.

   d **True**. After the signal peptide has been enzymatically cleaved from the pre-prohormone the remaining chain of amino acids may not be the final form of the secreted hormone. It is still a precursor, and is called the prohormone. The term is generally used for the final precursor stage; for example angiotensin I, which is formed from its own precursor angiotensinogen in the blood, can be considered to be the prohormone for the bioactive hormone angiotensin II.

   e **True**. This is generally where the final bioactive secretory product of an endocrine cell is produced.

P.3 a **False**. Steroid hormone synthesis does not *necessitate* initial gene activation in order to produce the molecule because precursors will be present in the cell. All that is actually required is activation of specific enzymes in the endocrine cells, accomplished by the appropriate stimulus. These enzymes then catalyse specific conversions of precursors to final product.

   b **False**. Most steroid hormone production in the endocrine cells actually starts with cholesterol or a cholesterol derivative as the initial precursor. However, it is true that endocrine cells generally have the capacity to synthesize *some* cholesterol from acetate (like most cells, in fact), in which case a certain proportion begins with acetate at the initial precursor.

   c **True**. The structure of all steroid hormones is based on the common cyclopentanoperhydro-phenanthrene nucleus.

   d **True**. This is the basis for the synthesis of all steroid hormones, the activity of the specific enzymes providing the regulatory points at which controlling factors exert their influence on the production process.

   e **False**. Relevant enzyme activity can be increased/decreased very rapidly so that the steroid hormones can be synthesized fast (in much less that 20 minutes). The proviso here is that sufficient precursor molecules are available for conversion at each stage of the synthesis process.

P.4 a **False**. It is very common for most protein and polypeptide hormones.

   b **True**. Storage of protein and polypeptide hormones within secretory granules in the endocrine cell cytoplasm is common. (The detection of secretory granules inside cells is a useful indicator of their possible endocrine function.)

   c **False**. This is unlikely to be a major storage form of these hormones, but it may occur. In some cases the protein/polypeptide hormones may be associated with other molecules or elements (e.g. insulin with zinc inside pancreatic β cells).

   d **False**. The synthesis process requires the switching on of specific genes, the transcription of mRNA, the translation to protein, and the ultimate transfer to secretory granules (or cytoplasm), all of which usually takes a certain time. The presence of stored hormone is therefore essential for rapid release.

   e **False**. The liver has many storage functions, it is an endocrine gland in its own right (e.g. somatomedins), and is an extremely important inactivation and excretory organ regarding hormone metabolism. It is *not*, however, a general storage organ for protein and polypeptide hormones, which this question implies.

P.5 a **False**. Probably because steroids are lipid-soluble (and therefore would rapidly diffuse out of their cells of synthesis immediately when synthesized) they are produced on demand.

   b **True**. It is likely that small quantities of steroid hormones, in the form of their esters, are stored in the phospholipid component of the endocrine cell membranes.

   c **False**. Adipose tissue *is* a source of certain steroid hormones following enzyme-catalysed conversion from circulating precursors (e.g. oestrogens from androgens) but it is not a general storage organ for them.

   d **True**. The plasma proteins, both specific globulins and relatively nonspecific albumins, bind steroid hormones thus providing an important storage form within the circulation. This also provides the hormones protection from being degraded by non-target tissues.

   e **False**. The only hormones known to be stored as colloid in cell-lined follicles are the thyroidal iodothyronines which are iodinated amino acid derivatives not belonging to either of the two main groups of hormones (the protein/polypeptide and steroid groups; see P.1b above).

P.6 a **True**. This is the most common way of releasing the previously synthesized and stored hormone from the endocrine cell.

   b **False**. It is found that hormone release is related to the *depolarization* of the plasma cell membrane ('excitation – secretion coupling').

   c **False**. Since protein and polypeptide molecules are not lipid-soluble, they would not be released into the extracellular medium simply by diffusion across the phospholipid component of the membrane.

   d **True**. Certainly, the process of exocytosis requires calcium ions. (Depolarization of the cell membrane, whether nerve terminal or endocrine cell, is associated with the movement of calcium ions from extracellular to intracellular fluids.)

e **True.** This has the effect of depolarizing the plasma cell membrane, and results in excitation of the secretory process.

P.7 a **True.** The steroids are lipophilic, unlike protein/polypeptide hormones.

b **True.** Since they are lipophilic, they would diffuse across the plasma cell membrane down their concentration gradient as soon as they were synthesized.

c **False.** They are not stored in granules hence they are not released by exocytosis.

d **False.** The microtubular network is involved in release processes associated with the protein/polypeptide hormones in particular (e.g. the movement of granules to the plasma membrane). Disruption of the microtubular network will not have any effect on the release of steroid hormones which occurs by simple diffusion.

e **False.** The hypothalamic releasing factors stimulate the release of specific protein/polypeptide hormones from the adenohypophysis (anterior pituitary) which may in turn stimulate the synthesis pathways of specific steroid hormones. However, they do not have any major *direct* effect on the release of steroid hormones.

P.8 a **False.** Although the unbound component may be large, and is the bioactive component, many (if not most) protein and polypeptide hormones have specific plasma protein 'carriers' to which a proportion is bound.

b **True.** Certain hormones may be transported partly in specific cells (e.g. in platelets, as for vasopressin).

c **True.** One example is the synthesis, in the circulation, of angiotensin II (an octapeptide) from its precursor prohormone angiotensin I (a decapeptide).

d **False.** The *contents* of the secretory granules (i.e. the hormone molecules) are released into the circulation; the granules only exist within the endocrine cells.

e **True.** While the liver and kidneys function as primary organs for inactivation (and excretion), plasma protease enzymes do exist for specific hormones. For example, oxytocin is rapidly inactivated by a circulating oxytocinase present during pregnancy.

P.9 a **True.** The major part of released steroid hormones is transported in the circulation bound to specific plasma proteins. An important role of the binding plasma proteins is to provide a storage form of the lipophilic steroid hormones, which otherwise would be continually removed from the circulation due to diffusion into (non-target) cells.

b **False.** Cholesterol is an important precursor for steroid hormones, but it has nothing to do with their transport in the blood.

c **False.** While some hormone is likely to be present in the lymph, it is mostly within the vascular circulation.

d **False**. Most of the circulating steroid hormones in the blood are not present as free (i.e. unbound molecules), but as molecules bound to plasma proteins which may have a high affinity for specific hormones (e.g. certain globulins such as transcortin, sex hormone binding globulin) or have a high binding capacity (i.e. albumins).

e **False**. There is no knowledge of any steroid hormone being transported in platelets, unlike certain protein/polypeptide molecules (see P.8b above).

SAQ Answers

P.10

Synthesis of protein/polypeptide hormones is similar to that for any other protein and involves gene activation, nuclear transcription, and translation processes. The latter process takes place on ribosomes on the rough endoplasmic reticulum since the final hormone molecule is for export from the cell. Initially, a precursor molecule is synthesized; this pre-prohormone contains a signal (or leader) peptide sequence which appears to be necessary in order for the molecule to enter the endoplasmic reticulum. Once the signal peptide has been removed, the resulting prohormone is usually incorporated into granules in the Golgi complex. Within the granule the final end-products including the bioactive hormone are produced from the prohormone by enzymatic cleavage. The hormone molecules are often stored within their cells of production within secretory granules, although some hormone may be present in the cytoplasm as free protein or in the form of complexes with other intracellular components (e.g. insulin with zinc atoms). Many polypeptide and protein hormones are transported as free (i.e. unbound) molecules. In addition, it is clear that many protein/polypeptide hormones are also present in the circulation bound to plasma proteins, the bound component in dynamic equilibrium with the free unbound hormone. The protein-bound hormone component provides a store of readily available molecules within the circulation.

P.11

Plasma proteins play an important role in the transport (and storage) of hormones in the circulation. Many hormones (H), once in the circulation, enter a dynamic equilibrium with various plasma proteins (P), as illustrated by the following equilibrium equation:

[H] [P] $<=>$ [HP], where HP is the hormone–plasma protein complex

$$Kd = \frac{[H] \, [P]}{[HP]}, \text{ where Kd is the dissociation constant}$$

These proteins transport hormones to varying degrees depending on (a) their affinity and (b) their capacity to bind them. Binding proteins with a high affinity for the hormone are usually specific globulins (e.g. thyronine binding globulin, transcortin, sex hormone binding globulin, etc.) which may not have a large capacity for transporting hormone because their concentration in the blood is low. Other proteins, particularly albumin, do not have a particularly high affinity for any specific hormone but their concentration in the blood is quite high (relatively) and so they have a larger capacity for binding hormones generally. Because plasma proteins preferentially bind hormone relative to non-target cells, they have a protective role which also provides a form of storage within the circulation. In the presence of higher affinity target cells (related to the presence of specific hormone receptors) free hormone is taken up and this upsets the equilibrium between bound and free hormone fractions and the plasma protein concentration. Thus, more bound hormone dissociates from plasma binding protein in the vicinity of the target cells.

P.12

Hormones can be transported in three ways:

1. As free (i.e. unbound) hormone; this component is biologically active and can bind to its specific receptors in its target cells. All hormones are present in the blood as free molecules to some extent, usually as a part of the total hormone concentration in the blood. The iodothyronines, tri-iodothyronine and thyroxine, are two examples of hormones which are present as free molecules in the blood, albeit as a minute proportion of their total concentrations in the blood.

2. Bound to its plasma binding protein concentrations (see answer to P.11 above). Examples of hormones bound to specific binding proteins are numerous; for example, the iodothyronine hormones (mentioned above) are bound to the specific plasma protein thyronine binding globulin (TBG).

3. Transported in a cell element (e.g. the polypeptide hormone vasopressin, present within platelets in the blood).

P.13

Steroid hormones are synthesized when required by the activation of enzymes already available within the cells, which convert precursors into intermediate and final, released forms. The chain of reactions is initiated when the endocrine cell is stimulated; once the lipid-soluble steroid hormone is synthesized it diffuses out of the cell into the general circulation. Very little, if any, steroid hormone is stored within the cells of production but there is some evidence for minor quantities being stored in the cell membrane as esters. Once in the circulation the steroid hormone enters a dynamic equilibrium with specific plasma proteins to which it binds. The binding of hormone protects the hormone from being immediately metabolized by non-target cells into which it could readily diffuse, and provides a circulating store of hormone available in areas of greater affinity for the hormone such as in the region of target cells. This bound component, which is biologically inactive, is in dynamic equilibrium with the small (usually minute) quantities of hormone present in the unbound—'free'—state. It is the latter component which is bioactive.

References

Physiology

Topic: Possible functions of plasma steroid-binding proteins.

Hammond, G. L. (1995). *Trends in Endocrinology and Metabolism*, **6**, 298–304.

Topic: Regulation of steroid hormone production.

Stocco, D. M. *et al.* (1996). *Endocrine Reviews*, **17**, 221–44.

2 Hormone mechanisms of action (Physiology)

Multiple Choice Questions

P.1 A protein or polypeptide hormone

a generally binds to receptors in target cell membranes

b can only bind to its one (unique) receptor

c produces its effects by stimulating an intracellular second messenger system

d cannot have a genomic effect on protein synthesis

e always exerts its effects by generating intracellular cyclic AMP

P.2 Receptors for a specific protein or polypeptide hormone

a have a high affinity for that hormone

b can also bind other molecules (ligands)

c are often associated with membrane-bound G proteins

d can have intrinsic tyrosine kinase activity

e are often present in the membranes of intracellular organelles (e.g. mitochondria)

P.3 The G proteins:

a consist of three subunits (α, β, and γ)

b are linked to catalytic units such as adenyl cyclase

c mediate the actions of steroid hormones

d may be stimulatory or inhibitory

e if abnormal, can prevent specific hormones from exerting their intracellular effects

P.4 Intracellular second messenger systems

a mediate the intracellular effects of protein hormones

b amplify the initial signal provided by the circulating hormone

c can induce the nuclear transcription process

d may be influenced by changes in the intracellular calcium ion concentration

e are specific for particular hormones

P.5 Intracellular receptors

a span the target cell membrane, with both intracellular and extracellular domains

b can be located within target cell nuclei
c are 'activated' when they bind to their hormones
d dissociate from heat-shock proteins in the presence of a ligand
e consist of different functional domains one of which binds to a nuclear gene sequence specific for that hormone–receptor complex

P.6 *Steroid hormones*

a bind to intracellular receptors
b form hormone–receptor complexes in cytoplasm or nucleus
c influence the gene transcription process
d generally exert their effects by stimulating intracellular second messenger systems
e can exert rapid effects (within minutes) indicating non-genomic actions

P.7 *Hormones*

a must enter their target cells in order to exert nuclear effects
b if steroids, can cross the cell membranes by diffusion
c cannot enter their target cells if they are proteins
d can stimulate protein synthesis by inducing the formation of active transcription factors
e may influence membrane transport mechanisms by initially stimulating protein synthesis

P.8 *Second messenger systems*

a are activated by iodothyronine and steroid hormones
b are generated following activation of membrane-bound G proteins
c include cytoplasmic calcium ions
d often involve cascades of protein phosphorylations
e link the hormone–membrane receptor binding process to the intracellular actions of that hormone

Short Answer Questions

P.9

Identify two hormones which activate the cyclic AMP second messenger system and *briefly* outline the principal features of this mechanism of action.

P.10

Identify the different regions of a typical steroid hormone receptor and *briefly* explain how hormone–receptor interaction can lead to stimulation of protein synthesis.

P.11

Briefly describe two mechanisms of action associated with polypeptide/protein hormones which can increase the intracellular calcium ion concentration.

MCQ Answers

P.1 a **True**. Protein and polypeptide hormones are lipophobic and are, generally, not able to simply diffuse through the lipid membrane, nor do they have specific channels through which they can enter the cell. In order to influence cell activity they (usually) have to first bind to cell membrane receptors.

b **False**. Any hormone can have more than one type of receptor molecule each one of which can be linked to a different intracellular second messenger system. For example, the neurohypophysial hormone, vasopressin, can bind to at least two different receptor subtypes (V_1 and V_2 receptors). Furthermore, one hormone may have a certain affinity for the receptor of another hormone. An example here would be the affinities of insulin-like growth factors for the insulin receptor.

c **True**. Binding of the hormone to its cell membrane receptor elicits the generation of the intracellular second messenger which then 'transmits' the message from membrane to within the cell cytoplasm, thus mediating the action of the hormone.

d **False**. Some second messengers activate intracellular transcription factors which can then stimulate protein synthesis. Growth hormone (somatotrophin) and insulin are examples of protein/polypeptide hormones which bind to membrane receptors but have genomic effects on protein synthesis.

e **False**. While cyclic AMP (cyclic adenosine monophosphate) is certainly *one* second messenger, there are many others including cyclic GMP (cyclic guanosine monophosphate), inositol triphosphate, calcium ions and tyrosine kinase.

P.2 a **True**. The affinity of a receptor for a specific protein or polypeptide hormone is a key determining factor determining whether a particular cell will respond, or not, to that hormone. The receptor affinity for the hormone must be greater than that of any circulating binding proteins in the blood.

b **True**. In addition to the specific hormone, other hormones and agonist/antagonist molecules can also bind to the same receptor, depending on the relative affinities of the receptor for these different ligands.

c **True**. The membrane receptors are usually associated with other molecules, in particular the various G proteins which link the receptor to the catalytic units (enzymes such as adenyl cyclase).

d **True**. Certain receptors have intracellular regions which act as tyrosine kinases and can, when activated, phosphorylate tyrosyl units in intra-cellular proteins. These phosphorylated proteins can then activate (phosphorylate) yet other proteins leading to intracellular cascades of activity within the cell.

e **False.** Since these hormones are lipophobic they do not usually enter their target cells. Consequently, their receptors are generally found spanning the cell membranes. There is some evidence to suggest that some protein/polypeptide hormones may enter their target cells to varying degrees (e.g. by endocytosis), so it is feasible that they bind to intracellular receptors. However, so far there is no evidence in support of this notion.

P.3 a **True.** When the hormone binds to its receptor molecule the G protein subunits dissociate. The α subunit binds guanine nucleotides; in the in-active state it binds guanosine diphosphate (GDP) but when activated, following hormone–receptor binding, it binds guanosine triphosphate (GTP). This activated form then dissociates from the β–γ subunits and in turn activates the catalytic unit in the membrane.

b **True.** Various catalytic units (sometimes called effectors) are linked to different G proteins. Adenyl cyclase, guanyl cyclase, phopholipase C, and phospholipase A2 are examples of catalytic units linked to G proteins. Indeed, more than one G protein may be activated by the initial hormone–receptor interaction at the cell membrane.

c **False.** Steroid hormones are lipophilic and usually diffuse through the cell membranes. They can then bind to their specific intracellular receptors.

d **True.** The various G proteins which have been cloned include G_s (stimulatory) and G_i (inhibitory) proteins for the catalytic unit adenyl cyclase.

e **True.** Certain endocrine disorders have been linked to defective G proteins (e.g. certain familial forms of type II diabetes mellitus).

P.4 a **True.** Protein hormones generally cannot diffuse through the lipid membrane of their target cells and therefore, in order to influence intracellular activity, have to attach to membrane receptors which then activate an intracellular second messenger system. This is how the message reaching the cell via the hormone is transmitted into the cell cytoplasm to produce the hormone's physiological effect.

b **True.** One hormone–receptor linkage can activate many catalytic units (e.g. adenyl cyclase molecules) which then induce the formation of a number of second messenger molecules (e.g. cyclic AMP) resulting in amplification of the initial signal.

c **True.** Certain activated (phosphorylated) intracellular proteins act as transcription factors and enter the cell nucleus, binding to specific recognition sites on genes.

d **True.** Intracellular control systems certainly exist; for instance, an increase in the cytoplasmic calcium ion concentration is associated with an inhibition of the cyclic AMP second messenger system and/or a stimulation of the cyclic GMP system.

e **False.** Cyclic AMP is a second messenger for many different hormones, for instance, as are many others including the inositol triphosphate and calcium ion systems.

P.5 a **False.** This is true for membrane receptors, *not* intracellular receptors. Membrane receptors belong to different families of receptor proteins which span the cell membranes. The extracellular domains (or regions) will contain loci for the binding of specific molecules (or ligands) such as hormones and their agonists/antagonists, while their intracellular domains may contain loci for the binding of catalytic units such as tyrosine kinase.

b **True.** The intracellular receptors are usually located in the cytoplasm, where they bind with their hormone molecules before entering the cell nucleus, or they may already be present within the nucleus.

c **True.** Once the hormone–receptor complex has been formed in the cytoplasm, it usually enters the nucleus where it can induce its genomic effect (i.e. it has become active).

d **True.** There are various heat-shock proteins in cells. They may act as protective elements which bind to the cytoplasmic receptors, preventing them from binding to their nuclear recognition sites in the absence of the hormone signal. When the hormone molecules enter the cell they bind to their receptors, releasing the heat-shock proteins.

e **True.** The intracellular receptors may have five or six different domains, the functions of each of which are not all understood presently. One of these domains (the C region) is a specific nuclear recognition site which binds to the DNA sequence called the hormone-responsive element. Other regions (A and B regions) incorporate the specific transcription elements which induce the transcriptive process.

P.6 a **True.** Steroid hormones such as the gonadal hormones (androgens, oestrogens, and progestogens) and the adrenocortical hormones (e.g. glucocorticoids, mineralocorticoids), as well as the iodothyronines which are amino acid derivatives, all cross cell membranes. In their target cells they bind to intracellular receptors which are usually located in the cytoplasm but may also be in the nucleus.

b **True.** The binding of steroid hormone to its intracellular receptor results in the formation of a complex which can enter the cell nucleus. The hormone–receptor binding process may also occur within the nucleus.

c **True.** Most of the known effects of steroids involve stimulation of RNA synthesis and subsequent new protein formation, as a result of gene transcription activation within the nucleus. New protein synthesis is a process that takes a finite time (around 40–50 minutes) so that most steral effects are not detectable within this minimum time span (increased RNA synthesis can be detected within 20 minutes, however).

d **False**. Second messenger systems are unnecessary for mediating steroid hormone actions since they can enter cells and influence their activity directly.

e **True**. Recent evidence supports the view that some steroid hormones exert rapid effects on cells which cannot be mediated by the longer-term activation of the gene transcription process. Such non-genomic effects (e.g. of aldosterone on some ion transport processes) have been usually, but not invariably, detected in cell cultures.

P.7 a **False**. Protein and polypeptide hormones can stimulate intracellular second messenger systems which may include the activation of cytoplasmic transcription factors. These factors can then enter the nucleus where they can stimulate (or inhibit) the gene transcription process.

b **True**. Steroids are lipophilic and can therefore diffuse through the lipid component of the cell membrane. However, it is possible that some hormones which are not steroids can also enter cells (e.g. iodothyronines); these hormones may have specific membrane transport systems which assist their entry into the cells.

c **False**. Some protein hormones, for example, somatotrophin (growth hormone), have been located inside cells and could have entered by endocytosis.

d **True**. Any hormone which stimulates protein synthesis by increased transcription in the nucleus has to either produce an intracellular transcription factor as a consequence of second messenger system activation (e.g. protein/polypeptide hormone mechanism), or by binding to intracellular receptors to enter the nucleus where the complex acts as the transcription factor (e.g. steroid hormone mechanism).

e **True**. If a hormone stimulates new protein synthesis it is quite possible that these new proteins are involved in specific membrane transport mechanisms. For example, aldosterone probably stimulates renal sodium ion reabsorption by stimulating Na^+/K^+-ATPase synthesis.

P.8 a **False**. Both the iodothyronines (e.g. thyroxine) and steroid hormones enter their target cells and bind to intracellular receptors, so their mechanisms of action do not involve second messenger system activation.

b **True**. Many membrane receptors are linked to G proteins of which there are at least five, including stimulatory and inhibitory (G_s and G_i) proteins which influence different catalytic units, or which influence the same catalytic units but in opposite ways. An example of the latter is the stimulation or inhibition of adenyl cyclase depending on whether the hormone–receptor linkage is associated with the activation of the G_s or the G_i protein.

c **True**. Cytoplasmic calcium ions are involved in many cells as second messengers, inducing enzyme activity within the cells and also influencing other second messenger systems (e.g. by inhibiting adenyl cyclase activity).

d **True**. Once the hormone has bound to its membrane receptor, protein phosphorylation cascades result in the activation of different intracellular pathways. Amplification of the initial signal thus becomes possible. Also, different effects can be produced by the same hormone, depending on which enzymes become phosphorylated.

e **True**. This is the purpose of intracellular second messengers.

SAQ Answers

P.9

Many protein and polypeptide hormones activate the adenyl cyclase–cyclic AMP system and these include hypothalamic releasing hormones such as thyrotrophin releasing hormone, adenohypophysial hormones such as corticotrophin, the neurohypophysial hormone vasopressin (via V_2 receptors), catecholamines (via β receptors), parathyroid hormones, and glucagon. The principal features to include in the answer are: hormone binds to membrane receptor; the associated G protein is activated; dissociation of α, β, and γ subunits takes place; consequently adenyl cyclase is activated; adenosine triphosphate is converted to cyclic AMP; this molecule acts as the intracellular messenger; it activates protein kinase A; there is a phosphorylation cascade and the various activated proteins produce the effects associated with the initial stimulus provided by the hormone. Finally, phosphodiesterase enzyme inactivates cyclic AMP. There is plenty of scope for amplification of the initial stimulus; many cyclic AMP molecules can be produced from the initial hormone–receptor binding, and each cyclic AMP can activate many kinases.

P.10

The different regions, or domains, of a typical steroid hormone receptor would be: (i) the A and B regions, with specific transcription activator components; (ii) the C region which corresponds to the DNA binding domain (commonly incorporating the two zinc 'fingers' which each consist of a zinc ion bound to cysteine-histidine structures and which are believed to play a role in DNA binding); (iii) D region, function still unclear; and (iv) the E region which has multiple functions including the hormone recognition element (HRE); (v) some receptors also have an F region, function also still unclear.

Once formed, the hormone-receptor complex binds to its hormone responsive element on the DNA in the cell nucleus and specific gene transcription is activated. The exon coding sequences are spliced into specific messenger RNA (mRNA) molecules which leave the nucleus through pores in the membrane. The mRNA is then translated into new protein molecules on the ribosomes in the cytoplasm.

P.11

Certain polypeptide and protein hormones bind to their membrane receptors and through their G proteins activate membrane-bound phospholipase C enzyme which initiates the formation of phosphatidylinositol diphosphate (IP_2) from membrane phospholipids. The IP_2 molecule is itself a precursor for phosphatidyl inositol triphosphate (IP_3), which can stimulate the movement of calcium from intracellular stores, such as microsomes, into the cytoplasm. The intracellular calcium ion concentration is normally kept very low in comparison with its concentration outside the cell (compare 10^{-7} M inside with 10^{-3} M outside). Calcium ions are themselves important mediators ('third' messengers) of intracellular activity, so an increase in its intracellular concentration results in activation of a variety of metabolic pathways.

Phospholipase C also initiates the synthesis of another molecule from IP_2 called diacylglycerol, which activates intracellular protein kinase C (which exists in a number of isomeric forms expressed in different tissues). Protein kinase C then activates other intracellular proteins which include transcription factors and other enzymes which can stimulate a variety of metabolic pathways within the cell as well as opening calcium channels in the outer (plasma) membranes, for example.

References

Physiology

Topic: Inositol phosphates, calcium ions and cell regulation.

Balla, T. *et al.* (1); Putney, J. W. *et al.* (2) (1994). *Trends in Endocrinology and Metabolism*, **5**, 250–5 (1) and 256–60 (2).

Topic: Isoforms of cyclic nucleotide phosphodiesterases.

Beavo, J. A. (1995). *Physiological Reviews*, **75**, 725–48.

Topic: Regulation of intracellular protein transport to the nucleus.

Jans, D. A. *et al.* (1996). *Physiological Reviews*, **76**, 651–86.

Topic: Signal transduction involving receptors, G-proteins and adenylate cyclases.

Posner, A. *et al.* (1996). *Clinical Science*, **91**, 527–37.

Topic: Nuclear hormone receptor genes.

Ralff, C. J. *et al.* (1995). *Annual Review of Medicine*, **46**, 443–54.

Topic: Non-genomic actions of steroids.

Wehling, M. (1994). *Trends in Endocrinology and Metabolism*, **5**, 347–53.

3 Control of the endocrine system (Physiology)

Multiple Choice Questions

P.1 The concentration of a hormone in the blood

a can consist of protein-bound and free hormone fractions
b is normally regulated within quite precise physiological limits
c if increased, invariably leads to the clinical hypersecretion state
d is independent of the rate of its metabolic removal from the blood
e is always maintained in a constant, basal state

P.2 A bioactive hormone can be removed from the circulation by

a endocytosis, after binding to its membrane receptors
b being filtered at the renal glomeruli and excreted into the urine
c being inactivated in the liver
d exhalation from the lungs
e being degraded by circulating enzymes

P.3 The free (unbound) plasma hormone concentration

a is directly regulated by the central nervous system, unlike the bound component
b when increased is usually inversely proportional to the secretion of that hormone
c is usually decreased during pregnancy
d is normally under negative feedback control
e will decrease initially, whenever there is an increase in plasma binding protein concentration

P.4 Feedback regulation

a is negative if the hormone secretion increases in response to a rise in its circulating concentration
b is negative when it applies specifically to protein/polypeptide hormones
c only operates between the circulating concentration of that hormone and its production from the relevant endocrine gland
d does not apply to any hormone secretion following a diurnal variation
e if disrupted can lead to clinical disease

P.5   *Negative feedback loops*

a   operate between circulating free hormone and its endocrine gland source
b   link all hormones to the adenohypophysis (anterior pituitary)
c   can relate changes in a plasma metabolite or ion concentration to the secretion of the hormone which influences it
d   do not operate between the endocrine gland and its hormone when the principal source of that hormone is ectopic
e   are sometimes called 'indirect' if they involve the central nervous system

P.6   *A positive feedback loop*

a   is one in which the production of a hormone is enhanced by increasing circulating levels of that hormone
b   is inherently chaotic if allowed to run unchecked
c   can be a local effect (autocrine) (i.e. a direct stimulation of the cell by its own hormonal secretion)
d   is more common than the alternative negative feedback loop
e   can be direct and/or indirect (i.e. acting back on the hypothalamus)

P.7   *Endocrine negative feedback*

a   is an important physiological action of all hormones
b   can be overridden by other, more potent, controlling factors
c   operates whether the hormone comes from an endogenous or an exogenous source
d   can operate even when the controlling factor is a hormone degradation product
e   switches into positive feedback before returning to its normal negative mode

P.8   *Clinical endocrine disease can result from each of the following*

a   the production of autoantibodies to hormone receptors
b   a mutation in the gene associated with the synthesis of a bioactive hormone
c   liver disease (e.g. cirrhosis)
d   chronically reduced calorific intake
e   an increase in hormone production following a reduction in the negative feedback loop controlling its synthesis and release

Short Answer Questions

P.9

Briefly explain the concept of negative feedback in an endocrine system using insulin as the hormone model.

P.10

Briefly identify three mechanisms by which a hormone (or more specifically its bioactivity) can be removed from the circulation.

P.11

Explain the term *positive feedback* as applied to endocrinology, giving an example to illustrate your answer.

MCQ Answers

P.1 a **True**. Many (if not most) hormones are to some extent transported in the blood either bound to circulating plasma proteins or free (i.e. unbound).

   b **True**. Otherwise conditions associated with hypo- and hypersecretion would be commonplace.

   c **False**. It is quite possible for there to be an increase in total circulating hormone concentrations without any clinical condition developing (e.g. during pregnancy), because usually most of the increase in circulating hormone is bound to the plasma proteins.

   d **False**. The concentration of hormone in the blood is a balance between its production (secretion) rate and rate of its metabolic removal (by inactivation and excretion).

   e **False**. Many hormones are released in pulses (e.g. those associated with the adenohypophysis), are stimulated by appropriate stimuli (e.g. increases in dietary substrates entering the blood after a meal), and/or follow diurnal variation patterns. Therefore, even though blood sampling may suggest a steady state due to the integration of pulses of released hormone, the concentrations usually do alter because of the effects of stimuli.

P.2 a **True**. This is certainly one way in which a hormone will be removed from the circulation.

   b **True**. Some small hormones can be filtered by the renal glomeruli, enter the tubular fluid, and are excreted in the urine.

   c **True**. The liver is the main organ in the body associated with the inactivation of hormones. Many metabolites or conjugated forms are then excreted into the duodenum via the bile ducts, or re-enter the circulation to be excreted by the kidneys.

d **False**. There is no knowledge of any hormone being removed from the body in expired air.

e **True**. There are circulating enzymes which can inactivate specific hormones (or convert one molecular form to a less active form, e.g. angiotensin II, to the less active angiotensin III by angiotensinase), sometimes particularly under specific conditions (e.g. oxytocin by oxytocinase during lactation).

P.3 a **False**. Although the central nervous system is associated with the control of synthesis and release of certain hormones it plays no part in determining the free component in the circulation specifically.

b **True**. Usually under these conditions any increase in free hormone concentration will inhibit further synthesis/release by negative feedback.

c **False**. During pregnancy most endocrine glands undergo hyperplasia and there is an increase in total circulating levels of many hormones (main exceptions being LH and FSH which are inhibited by the high concentrations of circulating oestrogens and progesterone). However, the free hormone concentration does not change much because there is a greater protein-bound fraction.

d **True**. It is the free, unbound component which is bioactive and one of its physiological actions will be to influence its own production by operating a negative feedback loop.

e **True**. This must be the case if there is an increase in plasma binding protein concentration, since the dynamic equilibrium between the free hormone and the plasma protein concentrations will be disturbed, initially.

P.4 a **False**. This would be a positive feedback effect.

b **False**. Negative feedback loops can operate for hormone systems independent of their molecular class, whether the hormone is a protein, a polypeptide, a steroid, a catecholamine, or any other molecular form.

c **False**. Some feedback loops involve the controlled metabolic product rather than the hormone itself (e.g. glucose on glucagon release, calcium ion concentration on parathormone release).

d **False**. Feedback regulation can still operate perfectly normally on a hormone which is also following diurnal variation imposed by the hypothalamus or higher centres of the brain (c.f. the adenohypophysial–adrenal axis with reference to corticotrophin and cortisol production).

e **True**. If the endocrine gland 'escapes' from the feedback regulation by its own hormone then clinical disease can follow (e.g. tertiary hyperparathyroidism).

P.5 a **True**. This is an important action of many hormones.

b **False**. Many hormones controlled by adenohypophysial hormones do indeed exert negative feedback effects on the adenohypophysis. However the term 'negative feedback' is a general one which refers to all hormones, and not simply to those linked in some way to the adenohypophysis.

c **True**. A negative feedback loop operates between the hormone and/or the metabolic product it controls and the endocrine gland producing that hormone.

d **False**. Providing that the ectopic hormone is truly bioactive, it will quite successfully switch off the normal site of production of that hormone (i.e. the specific endocrine gland) (The same is true if the circulating hormone level is raised as a result of exogenous administration of that hormone, e.g. iatrogenic Cushing's syndrome.)

e **True**. This term then allows use of the term 'direct' to apply to the negative feedback loops which operate between specific hormones and the adenohypophysis (cf. hypothalamo–adenohypophysial adrenal, thyroidal, and gonadal axes). Some endocrinologists refer to 'long' and 'very long' loops. 'Short' (or 'auro') feedback loops relate the adenohypophysial hormones to their hypothalamic releasing/inhibiting factors.

P.6 a **True**. It is worth remembering that it is the free, unbound hormone which is active in exerting the positive feedback control, as it is for negative feedback loops.

b **True**. Positive feedback loops only operate when the 'correct' conditions apply. As soon as those conditions are altered the normally operational negative feedback steps in.

c **True**. The granulosa cell of the developing follicle is an excellent example of such a local—autocrine—effect exerted by oestrogens.

d **False**. The positive feedback loops are relatively rare; the negative feedback loop, on the other hand, is a common feature of endocrine gland regulation.

e **True**. The same distinction applies to the positive feedback as to the negative feedback loops (see P.5e).

P.7 a **True**. All hormones have to be controlled and the negative feedback relating the concentration of (free) hormone is one important physiological effect that they can exert.

b **True**. Any endocrine cell is controlled by the integration of multiple influences, stimulatory and inhibitory. The inhibitory influence exerted by a negative feedback loop can therefore be overridden by a more powerful stimulus such as a stressor.

c **True**. An important example of the inhibitory influence of exogenously administered hormone is the use of steroids in clinical treatment. The endogenous production of the steroid can be inhibited by the negative feedback influence of exogenous hormone acting on the appropriate endocrine gland.

d **False**. Degradation products are generally biologically inactive.

e **False**. Negative and positive feedback effects are not normally linked in any routine way.

P.8 a **True**. Autoimmune diseases of various endocrine systems are now recognized as relatively common (e.g. thyroid diseases, etc).

b **True**. A mutated gene will be associated with an abnormal product lacking the biological effects of the normally produced hormone molecule.

c **True**. Liver disease such as cirrhosis will be associated with defective inactivation and excretion of hormones. In addition, a disturbance in plasma protein synthesis is likely, and this would affect the hormone binding capability of the blood resulting in altered hormone binding protein dynamics.

d **True**. Reduced caloric intake will affect various aspects of normal endocrine physiology. For example, reduced reproductive function is associated with starvation in both sexes.

e **False**. A decreased negative feedback on an endocrine gland will simply result in increased hormone production until the appropriate level of hormone has been restored.

SAQ Answers

P.9

Negative feedback is a common means of controlling an endocrine gland's production of a hormone. It relates the plasma concentration of the free (i.e. unbound) hormone—or of a metabolite, substrate, or ion regulated by that hormone—to the endocrine gland producing that hormone. For example, as the level of hormone in the blood rises it increasingly inhibits its own production, operating on its own endocrine gland cells to decrease synthesis and/or release of further hormone.

For insulin as the hormone model, the principal direct negative feedback loop operating on its cells of production, the β cells of the pancreatic islets of Langerhans, involves the energy substrate, glucose. An initial stimulus for insulin release is an increase in blood glucose levels. Insulin acts on muscle, adipose tissue, and liver to increase the removal of glucose from the blood. As the glucose concentration decreases as a consequence of the actions of insulin, the stimulus is reduced and less insulin is released (and synthesized). This is a negative feedback loop (see Fig. 3.1).

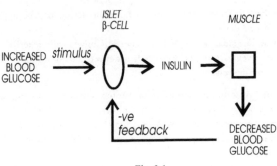

Fig. 3.1

P.10

It is necessary, for the stability of any endocrine control system, for there to be appropriate mechanisms for the inactivation or removal of the hormone released in response to the initial stimulus. A hormone (more specifically its bioactivity) can be removed from the circulation in various ways:

1. It can be removed by being taken up by its target cells (e.g. by endocytosis). The binding of a polypeptide/protein hormone to its membrane receptor can initiate the uptake process.

2. It can be inactivated by circulating enzymes; examples of hormones which are inactivated by enzymes in the blood are oxytocin (particularly during pregnancy and lactation) and glucagon.

3. It can be inactivated by the liver, which is by far the most important site of hormone (and other active molecules such as drugs, etc.), inactivation, and removal in the body. Some hydrophobic hormones such as steroids are first converted to water-soluble products by a conjugation process; an example is the conversion of cortisol to its glucuronide or its sulphate, both of which can then be excreted by the kidneys.

4. It can be excreted unchanged by the kidneys. In addition to the renal excretion of some hormones after conversion to water-soluble products, some hormones can be excreted directly (i.e. unchanged). Naturally, these have to be relatively small and water-soluble. One example is the nonapeptide, vasopressin, which is excreted in the urine at a concentration which is directly proportional to its concentration in the blood.

Any of these mechanisms for the removal of a hormone from the circulation would provide an answer to the question.

P.11

Positive feedback occurs when an increase in hormone concentration stimulates the further production of that hormone. This is in direct contrast to the far more common negative feedback loop, and requires specific conditions to prevail in order for it to operate. The only clear examples of positive feedback occur within the hypothalamo–adenohypophysial–ovarian axis. Normally, oestrogen (i.e. 17β-oestradiol) has a negative feedback effect on its own production by acting on the hypothalamus to inhibit gonadotrophin releasing hormone release, and on the adenohypophysis to inhibit luteinizing hormone (LH) and follicle stimulating-hormone (FSH) release (indirect and direct negative feedback loops, respectively) during the menstrual cycle. However, if oestradiol rises to a sufficiently high concentration in the blood for at least 36 hours, in the absence of high levels of circulating progesterone, then it stimulates hypothalamus and adenohypophysis culminating in increased LH and FSH production. This is a positive feedback effect resulting in the crucial LH and FSH surges which are necessary for the process of ovulation to occur.

References

Physiology.

Topic: Early glucocorticoid feedback inhibition on corticotrophin release.

Shipston, M. J. (1995). *Trends in Endocrinology and Metabolism,* 6, 261–6.

Topic: Gonadal hormone (steroid and peptide) feedback effects on the pituitary gonadotrophs.

Shupnik, M. A. (1996). *Trends in Endocrinology and Metabolism,* 7, 272–6.

4 The hypothalamo–hypophysial axis (Physiology)

Multiple Choice questions

P.1 The endocrine function of the hypothalamus

a is associated with neurones which terminate at the median eminence
b is associated with its link to the hypophysis (pituitary gland)
c is to influence directly 'higher' centres of the brain
d is provided by neurosecretions released into the blood
e is to provide a link between the central nervous and endocrine systems

P.2 The endocrine secretions from the hypothalamus

a are produced by glial cells
b are transported along nerve axons to their target cells
c are steroid hormones
d control the release of the adenohypophysial (anterior pituitary) hormones
e reach the neurohypophysis (posterior pituitary) via a local portal circulation

P.3 Thyrotrophin releasing hormone (TRH)

a is a glycoprotein
b is released from hypothalamic neurones
c acts by stimulating cyclic AMP generation in its target cells
d stimulates the release of prolactin from the adenohypophysis
e inhibits the production of iodothyronines from the thyroid

P.4 Gonadotrophin releasing hormone (GnRH)

a is a polypeptide
b is released into the hypothalamo–hypophysial portal circulation
c acts on adenohypophysial cells called gonadotrophs
d is released in pulses
e stimulates the release of both follicle-stimulating hormone and luteinizing hormone

P.5 Somatostatin

a is synthesized in hypothalamic neurones projecting to the median eminence b binds to membrane receptors on its target cells

c stimulates the production of the adenohypophysial hormone somato-trophin (growth hormone)

d inhibits the release of thyrotrophin (thyroid-stimulating hormone) from the adenohypophysis

e stimulates insulin release from pancreatic β cells

P.6 *Corticotrophin releasing hormone (CRH)*

a is present in various parts of the brain

b acts in synergy with the neurohypophysial hormone, arginine vasopressin

c stimulates the release of corticotrophin (adrenocorticotrophic hormone, ACTH)

d is released in response to various stressors

e has its release inhibited by glucocorticoids

P.7 *Dopamine:*

a is a hypothalamic neurosecretion

b is released into the hypothalamo–hypophysial portal blood

c is synthesized in chromaffin cells of the adrenal medulla

d stimulates the release of prolactin

e directly inhibits the release of somatotrophin (growth hormone)

P.8 *The pituitary gland (hypophysis)*

a is an endocrine gland

b lies within a bony cavity called the sella turcica

c consists of anterior, intermediate, and posterior lobes

d is derived entirely from an upwards growth of ectodermal tissue from the primitive pharynx

e produces hormones which regulate the activity of various endocrine glands

P.9 *The anterior lobe of the pituitary (the adenohypophysis)*

a is comprised of a single identifiable type of secretary cell

b is the source of various growth-stimulating (trophic) hormones

c receives a major part of its blood via a special portal system linking it to the hypothalamus

d is extensively innervated by fibres originating in the hypothalamus

e is an important regulator of other endocrine glands

P.10 *The adenohypophysial (anterior pituitary) hormones*

a are all polypeptide hormones

b are produced in greater quantities when the pituitary is transplanted under the renal capsule

    c are stored in intracellular secretory granules
    d are released in pulses
    e can operate negative feedback loops back to specific hypothalamic neurones

P.11 Control of adenohypophysial hormone release

    a is chiefly by paracrine influences from nearby cells
    b is lost following section of the pituitary stalk
    c is partly by the negative feedback effects of other hormones
    d depends entirely on hypothalamic neurosecretions
    e is lost during pregnancy

P.12 Somatotrophin (growth hormone)

    a is a protein
    b is synthesized in hypothalamic neurones
    c is partly transported in the blood bound to specific plasma proteins
    d enters its target cells through specific channels in the membrane
    e activates the inositol triphosphate second messenger system in its target cells

P.13 The release of somatotrophin

    a is mainly by exocytotic secretion (from granules)
    b is pulsatile
    c follows a circadian rhythm
    d is under dominant inhibitory control from the hypothalamus
    e is stimulated by hyperglycaemia

P.14 The effects of somatotrophin:

    a are initiated by the binding of hormone to its membrane receptor
    b are mediated at least partly by the insulin-like growth factors (IGF-I and IGF-II)
    c include the stimulation of lipolysis
    d are attenuated by androgens
    e are absent after puberty

P.15 Prolactin

    a is a hypothalamic neurosecretion
    b is a protein hormone
    c is released in a pulsatile manner
    d acts on receptors located on gonadal cells
    e actions are mediated by the intracellular messenger cyclic AMP

P.16 Prolactin synthesis

    a is stimulated by various stressors

b only occurs during pregnancy and lactation
c is increased in the presence of oestrogens
d is always basal in males
e increases when the pituitary is transplanted to another vascular site in the body

P.17 *Prolactin's actions*

a are primarily to stimulate milk ejection during lactation
b are similar to those of placental lactogen
c include participation in the body's overall immune response
d are potentiated by the hormone oxytocin
e to some extent overlap those of somatotrophin (growth hormone)

P.18 *Thyrotrophin (thyroid-stimulating hormone, TSH)*

a is a glycoprotein
b is synthesized in adenohypophysial cells called thyrotrophs
c production is partly regulated by negative feedback effects of calcitonin
d stimulates the uptake of iodide in its target cells
e in excess causes a goitre

P.19 *Follicle-stimulating hormone (FSH)*

a is synthesized in the adenohypophysis
b is a polypeptide
c consists of two chains of amino acids
d is located in cells which also contain luteinizing hormone
e is only produced in females

P.20 *Luteinizing hormone (LH)*

a structurally resembles the human placental hormone chorionic gonado-trophin (hCG)
b binds to its receptors on Leydig cells in the testes
c stimulates the aromatization of androgen to oestrogen
d induces ovulation
e is produced in increasing quantities during pregnancy

P.21 *Corticotrophin, also known as adrenocorticotrophic hormone (ACTH)*

a is synthesized initially as a prohormone called pro-opiomelanocortin (POMC)
b is synthesized by macrophages in the blood
c release is inhibited by mental and physical stressors
d stimulates the production of androgens from the adrenal cortex
e in excess can stimulate melanocytes to increase pigmentation

P.22 The neurohypophysis (posterior pituitary)

a develops as a down-growth of neural tissue from the hypothalamus
b contains cells called pituicytes
c is separated from the adenohypophysis by a pars intermedia
d produces hormones which are neurosecretions
e releases hormones into the hypothalamo–hypophysial portal circulation

P.23 Vasopressin

a is synthesized in cell bodies of the supraoptic and paraventricular nuclei
b is converted to a hormone called oxytocin in the neurohypophysis
c is released from large magnocellular neurones
d is released directly into the general circulation
e can be produced by certain tumours (ectopic production)

P.24 Vasopressin

a is synthesized in suprachiasmatic neurones in the hypothalamus
b is released as a neurotransmitter from terminals in the nucleus tractus solitarius
c is released in pulses
d follows a circadian rhythm
e production decreases with age

P.25 The hormone vasopressin

a is synthesized as part of a larger precursor called provasopressin
b is a nonapeptide differing from angiotensin II by only two of its amino acids
c has at least two different receptors
d can produce a profound tachycardia when present in high concentrations in the circulation
e is a powerful vasoactive molecule on isolated arterioles

P.26 Vasopressin acts

a first by binding to its G protein-linked receptors
b to increase renal water transport through a V_2 receptor-linked mechanism
c on all its target cells by generating the intracellular second messenger cyclic AMP
d on vascular smooth muscle as a constrictor
e as a corticotrophin releasing hormone

P.27 The production of vasopressin

a is stimulated by hypervolaemia
b is increased when osmoreceptors in the hypothalamus are stimulated
c will rise when the arterial baroreceptors are stimulated

d is increased by various stressors
e increases whenever oxytocin is released to stimulate milk ejection

P.28 In the kidneys vasopressin

a has an antidiuretic action
b increases proximal tubular water reabsorption
c stimulates the transfer of water channels to the apical membranes of its target cells
d acts as a natriuretic hormone
e can stimulate urea reabsorption in the collecting ducts

P.29 Oxytocin

a is synthesized in hypothalamic neurones
b is released from nerve endings in the median eminence
c is released following stimulation of tactile receptors around the nipples
d is released as a neurotransmitter within the central nervous system
e release is non-pulsatile

P.30 The synthesis of oxytocin

a is inhibited by prolactin
b is absent in males
c increases throughout pregnancy
d is essential for parturition
e is stimulated by increased stretch of uterine muscle at parturition

P.31 The actions of oxytocin

a involve its initial uptake by endocytosis in its target cells
b include the contraction of vascular smooth muscle
c include contraction of the myoepithelial cells lining the milk ducts in the breasts during lactation
d generally require the presence of ovarian steroids
e are absent when circulating vasopressin levels are reduced

Short Answer Questions

P.32

Draw a labelled diagram illustrating how the hypothalamus regulates adeno-hypophysial (anterior pituitary) function.

P.33

List the principal adenohypophysial hormones and their hypothalamic releasing/

inhibiting hormones, identifying whether the main influence is stimulatory or inhibitory in each case.

P.34

Illustrate by means of a simple diagram the concepts of negative and positive feedback involving the hypothalamo–adenohypophysial–ovarian axis.

P.35

By means of a labelled diagram indicate: (a) the source, and (b) the principal actions of, somatotrophin. Include the somatomedins (IGF-I and IGF-II) in your answer.

P.36

Illustrate by means of a simple diagram a neuroendocrine reflex arc using oxytocin in the efferent pathway.

P.37

Briefly describe the effects of vasopressin on water regulation and vascular smooth muscle, identifying which receptors are involved in each case.

P.38

Draw a diagram showing how changes in plasma osmolality (osmolarity) and blood pressure alter vasopressin release.

MCQ Answers

P.1   a **True**. Most of the hypothalamic hormones are neurosecretions released from neurone terminals in the median eminence. Two of them, vasopressin and oxytocin, are released mainly from nerve terminals in the neurohypophysis (posterior pituitary).

    b **True**. Most of the hormones produced by the hypothalamic neurones act on specific adenohypophysial (anterior pituitary) target cells to stimulate or inhibit the release of adenohypophysial hormones. Two hypothalamic hormones are actually released from the neurohypophysis (see a above).

    c **False**. While there are many direct connections between the hypothalamus and other 'higher' centres in the brain, these are associated with neurosecretions acting as transmitters (i.e. across synapses). It is possible, however, that certain hypothalamic hormones influence other parts of the brain but it is likely that indirect pathways would be involved (e.g. via an adenohypophysial hormone's actions, or by hormones released by peripheral endocrine glands in response to stimulation by the appropriate adenohypophysial hormone).

d **True**. The hypothalamic hormones are released either into the special hypothalamo–hypophysial portal system linking the median eminence to the adenohypophysis, or into the venous outflow from the neurohypophysis.

e **True**. Many stimuli which may originate in the higher centres of the brain (e.g. behavioural or environmental) influence body function through the endocrine system, the link being the hypothalamo–hypophysial axis.

P.2 a **False**. The hypothalamic secretions are produced by neurones, not by the glial cells whose functions remain largely unknown. (However, glial cells do produce cytokines, which may be important in mediating the hypothalamo–hypophysial response to an immune challenge, for example.)

b **False**. The hypothalamic secretions are all released from nerve endings, but the endocrine neurosecretions must, by definition, reach their target cells through the circulation.

c **False**. None of the hypothalamic endocrine neurosecretions is a steroid; they are *almost* all polypeptides (dopamine is strictly a catecholamine, i.e. an amino acid derivative).

d **True**. Most, if not all, hypothalamic neurosecretions influence target cells in the adenohypophysis, either stimulating or inhibiting their production of specific hormones.

e **False**. Two of the hypothalamic neurosecretions reach the neurohypophysis via the neurones of the hypothalamo–hypophysial nerve tract. From the nerve terminals in the neurohypophysis these neurosecretions, vasopressin and oxytocin, are released into the general circulation.

P.3 a **False**. It is a tripeptide. None of the hypothalamic neurosecretions is as large as a protein (or glycoprotein) hence the term 'peptidergic neurones' for the hypothalamic neuroendocrine cells.

b **True**. It is released by neurone terminals in the median eminence; it then enters the hypothalamo–hypophysial portal blood system which carries it to the adenohypophysis.

c **True**. Certainly in the adenohypophysis (its main target tissue) cyclic AMP is generated by TRH, and cAMP is associated with thyrotrophin release. However, it now seems likely that another important mechanism of action is via the phosphoinositol–protein kinase C pathway. (How TRH acts when released as a neurotransmitter in the brain is not yet established.)

d **True**. In addition to its important role as a thyrotrophin releasing hormone, TRH acts as a stimulator of prolactin synthesis and release. In addition it may have other peripheral and central (e.g. as a neurotransmitter) effects.

e **False**. There is no evidence for any direct action of TRH on the thyroid gland.

P.4 a **True**. GnRH is a decapeptide derived from the cleavage of a larger proGnRH precursor which itself is initially synthesized as an even larger pre-proGnRH molecule.

b **True**. It is a hypothalamic neurosecretion released from neurones originating in the medial preoptic area. From the nerve terminals in the median eminence it enters the hypothalamo–hypophysial portal system. It is then transported via this portal blood system to its major target organ, the adenohypophysis.

c **True**. The gonadotroph cells in the adenohypophysis produce the gonadotrophins in response to stimulation by GnRH. The two gonadotrophins, luteinizing hormone and follicle stimulating hormone, are produced in both sexes.

d **True**. All hypothalamic neurohormones are released in pulses; GnRH is normally released in pulses at a rate of approximately 3/hour. If administered as a chronic infusion GnRH has an inhibitory effect on gonadotrophin release, emphasizing the importance of the pulsatile nature of the hypothalamic secretion.

e **True**. GnRH stimulates the gonadotrophs which produce both follicle stimulating hormone (FSH) and luteinizing hormone (LH). While it is likely that subsets of gonadotroph cells exist, synthesizing one or the other of the two gonadotrophins, double immunostaining of the cells for FSH and LH clearly identifies a population which synthesizes *both* molecules.

P.5 a **True**. Somatostatin is a tetradecapeptide released from hypothalamic nerves terminating in the median eminence from where it enters the hypothalamo–hypophysial portal blood system which transports it to the adenohypophysis. Somatostatin is also synthesized in other parts of the body (e.g. intestinal tract, δ cells of the pancreatic islets of Langerhans) as well as in hypothalamic neurones projecting to other parts of the brain.

b **True**. It binds to G protein-linked membrane receptors and this then results in *decreased* cyclic AMP and intracellular free Ca^{2+} concentrations.

c **False**. Somatostatin reaches the somatotrophs of the adenohypophysis where it exerts an inhibitory effect on somatotrophin (growth hormone) release. This inhibitory influence is normally the lesser effect from the hypothalamus, the dominant effect being stimulatory via the 44 amino acid polypeptide somatotrophin releasing hormone (growth hormone releasing hormone, GHRH, also called somatoliberin).

d **True**. Somatostatin inhibits thyrotrophin and somatotrophin release from the pituitary. Indeed, somatostatin is generally an inhibitory hormone wherever it has an effect (in the intestinal tract, in the pancreatic islets, in the brain (where it functions as a neurotransmitter).

e **False.** In the pancreatic islets of Langerhans somatostatin is produced by the δ cells. It has a paracrine inhibitory effect on neighbouring α-cells and β cells which produce glucagon and insulin respectively (this is interesting, because glucagon and insulin have opposing effects on glucose metabolism).

P.6 a **True.** CRH has been found in the cerebral cortex and the limbic system, where it functions as a neurotransmitter, as well as in the hypothalamus. It coexists with arginine vasopressin in paraventricular neurones which release their neurosecretions into the hypothalamo–hypophysial portal system.

b **True.** Arginine vasopressin has relatively little CRH activity of its own, but markedly potentiates the activity of the hypothalamic 41 amino acid polypeptide called CRH (or corticoliberin).

c **True.** The stimulation of corticotrophin release from the adenohypophysial corticotrophs is the main action of CRH. However, it is associated with other effects, for instance inhibiting gonadotrophin release in acute stress.

d **True.** Activation of the hypothalamo–hypophysial–adrenal axis, which includes the release of hypothalamic CRH, is a key feature of the body's response to stressors.

e **True.** Negative feedback loops operated by glucocorticoids from the adrenal glands to the adenohypophysis (direct negative) and hypothalamus (indirect negative) are important in the control of the hypothalamo–hypophysial–adrenal axis. Interestingly, large amounts of CRH, for instance released in severe stress, can overcome the negative feedback of the glucocorticoids.

P.7 a **True.** Dopamine is found in many neurones in the brain, where it acts as a neurotransmitter; however some hypothalamic neurones release it as a neurosecretion into the hypothalamo–hypophysial portal system.

b **True.** Dopamine is released from nerve endings in the median eminence into the hypothalamo–hypophysial portal system which transports it to its target cells in the adenohypophysis where it acts as an inhibitory hormone.

c **True.** Dopamine is a catecholamine, and it is a precursor of adrenaline and noradrenaline in the chromaffin cells of the adrenal medulla. Other chromaffin cells of neural crest derivation also produce these catecholamines.

d **False.** Dopamine is a powerful inhibitor of prolactin release, and dopamine agonists such as bromocryptine are of use clinically in the treatment of prolactinomas.

e **False.** Dopamine, as well as being the main prolactin inhibitory hormone, is also associated with decreased somatotrophin release, for example. However, the latter effect is by a central action as a neuro-transmitter, probably acting at least partly directly on the hypothalamic neurones producing somatotrophin releasing hormone.

P.8   a   **True**. The pituitary gland produces various hormones which have effects on various tissues. Some of the hormones act specifically as stimulatory hormones on other endocrine glands.

b   **True**. This is particularly relevant when considering the growth of pituitary tumours when downward growth is restricted by the bony fossa, increasing the likelihood of growth upwards towards the optic chiasma.

c   **True**. In many vertebrates the intermediate lobe is the source of specific hormones such as melanocyte stimulating hormone. In humans the intermediate lobe is almost non-existent except during pregnancy, when it develops markedly.

d   **False**. It is actually a fusion of tissue derived from an upwards growth of tissue from the primitive pharynx (which becomes typical endocrine secretory cell tissue—the adenohypophysis) and neural tissue growing downwards from the developing brain (the neurohypophysis).

e   **True**. Various 'trophic' (i.e. stimulating growth of) hormones which stimulate other endocrine glands such as thyroid, adrenal cortex, and gonads are produced by the adenohypophysis (which is sometimes described as the 'leader of the endocrine orchestra', the 'conductor' presumably being the hypothalamus!)

P.9   a   **False**. It is comprised of several clearly defined types of secretory cell. Using simple staining techniques three types of cell were originally identified: eaosinophilic, basophilic, and chromophobe cells. With more recent immunostaining techniques cells associated with the synthesis of specific adenohypophysial hormones can be identified, these being gonadotrophs (producing the gonadotrophins), corticotrophs (producing corticotrophin), thyrotrophs (producing thyrotrophin), lactotrophs (producing prolactin), and somatotrophs (producing somatotrophin).

b   **True**. Most (if not all) pituitary hormones are trophic, i.e. they stimulate the growth of other tissues, whether these be specific endocrine gland cells (e.g. of the thyroid, the adrenal cortex and the gonads) or more general tissues (e.g. by somatotrophin).

c   **True**. This link, the hypothalamo–hypophysial portal system, is central to the control of adenohypophysial function by the hypothalamus. It consists of a primary capillary network in the hypothalamic median eminence which receives blood from the superior hypophysial artery, portal vessels (sinusoidal) which collect the blood from the primary capillary plexus and which descend through the pituitary stalk, and a secondary capillary network within the adenohypophysis.

d **False**. There is some autonomic innervation of the adenohypophysis but little evidence for much direct innervation originating in the hypothalamus.

e **True**. The thyroid, the cortex of each adrenal, and the gonads are the principal examples of peripheral endocrine glands which produce hormones under the primary controlling influence of specific adenohypophysial hormones.

P.10 a **False**. A polypeptide is a chain of less than 100 amino acids. Most adenohypophysial hormones are proteins (somatotrophin and prolactin) or glycoproteins (thyrotrophin and the two gonadotrophins). Only corticotrophin is a polypeptide, consisting of 39 amino acids.

b **False**. The connection with the hypothalamus is lost when the pituitary gland is transplanted to the renal capsule, so the adenohypophysis no longer receives the stimulatory effect of the hypothalamic releasing hormones. Note, however, that prolactin secretion would increase because, unlike all other adenohypophysial hormones, it receives a dominant *inhibitory* influence from the hypothalamus which will be lost following pituitary section.

c **True**. The adenohypophysial cells are typical endocrine cells with obvious secretory granules which contain synthesized hormones.

d **True**. All adenohypophysial hormones are released in pulses. This is because they are mainly controlled by the hypothalamic hormones which themselves are released in a pulsatile fashion. A pulsatile release pattern is often crucial for the physiological effects of the adenohypophysial hormones, particularly the gonadotrophins.

e **True**. There is evidence for short (or auto) negative loops operating between specific adenohypophysial hormones and the hypothalamic neurones which produce the relevant releasing, or inhibitory, hormones.

P.11 a **False**. The *chief* influence has to be the hormonal control exerted by the hypothalamus; the negative feedback influence on the adenohypophysis is also very important. Paracrine effects undoubtedly exist but they are more of a modulatory influence only.

b **True**. Consequently, the production of most adenohypophysial hormones decreases and the adenohypophysis generally atrophies. The lactotroph cells which produce prolactin thrive, however, and prolactin synthesis actually increases because of the loss of the dominant inhibitory influence of hypothalamic dopamine.

c **True**. The hormones produced by those peripheral endocrine glands controlled largely by adenohypophysial hormones exert important (direct) negative feedback control on the adenohypophysis (e.g. thyroidal iodothyronines on thyrotrophin production, cortisol on corticotrophin production, oestrogens or androgens on gonadotrophin production). In addition, negative feedback loops (indirect) operate between the peripheral endocrine gland hormones and the hypothalamic releasing and inhibitory hormones.

d **False**. Hypothalamic neurosecretions are generally the most important controlling influences on adenohypophysial hormone production, but they are most definitely not the entire story (e.g. see c above).

e **False**. Control of adenohypophysial hormone production continues throughout pregnancy although there may be certain changes in sensitivity to particular stimuli. However, the pituitary gland does hypertrophy during pregnancy and most adenohypophysial hormones are produced in greater quantities, the exceptions being luteinizing hormone and follicle-stimulating hormone (which are inhibited by the negative feedback effects of rising levels of oestrogens).

P.12 a **True**. Somatotrophin is a single chain protein of 191 amino acids (in humans) which has a high homology with another adenohypophysial hormone, prolactin. It is mainly synthesized as a molecule of approximately 22 kD from a 27 kD prosomatotrophin precursor, which in turn is cleaved from the initial pre-prosomatotrophin molecule.

b **False**. Somatotrophin is synthesized in specific cells of the adeno-hypophysis called somatotrophs. Its production is under the control of the hypothalamus however via hypothalamic neurosecretions, particularly somatotrophin releasing hormone (SRH, also known as growth hormone releasing hormone, GHRH) and somatotrophin inhibitory hormone (better known as somatostatin).

c **True**. Various binding proteins are associated with somatotrophin in the blood, and approximately 70% of the hormone is estimated to be present in the bound form. Interestingly, the main binding protein (GHBP) has an amino acid sequence which is almost identical to the extracellular sequence of the somatotrophin receptor. The role of the binding proteins for this large protein hormone is unclear.

d **False**. Somatotrophin binds to membrane receptors; however, there is evidence that some somatotrophin may enter target cells, probably by endocytosis.

e **False**. Somatotrophin activates membrane receptor-bound tyrosine kinase, and consequently various intracellular proteins are phosphorylated, some of which induce gene transcription resulting in new protein synthesis.

P.13 a **True**. Most protein (and polypeptide) hormones are stored within secretory granules, and their release into the extracellular fluid by exocytosis is the principal mechanism by which these molecules (such as the large 191 amino acid protein somatotrophin) can be secreted.

b **True**. A pulsatile form of release is characteristic of all adeno-hypophysial hormones, and is related to their control from the hypothalamus since the hypothalamic releasing and inhibiting hormones are themselves released in pulses.

c **False**. It is certainly released in more prominent bursts of pulses during slow wave sleep (stages III and IV) but many other factors (e.g. hormonal and metabolic) also influence the pattern of release and no clearly defined circadian rhythm has so far been identified.

d **False**. The dominant influence from the hypothalamus is by the pulsatile release of somatoliberin (somatotrophin releasing hormone). The inhibitory hormone somatostatin is of lesser importance.

e **False**. *Hypoglycaemia*, not hyperglycaemia, is a powerful stimulus for somatotrophin release. (Somatotrophin's actions will tend to increase blood glucose, for instance when released by stressors.) A clinical stimulation test for pituitary somatotrophin function (carried out under carefully supervised conditions) is to administer insulin which induces a hypoglycaemia which, in turn acts as a powerful stimulus for somatotrophin release.

P.14 a **True**. Somatotrophin is a (relatively) large protein hormone which binds to a membrane receptor in its target cells. Tyrosine kinase phosphorylation following hormone–receptor binding is the initial step in a cascade of intracellular protein phosphorylations which mediate the actions of the hormone.

b **True**. One of the principal actions of somatotrophin is to stimulate the synthesis of insulin-like growth factors IGF-I and IGF-II (also known as the somatomedins) which mediate various effects once attributed directly to somatotrophin.

c **True**. Somatotrophin stimulates lipolysis in adipose tissue, and consequently plasma non-esterified fatty acid levels increase.

d **False**. The combined effects of somatotrophin and increased circulating levels of gonadal steroids (androgens and oestrogens) give rise to the pubertal growth spurt. Gonadal steroids probably exert much of their effect by stimulating somatotrophin release.

e **False**. The precise role of somatotrophin in the adult is not yet clearly defined, and plasma levels do decline with age. However, there is evidence that somatotrophin does have effects in adults which are not necessarily easily quantifiable (e.g. on the quality of life—perhaps a 'feel good' factor!) and current therapies with this hormone indicate that it exerts various beneficial effects.

P.15 a **False**. Prolactin is an *adenohypophysial* hormone released from lactotrophs in the anterior pituitary tissue. While its production is under the control of the hypothalamus it is not produced by any neurones (indeed, this would be unlikely since it is a large protein).

b **True**. The structure of prolactin is similar to that of somatotrophin (and human placental lactogen). It consists of 199 amino acids, and as for other similar hormones it is cleaved from a larger precursor proprolactin molecule.

    c **True**. All adenohypophysial hormones are released in pulses directed by the pulsatile release of the hypothalamic releasing and inhibiting hormones, in the case of prolactin mainly by the inhibitory dopamine (thyrotrophin releasing hormone normally having a lesser influence as a releasing hormone for prolactin).

    d **True**. Prolactin receptors have been located on Leydig cells in the testis and corpus luteal cells in the ovary. The functions of prolactin in the gonads (particularly in humans) remain unclear. One action may be to stimulate the synthesis of LH receptors in these target cells. It is important to remember that hyperprolactinaemia is associated with *decreased* gonadal function, however.

    e **False**. Binding of prolactin to its membrane receptor is associated initially with activation of a tyrosine kinase (called JAK2) which then promotes the activation of other molecules (including phospholipase C which stimulates the formation of inositol triphosphate and diacylglycerol). Cyclic AMP does not seem to be involved.

P.16 a **True**. Prolactin is indeed a 'stress hormone', being released as part of the body's adaptive response to various stressors. Its release by stressors may be mediated partly by VIP (vasoactive intestinal peptide).

    b **False**. Prolactin exerts its main physiological effects during pregnancy and lactation, but it is produced throughout life, in males as well as in females, and has various effects on target tissues in addition to the breasts (e.g. possible effects include actions on the immune system and on renal function).

    c **True**. Oestrogens have an important influence on prolactin release, this effect probably occurring both at pituitary and hypothalamic levels (oestrogen receptors have certainly been located in both the pituitary and central nervous system).

    d **False**. Stimuli such as stressors (for instance) can increase prolactin release in both sexes. Furthermore, there is evidence for a diurnal variation in both sexes (although the amplitude of the pulses is generally smaller in males than in females).

    e **True**. Prolactin is the only adenohypophysial hormone which is normally subject to a dominant inhibitory influence from the hypothalamus. More than one hypothalamic prolactin inhibitory factor has been suggested, but the main inhibitory influence is by dopamine. Remove the lactotrophs from this influence and prolactin secretion increases, as occurs when the pituitary is transplanted to another part of the body.

P.17 a **False**. Prolactin stimulates milk synthesis and secretion from the alveolar cells into the ducts. It does not have any contractile effect on the myoepithelial cells lining the ducts and does not have any influence on milk ejection, this being an action associated with another hormone (cf. oxytocin).

b **True.** There is certainly an overlap between the actions of prolactin and human placental lactogen, a hormone which is synthesized by the placenta (i.e. only during pregnancy, normally). Both hormones stimulate the growth and development of the breasts in the presence of other necessary hormones such as the oestrogens and progesterone.

c **True.** There is increasing interest in the role of prolactin on cells of the immune system. It stimulates lymphocyte proliferation, for example.

d **False.** The actions of the two hormones are quite different although they are both released by the same tactile stimulus on mechanoreceptors (tactile, or stretch, receptors) around the nipple.

e **True.** There is a small 16% homology (i.e. approximately 16% of the amino acid sequences are identical) between somatotrophin and prolactin. There is a similar, minor, overlap between the actions of the two hormones which is probably of little physiological relevance.

P.18 a **True.** The other glycoprotein hormones from the adenohypophysis are the two gonadotrophins, luteinizing hormone and follicle-stimulating hormone.

b **True.** These cells can be identified by appropriate immunostaining techniques.

c **False.** Calcitonin comes from the thyroid parafollicular cells which lie between the thyroid follicles. It is a polypeptide hormone involved in calcium regulation and has nothing whatsoever to do with the hypothalamo–adenohypophysial–thyroid axis.

d **True.** Thyrotrophin stimulates many aspects of iodothyronine synthesis in the thyroid follicular cells, including stimulation of the iodide pump in the apical membranes which allows iodide to enter the cells against an electrochemical gradient. Other actions of thyrotrophin include the stimulation of thyroglobulin synthesis, the activation of iodide to a more reactive form ('activated iodine', maybe iodine radicals), the iodination of tyrosyl groups which comprise approximately 8% of the thyroglobulin molecule, the coupling reaction which results in tri- and tetra-iodothyronine formation on the thyroglobulin molecule, the exocytosis of the iodinated thyroglobulin into the central follicle, and the endocytosis of colloid from the follicle back into the follicular cells.

e **True.** Thyrotrophin, as its name suggests (trophin means 'nourishes, stimulates growth of'), stimulates growth of the follicular cells which can result in increased size of the thyroid (i.e. goitre). One cause of goitre (endemic goitre) is the lack of iodide in the diet resulting in decreased iodothyronine production. The negative feedback normally exerted by the circulating iodothyronines on the hypothalamo–hypophysial axis is diminished and consequently the increased release of thyrotrophin stimulates the follicular cells in an attempt to increase iodothyronine production. One effect of thyrotrophin is to stimulate hypertrophy of the follicular cells while another is to produce more follicular colloid.

P.19 a **True**. FSH is one of the two gonadotrophins synthesized by gonadotrophs in the adenohypophysis in response to stimulation by gonadotrophin releasing hormone (GnRH).

b **False**. FSH is a glycoprotein, not a polypeptide. Glycoproteins consist of chains of amino acids with carbohydrate branches.

c **True**. Like the other two adenohypophysial glycoprotein hormones (LH and thyrotrophin) FSH consists of two chains of amino acids (α and β), the α chain being common to all three molecules. The individual characteristics of the different hormones are related to the β chain.

d **True**. There is no doubt that some of the gonadotroph cells contain both FSH and LH, although it is quite probable that other gonadotroph cell populations containing either one of the hormones also exist within the adenohypophysis.

e **False**. Both gonadotrophins are produced in males and females. FSH stimulates the Sertoli cells in the testes and stimulates follicular growth in the ovaries.

P.20 a **True**. There is a similarity between LH and hCG; in addition to having identical α chains, the β chains are quite similar (hCG having an additional 32 amino acids).

b **True**. The Leydig cells in the testes produce androgens (chiefly testosterone) when stimulated by LH.

c **False**. LH stimulates androgen (i.e. mainly testosterone) production in the Leydig cells of the testes in males, and in ovarian thecal cells (mainly androstenedione and some testosterone) in females. Some (limited) aromatization of androgen to oestrogen occurs in males (e.g. in Sertoli cells) while aromatization of androgen (mainly 17β-oestradiol) by the ovarian granulosa cells is the principal pathway of oestrogen synthesis during the follicular phase of the menstrual cycle. The aromatase enzymes involved in the conversion of androgen to oestrogen are stimulated mainly by FSH.

d **True**. Towards day 13 of the typical menstrual cycle, the 17β-oestradiol concentration in the blood has risen sufficiently high for it to exert a positive feedback effect on LH production from the adenohypophysis. The subsequent LH surge is necessary for the final maturation of the ripening ovum and its release from the Graaffian follicle (ovulation).

e **False**. During pregnancy, oestrogen and progestogen levels in the blood increase markedly, and these steroids exert a negative feedback effect on LH (and FSH) secretion by the maternal adenohypophysis. (They are, in fact, the only hormones whose levels in the blood *decrease* during pregnancy.) The stimulatory effect of LH on steroid production is taken over by hCG produced by the implanting blastocyst and later the feto-placental unit.

P.21 a **True**. In the adenohypophysis POMC is broken down to corticotrophin and β-lipotrophin.

b **True**. Corticotrophin is synthesized in, and released by, macrophages in response to an immune challenge. This corticotrophin, like adeno-hypophysial corticotrophin, stimulates the adrenal cortex to produce the glucocorticoid hormone cortisol. Cortisol in turn inhibits the actions of macrophages (including the production of corticotrophin) by a typical negative feedback loop. This is one indication of the important inter-actions which occur between endocrine and immune systems, particularly with respect to the hypothalamo–adenohypophysial–adrenal axis.

c **False**. All stressors stimulate the hypothalamo–adenohypophysial–adrenal axis. The endocrine cascade begins with the increased release of the hypothalamic corticotrophin releasing hormone (and vasopressin usually), the subsequent stimulation of corticotrophin release and the resulting increased production of cortisol by the adrenal cortex. The release of cortisol as part of the stress response is tantamount to the definition of the endocrine response to stress.

d **True**. Corticotrophin stimulates the enzymes in zonae fasciculata and reticularis which are involved in the synthesis not only of gluco-corticoids but also androgens.

e **True**. Increased pigmentation, particularly in the creases of the skin, can be a presenting sign of Cushing's syndrome (excess cortisol production) when caused by excessively raised corticotrophin concentrations in the circulation. However, whether the pigmentation is entirely caused by excessive quantities of circulating corticotrophin or whether another molecule released with the corticotrophin is a contributing factor is still unclear. Certainly β-MSH (melanocyte stimulating hormone) which induces pigmentation is not normally produced by the adenohypophysis, but β-lipotrophin which is released with corticotrophin may be involved.

P.22 a **True**. This occurs during embryonic development. The downwards growth of neural tissue, which forms the neurohypophysis, ultimately fuses with the upwards growth of ectodermal tissue from the primitive buccal cavity which forms the anterior lobe of the pituitary (the adenohypophysis).

b **True**. The function of these glial-type cells is unclear, but bioactive molecules such as endorphins are secreted by them. A possible paracrine role, whereby these endorphins may influence the release of neuro-hypophysial hormones, has been proposed.

c **True**. In humans the pars intermedia is normally reduced to a thin, relatively avascular, band of tissue which appears to be relatively inactive. However, in lower vertebrates, and interestingly during pregnancy in humans, this area is increased in size and activity. Melanocyte-stimulating hormone is one molecule synthesized by the pars intermedia in amphibia, for example. Its function during pregnancy is unclear.

d **True**. Most of the neurohypophysis consists of nerve axons. Their neurosecretions are released into the general circulation and are the neurohypophysial hormones vasopressin and oxytocin.

e **False**. The neurosecretions from the neurohypophysis enter the systemic circulation directly, and not into the localized hypothalamo–hypophysial portal system which links the hypothalamic median eminence to the adenohypophysis. (Note that it has been suggested that some of the neurosecretions can reach the adenohypophysis via short portal vessels linking the two lobes.)

P.23 a **True**. Vasopressin is also synthesized in cells in other parts of the body such as the chromaffin cells of the adrenal medulla, the sympathetic ganglia, and the gonads of both sexes. There is even a reported synthesis of vasopressin by cultures of pancreatic islet cells.

b **False**. Vasopressin and oxytocin are synthesized in different neurones in the hypothalamic supraoptic and paraventricular nuclei, and no conversion between the two molecules occurs.

c **True**. The neurones producing vasopressin (and oxytocin) which descend into the neurohypophysis are characteristically large (magnocellular). These magnocellular neurones are also characterized by swellings called Hering bodies which are present along the axons. Vasopressin is also synthesized in smaller parvocellular neurones which also originate in the paraventricular nuclei. In these neurones vasopressin is co-localized with other molecules, particularly corticotrophin releasing hormone.

d **True**. The neurosecretions of the neurohypophysis are released directly into vessels which drain into the jugular veins.

e **True**. Historically, vasopressin was one of the first hormones shown to be produced by non-endocrine (i.e. ectopic) tumours (in this case from oat cells of a carcinoma of the bronchus).

P.24 a **True**. This is another hypothalamic site of vasopressin synthesis. (Note that the suprachiasmatic nucleus is associated with biological rhythmicity.)

b **True**. Some vasopressinergic neurones from the hypothalamic nuclei pass to other parts of the brain, such as the nucleus tractus solitarius (involved in central cardiovascular regulation) and the hippocampus (an area of the brain associated with aspects of behaviour).

c **True**. The nature of the pulsatile release of vasopressin is characteristic (discrete pulses at regular intervals) and allows for differentiation between vasopressinergic and oxytocinergic neurones in electro-physiological studies.

d **False**. Many hormones associated with the hypothalamus follow diurnal (circadian) rhythms but so far this has not been shown for vasopressin.

e **True**. This may be one of the factors associated with the deteriorating control of water balance which occurs with age.

P.25 a **True**. However, initially it is transcribed containing a signal peptide sequence, at which stage it is called pre-provasopressin

b **False**. Angiotensin II is an octapeptide which differs markedly from vasopressin. The other neurohypophysial hormone oxytocin, however, is remarkably similar to vasopressin only differing by two of the amino acids.

c **True**. The two main receptor types for vasopressin are called V_1 (associated with vasoconstrictor and other actions of the hormone) and V_2 (associated with the principal physiological effect of vasopressin in the kidneys) receptors. A receptor similar, but not identical to, the V_1 receptor has been identified in the adenohypophysis. This has led to the V_1 receptor being classified as either V_{1a} or V_{1b} (the latter being the adenohypophysial receptor).

d **False**. The cardiovascular effects observed with high concentrations of vasopressin normally include a *bradycardia*. This may be at least partly due to a direct vasoconstrictor effect on the coronary vessels, and partly due to a reflex bradycardia initiated by the increase in arterial blood pressure induced by vasopressin at these high concentrations.

e **True**. Vasopressin appears to be the most potent naturally occurring vasoconstrictor molecule known, on isolated arteries at least. Interestingly, it is not associated with hypertension in cases of chronically raised vasopressin concentrations in the blood (syndrome of inappropriate antidiuretic hormone, SIADH), nor is it associated with hypotension in the absence of circulating hormone (as in central diabetes insipidus). A likely explanation is that vasopressin elicits a powerful reflex brady-cardia and a decrease in cardiac output which compensates largely for any increase in arterial blood pressure.

P.26 a **True**. Both V_1 and V_2 receptors, members of a family of similar proteins consisting of seven transmembrane domains, four extracellular and three intracellular regions, are associated with G proteins.

b **True**. This is the principal physiological effect of vasopressin, and accounts for its alternative name of antidiuretic hormone (nomenclature still commonly used, particularly by renal physiologists).

c **False**. The V_1 receptor is coupled to the inositol triphosphate–diacylglycerol mechanism which is associated with increasing intra-cellular calcium ion levels. However the V_2 receptor is associated with adenyl cyclase, activation of which results in generation of cyclic AMP.

   d **True**. This is the main vascular effect (V_1 receptor-mediated) of vasopressin. An additional V_2 receptor mechanism involving endothelial
cells and arteriolar vasodilation is the subject of current research in this
field. (The release of the vasodilator nitric oxide has been implicated.)

   e **True**. Vasopressin released from parvocellular neurones in the median
eminence has direct corticotrophin releasing activity of its own, but its
main effect is to act synergistically with the main hypothalamic corticotrophin releasing hormone CRH-41. This molecule is co-localized
(and usually released) with vasopressin.

P.27 a **False**. *Hypovolaemia* (and the associated decrease in arterial blood
pressure) is a potent stimulus of vasopressin production, acting via a
decreased stimulation of the baroreceptors in the carotid sinus and aortic
arch, and the volume receptors found mainly in the atria of the heart.
Note that a *decreased* stimulation of these receptors results in a reduction
in the tonic *inhibitory* influence exerted by this reflex pathway on
vasopressin release and the sympathetic nervous system.

   b **True**. An increased concentration of osmotically active molecules in the
blood activates osmoreceptors in the hypothalamus which, in turn,
stimulate vasopressin release from the neurohypophysis. Since over 95%
of the osmotically active particles in the blood are sodium and chloride
ions, an increase in the extracellular sodium chloride concentration is a
particularly important stimulus.

   c **False**. Increased stimulation of arterial baroreceptors (and atrial volume
receptors) results in an *inhibition* of vasopressin release.

   d **True**. Various stressors (e.g. surgery, anaesthesia, restraint) are potent
stimulators of vasopressin release.

   e **False**. The release of oxytocin following stimulation of tactile (stretch)
receptors around the nipple of the breast during lactation is the efferent
pathway of a neuroendocrine arc specifically associated with oxytocin
release.

P.28 a **True**. This is the main physiological effect of vasopressin, and it takes
place in the collecting ducts, particularly the medullary segment.

   b **False**. Vasopressin does not have any effect on proximal tubular
function. Water reabsorption in this early segment of the nephron
passively follows the reabsorption of solutes (particularly sodium
chloride) so that the fluid leaving the proximal tubule is isosmotic but
greatly reduced in volume.

   c **True**. This is believed to be how vasopressin stimulates water transport
in the collecting ducts. The vasopressin-sensitive water channels are
called aquaporin-2 proteins, and are members of a family of at least four
aquaporins involved in water transport across a variety of cell
membranes.

   d **False**. Vasopressin tends to stimulate sodium reabsorption (e.g. in the ascending limb of the loop of Henle and in the collecting duct) so would be antinatriuretic.

e **True**. Vasopressin may, by stimulating urea and sodium (chloride) reabsorption, have an important role participating in the maintenance of the medullary osmotic gradient. In the absence of a medullary gradient vasopressin is not effective in stimulating water reabsorption along the collecting ducts. For example, in central (cranial) diabetes insipidus, hormone replacement may be associated initially with a reduced anti-diuretic action until the medullary gradient has been restored.

P.29 a **True**. The cell bodies where oxytocin is synthesized are found in the supraoptic and paraventricular nuclei—the same nuclei associated with vasopressin synthesis.

b **False**. There is no evidence to support the view that oxytocin is released from parvocellular nerve endings in the median eminence, unlike vasopressin.

c **True**. This is a major afferent (neural) pathway which leads to the release of oxytocin as part of a neuroendocrine milk ejection reflex arc. Note that the endocrine milieu regarding the concentrations of other hormones (particularly gonadal/placental steroids) has to be appropriate for milk secretion, and therefore ejection, to occur.

d **True**. Various oxytocinergic fibres have been traced back to other parts of the brain where it presumably acts as a neurotransmitter. Various behavioural effects associated with oxytocin would be associated with these pathways, for instance. Indeed, some areas of the brain receive a greater oxytocinergic than a vasopressinergic innervation; one example is the nucleus tractus solitarius (associated with cardiovascular regulation).

e **False**. The pulsatile release of oxytocin is likely to be associated with the characteristic pattern of electrical activity seen in the neurones.

P.30 a **False**. There is no evidence, so far, for any inhibitory effect by prolactin. Indeed, the two hormones will be released simultaneously by the stimulus of suckling, both being efferent limbs of neuroendocrine reflex arcs.

b **False**. Oxytocin is produced in both sexes; this certainly suggests that oxytocin has effects other than during parturition and lactation in females. One possibility that has been suggested is that oxytocin is associated with the ejaculatory process in males.

c **False**. But its (pulsatile) release is stimulated towards term, and is associated with contractions of the uterine myometrium at labour.

d **False**. The key word here is 'essential'. While oxytocin is released at term and is certainly beneficial in promoting parturition, it is clear that a normal delivery can occur in the absence of this hormone. Other bioactive molecules (e.g. certain prostaglandins) probably play an equally important role in stimulating myometrial contractions.

e **True**. This is an important physiological stimulus for oxytocin release at parturition. Stretch receptors (i.e. mechanoreceptors) are located in the vagina and uterine wall.

P.31 a **False**. Oxytocin binds to specific membrane receptors following which intracellular second messenger systems (associated with an increased intracellular calcium ion concentration) operate to bring about its actions.

b **False**. Oxytocin has no major effect on vascular smooth muscle, although a slight vasodilatory effect has been observed when the hormone is administered intravenously.

c **True**. This is how milk ejection arises, following the secretion of milk into the ducts (brought about by prolactin).

d **True**. The actions of oxytocin (at least with respect to the milk ejection and uterine contraction reflexes) are dependent on the presence of sufficient quantities of circulating oestrogen.

e **False**. There is no known relationship between vasopressin and the actions of oxytocin.

SAQ Answers

P.32

Figure 4.2 shows the hypothalamo–adenohypophysial portal system linking median eminence and adenohypophysis. Also indicated are the hypothalamic neurones and their neurosecretions, the releasing and inhibiting hormones (RH and IH), which are transported to the anterior pituitary by the portal system. The hypothalamic hormones stimulate or inhibit the release of the adenohypophysial hormones.

P.33

Adenohypophysial hormones	*Hypothalamic hormones*	*Influence*
Prolactin	Dopamine	Inhibitory (dominant)
	Thyrotrophin RH (TRH)	Stimulatory
Somatotrophin (i.e. growth hormone, GH)	Somatotrophin RH (SRH) (GHRH, somatoliberin)	Stimulatory (dominant)
	Somatostatin	Inhibitory
Thyrotrophin (thyroid-stimulating hormone, TSH)	Thyrotrophin RH (TRH)	Stimulatory (dominant)
Gonadotrophins (LH and FSH)	Gonadotrophin RH (GnRH)	Stimulatory (dominant)
Corticotrophin (adrenocortico-trophic hormone, ACTH)	Corticotrophin RH (CRH) (Corticoliberin)	Stimulatory (dominant)
	Vasopressin	Stimulatory

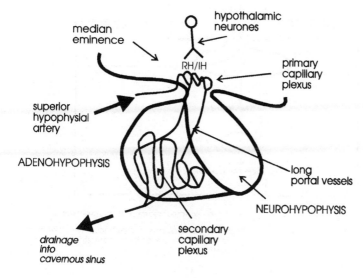

median
eminence

hypothalamic
neurones

RH/IH

primary
capillary
plexus

superior
hypophysial
artery

ADENOHYPOPHYSIS

long
portal vessels

NEUROHYPOPHYSIS

drainage
into
cavernous sinus

secondary
capillary
plexus

Fig. 4.1

P.34

Relevant points to include in the figure are: the hypothalamus, the adenohypophysis, gonadotrophin releasing hormone (GnRH), luteinizing hormone (LH),
follicle-stimulating hormone (FSH), an ovary, oestrogens (i.e. 17β-oestradiol),
negative feedback loops (direct and indirect), positive feedback loops (direct and
indirect, specifying that they only operate under very specific conditions) (see
Fig. 4.2.) *Note* that progesterone and inhibin have negative feedback loops, the
latter specifically on FSH release.

P.35

The diagram should include the following: somatotrophin (growth hormone, GH),
liver, somatomedins (i.e. insulin-like growth factors, IGF-I and IGF-II), metabolic
effects (protein synthesis, lipolysis, increase in blood glucose concentration),
stimulation of growth (e.g. linear, on cartilage, bone), interaction with the immune
system. (See Fig. 4.3.) (NEFA = non-esterified fatty acids.)

P.36

The neuroendocrine reflex arc involving oxytocin which you describe in your
answer could have a neural afferent pathway beginning with tactile receptors either
around the nipple of the breast or in the uterine myometrium. Oxytocin acts on
smooth muscle (myoepithelial and myometrial) cells causing constriction (See
Fig. 4.4.) (*Note* that raised ovarian steroid concentrations are necessary for the
normal milk ejection or myometrial contraction reflexes to operate.)

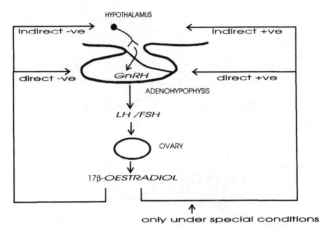

Fig. 4.2

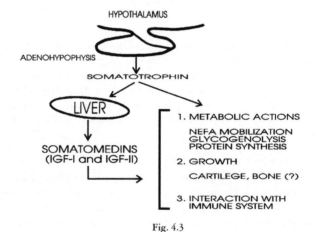

Fig. 4.3

P.37

The neurohypophysial hormone vasopressin has various physiological effects, the principal one being the stimulation of water reabsorption in the collecting ducts of the renal nephrons. This effect involves a specific receptor called the V_2 receptor found on the serosal (basal) membranes of the collecting duct cells. The receptor is associated with a G protein and a catalytic unit which is adenyl cyclase. When activated, adenosine triphosphate is converted to the second messenger cyclic

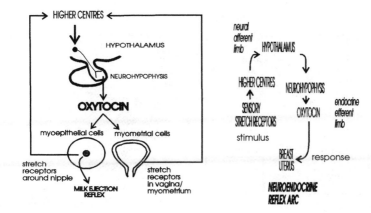

Fig. 4.4

adenosine monophosphate (cyclic AMP) which activates protein kinase A. This activated kinase is linked to the movement of water channels, proteins called aquaporins, to the apical membranes. The specific vasopressin-sensitive water channel in the collecting duct cells is called aquaporin-2. Vesicles containing aquaporin-2 molecules are called aggraphores; they are circulated to and from the apical membranes in the presence of vasopressin, and the water channels are inserted into the membranes. How the water actually crosses the cells is still unclear, but the cytoskeleton framework of microtubules may be involved, as may be actin filaments located along the lateral membranes. Certainly, an osmotic gradient across the collecting duct epithelium is necessary for successful water transport.

Vasopressin also has a powerful constrictor effect on vascular smooth muscle, as seen in isolated tissue studies. (It would appear to be the most potent, naturally occurring molecule known.) This effect is mediated by a different receptor called the V_1 receptor. It is located in the smooth muscle membranes and is linked to a G protein which, in turn, is linked to phospholipase C (PLC). This enzyme, when activated, converts membrane phosphatidylinositol 4,5-biphosphate to inositol 1,4,5-triphosphate which liberates calcium ions from intracellular stores. [Diacylglycerol is also formed, and this molecule activates protein kinase C which in turn phosphorylates (i.e. activates) various other intracellular proteins acting on a wide variety of metabolic pathways]. Membrane calcium channels may also be activated. In the case of vascular smooth muscle the rise in intracellular free calcium ions will result in increased actin and myosin linkage; consequently the muscle contracts.

P.38

Principal features to identify in your diagram are: hypothalamus (supraoptic and paraventricular nuclei can be specified), osmoreceptors, baroreceptors and volume

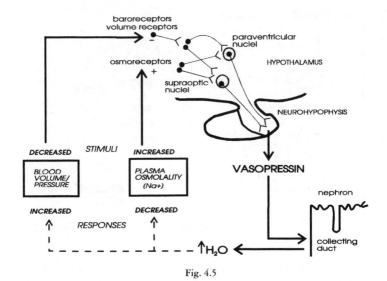

Fig. 4.5

receptors, neurohypophysis, vasopressin, tonic inhibition on vasopressin release via baroreceptors and volume receptors (note inhibitory neurone), stimulation of osmoreceptors by increased plasma osmolality. (See Fig. 4.5.)

The hypothalamo–hypophysial (Clinical)

Multiple Choice Questions

C.1

Which of the following groups of clinical features are found with increased frequency in patients with acromegaly?

a   Bilateral carpal tunnel syndrome and headache
b   Daytime somnolence and muscle weakness
c   Homonymous hemianopia and concomitant squint
d   Postural hypotension and Raynaud's phenomenon
e   Hyperextensible joints and gout

C.2

Which of the following conditions, known to cause sudden death, occur with increased frequency in acromegaly?

a Ventricular tachycardia
b Pituitary infarction/apoplexy
c Carotid artery aneurysm rupture
d Aortic aneurysm rupture
e Cerebral haemorrhage

C.3

A man age 55 is suspected of having acromegaly on the basis of coarsening facial features. Which of the following investigations would be consistent with this diagnosis?

a Fasting hypoglycaemia
b Low serum levels of IGF-I (somatomedin-C)
c A rise of growth hormone in response to intravenous thyrotrophin releasing hormone (TRH) 200 μg
d A serum growth hormone level of 2 mU/litre 1–2 hours after 75 g oral dextrose.
e Hypercalcaemia with undetectable serum parathormone levels

C.4

Which of the following is true in relation to the treatment of acromegaly?

a The condition may cure itself spontaneously
b Trans-sphenoidal pituitary surgery mostly normalizes growth hormone levels
c Dopamine agonist drugs are more effective than somatostatin analogues in reducing growth hormone levels
d External pituitary irradiation will usually normalize growth hormone levels in 5 years
e Restoration of normal growth hormone levels may reverse acromegalic cardio-myopathy

C.5

A 9-year-old boy has a height less than 3 standard deviations (SD) below the mean for his age (4 cm below 3rd centile). Serum-free T4 is 5 pmol/litre (NR 12–24) and serum TSH 1.5 mU/litre (NR 0.5–2.5 mU/l). Which of the following diagnoses would be consistent with these findings? (NR = normal range.)

a Idiopathic growth hormone deficiency
b Primary juvenile hypothyroidism
c Craniopharyngioma
d Malabsorption syndrome (gluten-sensitive enteropathy)
e Psychosocial deprivation syndrome/dwarfism

C.6

A 13-year-old boy with stage 1 puberty has a growth velocity of 3 cm per annum and a height 2 SD below the mean for his age. He is being investigated for possible growth hormone deficiency. Exercise to exhaustion induces a serum growth hormone peak of 6 mU/litre (N > 20) during multiple sampling over the following 30 minutes. Which of the following is/are true? (N = normal.)

a Testosterone 'priming' prior to exercise may result in a normal growth hormone response
b The result may be explained by a growth hormone resistance syndrome
c The findings are sufficient to justify commencement of growth hormone therapy
d Assessment of serum growth hormone response to GHRH infusion will confirm or refute growth hormone deficiency
e Insulin-induced hypoglycaemia is the most appropriate next step for identifying growth hormone deficiency

C.7

Which of the following features is/are consistent with the diagnosis of a pituitary tumour?
a Diplopia due to a third cranial (oculomotor) nerve lesion
b A temporal visual field defect in one eye
c CSF rhinorrhoea
d Normal pituitary function tests (in terms of gonadotrophin, TSH, and ACTH secretion)
e Normal size sella turcica on plain lateral skull radiography

C.8

Which of the following groups of biochemical findings would support a diagnosis of hypopituitarism in a 68-year-old woman?

a Normal range LH and FSH serum levels
b A serum-free T_4 of 7 pmol/litre (NR 12–24) and serum TSH of 1.6 mU/litre (NR 0.5–5.5)
c A serum cortisol of 150 nmol/litre rising to 580 nmol/litre 30 minutes after 250 μg IV tetrocosactrin (Synacthen) (normal maximum 550 nmol/l)
d A serum prolactin of 1550 mU/litre (NR 0–450)
e A random growth hormone level of 2 mU/litre (NR 2–30)

C.9

A 25-year-old woman complaining of fatigue and amenorrhoea is found to have a serum prolactin level of 3250 mU/litre (NR 50–450). Which of the following is/are consistent with this presentation?

a The use of antidepressants
b Anxiety associated with imminent loss of employment

c Primary hypothyroidism (Hashimoto's disease)
d Prolactinoma
e Pregnancy

C.10

Which of the following non-endocrine disorders may result in hypopituitarism?

a Sarcoidosis
b Carcinoma of the breast
c Postpartum haemorrhage
d Head injury following a motor vehicle accident
e Whole brain irradiation for meningeal lymphoma

C.11

A 21-year-old woman with primary amenorrhoea and infertility is found to have a serum 17 β-oestradiol level of 25 pmol/litre (normal follicular phase range 75–300 pmol/l) and a serum LH of 2.0 units/litre (NR 2.5–15). Which of the following conditions are consistent with these findings?

a Premature menopause
b Anorexia nervosa
c Kallman's syndrome
d Polycystic ovarian syndrome (PCO)
e Gonadal dysgenesis (Turner's syndrome)

C.12

A 50-year-old male presents with a history of moderate endogenous depression and hypertension. He gives a one-year history of increasing polyuria and polydipsia (approximately 5 litres daily output). Blood glucose is normal and there are no other abnormal clinical findings. After 6 hours fluid deprivation, serum osmolality is 302 mmol/kg (NR 284–295), and simultaneous urinary osmolality is 205 mmol/kg. Which of the following conditions would be consistent with these findings?

a Compulsive water drinking (psychogenic polydipsia)
b Hypokalaemic nephropathy
c Diabetes insipidus due to a hypothalamic tumour
d Toxicity relating to lithium carbonate treatment for his depression
e Surreptitious self-administration of a thiazide diuretic

C.13

Hypothalamic disorders may induce a variety of clinical endocrine syndromes. Which of the following entities is/are recognized as falling into this category?

a Delayed puberty due to pineal tumours
b Diabetes insipidus due to hypothalamic tumour

c Precocious puberty due to craniopharyngioma
d Hyperthyroidism due to aqueductal stenosis
e Acromegaly secondary to hypothalamic gangliocytoma

Short Answer Questions

C.14

Acromegaly may involve almost all body systems. For each of five systems, indicate one symptom or one sign reflecting this involvement.

C.15

List the key hormonal deficits resulting from destructive anterior lobe (adenohypophyseal) pituitary lesions. For each deficit, write *brief* notes on relevant replacement therapy.

C.16**

Write *brief* notes on the treatment of idiopathic (neurohypophyseal) diabetes insipidus.

C.17**

'Surgery is logical first-line treatment for a prolactinoma 1 cm in diameter, responsible for amenorrhoea and infertility in a 23-year-old woman'. Indicate in *concise* notes, why this approach may not be in the woman's best interests.

MCQ Answers

C.1 a **True**. These symptoms represent entrapment of the median (occasionally ulnar) nerve and occipital/frontal nerves, respectively, due to bone expansion and soft tissue hypertrophy. Headache in acromegaly may also be due to sinusitis, but is only very rarely attributable to pituitary gland enlargement.

b **True**. Acromegaly causes obstructive sleep apnoea because of palatopharyngeal hypertrophy. Consequent poor sleep patterns cause daytime somnolence. Muscle weakness represents myopathy.

c **False**. The usual field defect in pituitary tumours is a bitemporal (dominantly upper quadrantic) hemianopia. A squint can occur due to involvement of 3rd, 4th, or 6th nerves from cavernous sinus extension of the tumour: this squint is not concomitant.

d **False**. Hypertension is frequent in acromegaly, and together with acromegalic cardiomyopathy causes cardiac failure. The prevalence of Raynaud's phenomenon is not increased.

e **False**. Joints usually show reduced range of movement due to ligamentous thickening and degenerative joint disease. Uric acid excretion is actually increased in acromegaly.

C.2 a **True**. Ventricular and (less often) atrial arrythmias result from acromegalic cardiomyopathy; a major cause of death.

b **True**. As with any pituitary tumour, this syndrome may occur, marked by meningism and cardiovascular collapse. Following recovery, acromegaly may regress with undetectable growth hormone levels. There may also be variable destruction of the remaining pituitary with partial or panhypopituitarism.

c **True**. Carotid arery aneurysms are more frequent in patients with pituitary tumour than in the general population. This highlights the importance of contrast radiography with either CT or MRI scanning to characterize any intrasellar mass.

d **False**. Aortic aneurysms are no more common in acromegaly than in the general population, although there may be a marginal increased risk secondary to hypertension.

e **True**. This is due to hypertension coupled to increased severity of atherosclerosis.

C.3 a **False**. Hyperglycaemia is more likely, due to enhanced hepatic gluconeogenesis resulting from growth hormone excess. Frank diabetes is also more common, and reverts following successful treatment of acromegaly.

b **False**. IGF-I levels are usually raised, but may be falsely normal in the presence of infection, cardiac, hepatic, or renal disease, which decrease its hepatic synthesis. Serum IGF-I levels fall following treatment, but are not as reliable as suppressability of circulating growth hormone when evaluating remission of acromegaly.

c **True**. A rise of serum growth hormone after IV TRH is characteristic of acromegaly, often persisting even after correction of growth hormone hypersecretion: its mechanism is unclear.

d **False**. Suppression of growth hormone to 2 mU/litre absolutely excludes the diagnosis of active acromegaly.

e **True**. Hypercalcaemia is present in 10% of acromegalics, due to increased bone turnover and decreased calcium excretion: suppression of iPTH is a consequence. Rarely, in multiple endocrine neoplasia (MEN-1 syndrome), primary hyperparathyroidism may coexist with acromegaly.

C.4 a **True**. Acromegaly 'burns out' in 10–20% of cases, probably due to pituitary infarction which may be silent: sometimes this is referred to as 'fugitive' acromegaly.

    b **False**. Growth hormone levels often fall by 50–80%. However, except with the smallest tumours incompletely suppressible growth hormone levels are much more likely than biochemical cure, due to tumour cell rests in the wall of the sella.

    c **False**. Dopamine agonists often result in a fall of growth hormone, but rarely to non-acromegalic levels. Somatostatin analogues, however, are capable of normalizing growth hormone levels.

    d **False**. External irradiation alone, either by conventional (cobalt) or proton beam source rarely normalizes growth hormone within 5 years: only 10–30% achieve normal values even at 10 years.

    e **True**. Acromegalic cardiomyopathy may benefit from normalizing (or even reducing) growth hormone levels: a reduction in the transverse diameter of the heart is commonly seen in routine X-rays following successful treatment.

C.5 a **False**. (Idiopathic) growth hormone deficiency in children is only rarely accompanied by other pituitary hormone deficiencies.

    b **False**. In primary hypothyroidism, serum TSH would be elevated.

    c **True**. TSH deficiency quite often accompanies growth hormone deficiency in craniopharyngioma, due either to destruction/compression of the remaining pituitary or to interference with its blood supply.

    d **False**. The sick euthyroid syndrome, which may accompany the metabolic disturbance of serious malabsorption, can result in minor reductions of free T_4; but not to this extent.

    e **False**. Psychosocial dwarfism uniquely affects growth hormone secretion, which rapidly returns to normal when such children are 'rehoused' away from their socially stressful environment.

C.6 a **True**. Between 10% and 40% of (normal) prepubertal boys will have defective growth hormone response to physiological (and even pharmacological) growth hormone releasing stimuli.

    b **False**. Growth hormone resistance is due (mostly) to defective IGF-I production secondary to a mutation in the hepatic growth hormone receptor gene(s): circulating growth hormone levels are usually elevated.

    c **False**. The exercise test may fail to give an adequate growth hormone response in the small-delay syndrome (delayed puberty) or other causes of short stature: it is only a screening test. 'Priming' the boy with a testosterone injection of 100 mg (propionate) reduces the likelihood of false negative responses in this setting.

    d **False**. The response of serum growth hormone to GHRH infusion does not represent a diagnostic test for the presence of growth hormone deficiency: among other reasons, the primary lesion may be at the hypothalamic level: growth hormone responsiveness would be maintained.

    e **True**. The insulin stress test (sometimes preceded by arginine infusion) remains the mainstay of diagnosis, although there are potential complications resulting from the induced hypoglycaemia if the test is inadequately supervised.

C.7   a   **True**. Lateral extension of a pituitary tumour into the cavernous sinus often involves the 3rd (and sometimes the 4th or 6th) cranial nerve as they pass along the lateral wall of the sinus.

b   **True**. The optic chiasma is frequently involved by suprasellar extension of pituitary tumours, causing a bitemporal (often initially upper quadrantic) hemianopia. 'Post-fixed' chiasmata may result in a pituitary tumour causing a monocular field defect, since pressure is then dominantly on the optic nerve.

c   **True**. Extensive erosion of the sella floor may occur with pituitary tumours, which then extend into sphenoidal and less frequently ethmoidal sinuses.

d   **True**. Pituitary function may be totally unimpaired, even by large tumours extending beyond the confines of the sella. Even with the largest tumours, only growth hormone secretion may be impaired. Nevertheless, growth hormone and gonadotrophin tend to be affected earlier, and TSH and ACTH only later in the natural history of pituitary tumour growth.

e   **True**. Conventional lateral skull radiography (as distinct from CT or MRI imaging) is a very imprecise assessment. Tumours up to 12 mm diameter, even with suprasellar extension may occur without radiological bone involvement.

C.8   a   **True**. Gonadotrophin levels are high in normal postmenopausal women. Except in the presence of severe or chronic physical or psychological illness, which induces hypothalamic 'turn-off', this result is diagnostic of gonadotrophin deficiency.

b   **True**. Normal range (rather than low) TSH levels are often seen in hypopituitarism: the reason is unclear. The phenomenon appears to occur more frequently in pituitary rather than hypothalamic disease, and may relate to negative feedback stimulation of hypothalamic TRH release (i.e. maximally stimulated but defective thyrotroph function).

c   **False**. In hypopituitarism (other than within 2 weeks of pituitary surgery), tetracosactrin response is attenuated. This is due to adrenal atrophy secondary to prolonged ACTH understimulation.

d   **True**. Destructive pituitary lesions of the pituitary cause low levels of prolactin. Hypothalamic or partially destructive pituitary or stalk lesions result in high serum prolactin due to loss of dopaminergic inhibition ('pituitary disconnection'): values as high as 4000 mU/litre may occur.

e   **False**. Random growth hormone levels are of rarely of value in diagnosis of hypopituitarism. In normal subjects, undetectable levels may be found especially after food. Provocation tests (i.e. insulin hypoglycaemia stress) are potentially dangerous in this age group. In the absence of systemic illness, a low serum IGF-I level strongly supports hypopituitarism. When available, urine growth hormone may be the most appropriate assay in this age group.

C.9 a **True**. A wide variety of antidepressant (tricyclic, phenothiazine) and antipsychotic drugs as well as metoclopramide (all with dopaminergic blocking activity) cause hyperprolactinaemia, sometimes resulting in amenorrhoea with or without galactorroea.

b **False**. Anxiety can cause amenorrhoea (hypothalamic inhibition) and may raise prolactin levels as high as 1800 mU/litre. Levels above 2000 mU/litre must have other explanations.

c **True**. Primary hypothyroidism may elevate serum prolactin to this level (and may induce galactorrhoea). A possible mechanism is increased TRH secretion.

d **True**. Prolactinomas usually result in prolactin levels in the range 1200–500 000 mU/litre: non-functioning macroadenomas may also elevate serum prolactin to around 4000 mU/litre, by interfering with normal dopaminergic inhibition of prolactin secretion.

e **True**. Pregnancy alone may result in a level of serum prolactin as high as 15 000 mU/litre.

C.10 a **True**. As well as sarcoidosis, hypopituitarism may be caused by tuberculosis and a variety of other infiltrates including amyloidosis, Hand–Schüller–Christian disease, histiocytosis, eosiniphilic granuloma, and haemochromatosis.

b **True**. Metastases to the hypothalamic–pituitary area are common, probably based on its rich blood supply.

c **True**. Sheehan's syndrome (post-partum pituitary infarction) may follow severe post-partum haemorrhage. Surprisingly, despite usual involvement of all pituitary trophic hormones, clinical recognition may be delayed by years, unless amenorrhoea prompts early assessment.

d **True**. Although diabetes insipidus (often temporary) may follow head injury, either temporary or permanent anterior lobe damage is also well recognized after more severe injury.

e **True**. External brain irradiation for any indication frequently involves the hypothalamic area, which is more radiosensitive than the pituitary itself. Prevalence of ACTH or TSH deficiency approaches 50% within 10 years: gonadotrophin and growth hormone deficiency is present in up to 80% of cases.

C.11 a **False**. In premature ovarian failure, there are likely to have been some menstrual periods before onset of amenorrhoea. More importantly, serum LH would be raised.

b **True**. Anorexia and bulimia nervosa, as well as (stress-related) hypothalamic anovulation all represent 'functional' and reversible hypogonadotrophic hypogonadism.

c **True**. The amenorrhoea is due to a genetic hypothalamic defect, sometimes associated with anosmia, cleft palate or hare lip, and defects in renal development.

d **False**. Oestradiol and LH levels are normal or high in PCO syndrome: the amenorrhoea is due to anovulation and not to oestrogen deficiency.

e **False**. Because this is a primary gonadal disorder, negative feedback of low oestradiol would result in very high LH levels.

C.12 a **False**. In this condition, serum osmolality would be low or low–normal, accompanied by low urine osmolality of similar order to this patient. Some patients with this (functional) disorder acquire a reversible renal tubular concentration defect. This can cause confusion in interpreting the result of fluid deprivation testing, by simulating genuine diabetes insipidus.

b **True**. Chronic hypokalaemia produces a partially reversible tubular nephropathy, causing vasopressin non-responsiveness: nephrogenic diabetes insipidus. Chronic hypercalcaemia has similar consequences. Permanent renal tubular (and glomerular) damage in the latter situation is sometimes associated with nephrocalcinosis.

c **True**. The presentation and findings are typical with urine hypo-osmolality in the face of serum hyperosmolality: borderline cases sometime require a longer period of fluid deprivation, or more sophisticated testing assessing plasma ADH response to hypertonic saline infusion.

d **True**. Lithium frequently induces a polyuric syndrome due to a totally reversible vasopressin resistance at the renal tubular level.

e **False**. Serum osmolality would be low due to sodium depletion and consequent hyponatraemia.

C.13** a **False**. Only rarely. Although many pineal tumours are non-secretory, precocious puberty can be induced by some tumours (teratomas) by secretion of hCG, and others by pressure/destructive effects on the posterior hypothalamic nuclei.

b **True**. Any hypothalamic tumour—craniopharyngioma, hamartoma, meningioma, or glioma can produce diabetes insipidus (DI). Most patients with DI have no macroscopically apparent hypothalamic disorder, although neuronal degeneration can be microscopically identified in the supraoptic and/or paraventricular nuclei.

c **False**. Although very rare cases of this association have been described, the gonadal syndrome most often associated with craniopharyngioma is hypogonadism or delayed puberty.

d **False**. By causing third ventricle dilatation, aqueductal stenosis induces a variety of secondary hypothalamic deficits, particularly of growth hormone and gonadotrophin. Hypothyroidism may also occur.

e **True**. A possible primary hypothalamic origin of classical acromegaly continues to be debated. However GHRH-producing gangliocytomas (and bronchogenic and other carcinomas) have also been identified as rare causes of acromegaly.

SAQ Answers

C.14

CVS: (SY)) palpitations (arrhythmias): (SI) cardiomegaly, hypertension.

RS: (SY) breathlessness (cardiomyopathy): (SI) deep voice (laryngeal hypertrophy).

CNS: (SY) diplopia (cavernous sinus involvement by tumour), reduced visual acuity, paraesthesiae, headache, somnolence (obstructive sleep apnoea): (SI) bitemporal hemianopia.

MSS: (SY) back pain, arthralgia (osteoarthritis), weakness (myopathy): (SI) acral enlargement, muscle hypertrophy.

GIS: (SI) hepatomegaly, splenomegaly.

Skin: (SY) greasy skin, excessive sweating: (SI) thickened skin, papillomata, and other benign skin tags.

Repro: (SI) reduced libido, infertility.

C.15

TSH: thyroxine replacement with 50–200 μg thyroxine daily. Doses incremented no more frequently than 6-weekly, based on clinical state and serum-free thyroxine levels; serum TSH cannot be used as an indicator in hypothalamic–pituitary disease. Treatment may 'unmask' ACTH deficiency by inducing an adrenal crisis if coexistent ACTH (cortisol) deficiency unrecognized.

ACTH: cortisol used rather than synthetic steroid; doses 15–30 mg daily in divided dose, incremented 2–3fold with any stress. Replace with parenteral hydrocortisone 100 mg if vomiting or seriously unwell. Identification by bracelet/pendant.

LH, FSH: oestrogen (ethinyloestradiol 20–50 μg daily or equivalent with or without progestogen (e.g. medroxyprogesterone 5 mg on days 17–21) or androgen by injection (250 mg testosterone oenanthate, 3–4 weekly) or equivalent in patch or pellet form: oral therapy usually less effective. For fertility induction, either gonado-trophin or pulsed GnRH (for ovulation induction in hypothalamic disease only).

hGH: principal indication is restoration of growth in deficient children. Relative indication in adult growth hormone deficiency, balancing cost against mild to moderate clinical benefits.

C.16**

Standard treatment with desmopressin spray 10–20-μg intranasally twice daily: monitoring of dose symptomatically. For peri-operative management, parenteral desmopressin 5–20 μg, 6–12 hourly: monitoring by fluid balance, weight checks, and serum electrolyte and osmolality. Oral desmopressin 100–200 μg twice to thrice daily: not all patients controllable. Other oral drugs enhancing renal tubular cyclic AMP response to ADH (clofibrate, chlorpropamide) are no longer used.

C.17**

Surgery not always effective in normalizing elevated serum prolactin in adenomas; due to cell rests. Significant risk of hypopituitarism following incidental surgical damage to normal pituitary, rendering patient cortisol/thyroxine-dependent, perhaps with complex ovulation induction requirement if fertility desired. By contrast, no endocrine risk with dopamine agonist therapy, with 80–90% likelihood of restoration of fertility. Significant pregnancy-associated tumour enlargement unlikely, but if necessary controllable with dopamine agonist or surgery as a second-line approach.

References
Physiology
Topic: Endocrine regulation of salt and water balance.
Breyer, M. D. *et al.* (1994). *Annual Review of Physiology*, **56**, 711–39.
Topic: GHRH and somatostatin mechanisms of action.
Chen, C. *et al.* (1994). *Trends in Endocrinology and Metabolism*, **5**, 227–33.
Topic: Thyrotrophin-releasing hormone receptors.
Gershengorn, M. C. *et al.* (1996). *Physiological Reviews*, **76**, 175–92.
Topic: Lactotrophs and the changes in intracellular calcium in response to thyrotrophin releasing hormone.
Hinkle, P. M. *et al.* (1996). *Trends in Endocrinology and Metabolism*, **7**, 370–3.
Topic: Aquaporins (physiology and pathophysiology).
King, L. S. *et al.* (1996). *Annual Review of Physiology*, **58**, 619–48.
Topic: Growth hormone deficiency in adult life.
Shalet, S. M., *et al.* (1996) *Trends in Endocrinology and Metabolism*, **7**, 287–90.

Clinical
Topic: Replacement treatment of adults with growth hormone.
Beshyah, S. A. *et al.* (1995). *Clinical Endocrinology*, **42**, 73–84.
Topic: Pituitary tumours: diagnosis and management.
Faglia, G. (1993). *Acta Endocrinologica*, **129**(suppl.1), 1–40.
Topic: Diagnosis and treatment of acromegaly.
Soskin, A. *et al.* (1995). *Clinical Endocrinology*, **42**(suppl.1), 1–33.
Topic: Prolactinoma.
Soule, S. (1995). *British Journal of Obstetrics and Gynaecology*, **182**, 178–81.
Topic: Pituitary incidentaloma.
Soule, S. *et al.* (1996). *Postgraduate Medical Journal*, **72**, 256–62.
Topic: Hypopituitarism.
Vance, M. L. (1994). *New England Journal of Medicine*, **330**, 1651–62.
Topic: Investigation of pituitary enlargement.
von Werder, K. (1996). *Clinical Endocrinology*, **44**, 299–304.

5 The adrenals (Physiology)

Multiple Choice Questions

A. Adrenal medulla

P.1 The adrenal medulla

a is the central part of the adrenal gland

b is composed of cells embryologically derived from the neural crest

c receives part of its blood supply via drainage through the adrenal cortex

d is the source of adrenal steroids

e is innervated by postganglionic sympathetic nerve fibres

P.2 The adrenomedullary hormones

a are synthesized in chromaffin cells

b are derived from the amino acid, tyrosine

c include dopamine

d are released by acetylcholine

e are released when the sympathetic nervous system is activated

P.3 The catecholamines from the adrenal medulla

a are stored in secretory granules

b are transported to their target cells along specialized nerve axons

c bind to intracellular receptors

d bind to a variety of receptors classified into α and β subtypes

e exert some of their effects through the cyclic AMP second messenger system

P.4 Adrenaline

a is synthesized from the precursor noradrenaline

b is the main secretion from the adrenal medulla

c is present in the circulation in greater concentrations than noradrenaline

d stimulates glycogenolysis

e decreases heart rate

B. Adrenal cortex

See also Chapter 4 (Qs 6, 21, 26); Chapter 12 (Qs 2)

P.5 *The adrenal cortex*

  a surrounds the central medulla
  b comprises three histologically identified zones
  c produces steroid hormones
  d receives some autonomic innervation
  e is a source of androgens

P.6 *Aldosterone*

  a is a vital hormone
  b is only synthesized in the zona glomerulosa
  c is the principal mineralocorticoid in humans
  d is derived from cholesterol
  e is stored in intracellular granules

P.7 *Aldosterone*

  a is transported in the blood partly associated with plasma proteins
  b stimulates the nuclear transcription process in its target cells
  c acts on the salivary glands
  d stimulates renal potassium reabsorption
  e increases water reabsorption in the proximal tubule

P.8 *The production of aldosterone*

  a is mainly under the control of the hypothalamo–adenohypophysial axis
  b is stimulated by angiotensin II
  c increases when the plasma socium ion concentration rises by more than
     10 mmol/litre
  d is usually associated with increased plasma renin activity
  e increases when salt appetite is stimulated

P.9 *The renal actions of aldosterone*

  a can be induced by glucocorticoids if the enzyme 11β-hydroxysteroid
     dehydrogenase is inhibited
  b in the presence of vasopressin are associated with a modest expansion of
     the extracellular fluid volume
  c in conditions of mineralocorticoid excess can result in hypertension
  d are counteracted by atrial natriuretic hormone
  e are fundamental to the maintenance of the medullary gradient

P.10 *The glucocorticoid cortisol*

  a is synthesized in the zonae fasciculata and reticularis of the adrenal cortex

  b is derived from the precursor aldosterone
  c diffuses out of the adrenocortical cells into the blood
  d is produced in far greater quantities than aldosterone each day
  e is released as part of the normal response to stressors

P.11 Cortisol

  a is the main glucocorticoid in humans
  b is transported mainly in dynamic association with the plasma protein transcortin
  c production is stimulated by corticotrophin (adrenocorticotrophic hormone, ACTH)
  d can exert mineralocorticoid effects
  e binds to intracellular glucocorticoid receptors

P.12 Cortisol

  a is converted to biologically inactive cortisone in the liver
  b normally controls sodium reabsorption by the distal nephrons
  c stimulates protein catabolism
  d promotes gluconeogenesis
  e can be produced by non-endocrine tumours

P.13 Cortisol

  a is released in pulses from the adrenal cortex
  b reaches peak levels in the blood around midnight
  c exerts a positive feedback on the hypothalamo–hypophysial axis
  d inhibits the release of corticotrophin releasing hormone from the hypothalamus
  e stimulates aldosterone synthesis

P.14 The adrenal androgens

  a are synthesized in the innermost zona reticularis
  b consist mainly of dehydroepiandrosterone
  c are precursors for oestrogen synthesis
  d are produced in increasing quantities during adrenarche
  e stimulate the synthesis of pubic hair at puberty

Short Answer Questions

P.15

Briefly explain why intravenously administered noradrenaline, but not adrenaline, can produce a reflex bradycardia

P.16

Name the principal mineralocorticoid in humans and *briefly* describe its renal actions with the aid of a labelled diagram

P.17

Briefly explain how aldosterone and vasopressin actions combine to increase the extracellular fluid volume. (Use a labelled diagram if you wish.)

P.18

By means of a labelled diagram explain how aldosterone production is controlled

P.19

List four actions of cortisol and the clinical signs and symptoms which they are associated with in Cushing's syndrome (overproduction condition)

P.20

By means of a labelled diagram explain how cortisol production is controlled

MCQ Answers

A. Adrenal medulla

P.1   a   **True**. Each adrenal gland consists of an outer cortex and an inner medulla.
     b   **True**. The adrenal medullary cells are, in effect, specialized post-ganglionic sympathetic nerve fibres called chromaffin cells.
     c   **True**. The adrenal gland receives arterial blood directly via small arteries branching off from the aorta and the inferior, phrenic, and renal arteries. Blood drains from an arteriolar plexus present below the adrenal capsule into a capillary network in the outer cortex, which becomes sinusoidal as it reaches the inner zones. This arterial blood drains through the adrenal cortex and hence is partly deoxygenated when it reaches the innermost cells, including those of the adrenal medulla.
     d   **False**. The adrenal cortex produces steroids; the adrenal medulla produces amines (catecholamines).
     e   **False**. The adrenal medulla receives a *pre*ganglionic sympathetic inner-vation. The chromaffin cells are stimulated by acetylcholine, the neuro-transmitter released from preganglionic sympathetic nerve endings.

P.2   a   **True**. The cells of the adrenal medulla are called chromaffin cells because they have an affinity for chromic salts. When stimulated the cells release catecholamines into the general circulation.

b **True**. Tyrosine is hydroxylated to L-dopa which is decarboxylated to dopamine. Dopamine is then hydroxylated to noradrenaline, and the synthesis pathway up to this point is similar to the one present in post-ganglionic sympathetic nerve fibres. From here, however, the chromaffin cells are unusual because they contain the enzyme phenylethanolamine-N-methyl transferase which methylates noradrenaline to adrenaline.

c **True**. L-Dopa is decarboxylated to form dopamine which is a catecholamine found in many neurones in the central nervous system in addition to other cells of neural crest derivation such as the adrenal medullary cells.

d **True**. Acetylcholine is the neurotransmitter released from preganglionic sympathetic fibres such as those innervating the chromaffin cells. Activation of the preganglionic sympathetic fibres (in the splanchnic nerve) innervating the adrenal gland is the principal stimulus for the release of the adrenomedullary catecholamines

e **True**. The adrenal medulla releases its hormones directly into the general circulation as part of the general response to sympathetic system activation. It is possible that the adrenal medulla can be stimulated on its own, independent of the rest of the sympathetic nervous system.

P.3 a **True**. The chromaffin cells contain typical secretory granules which contain the catecholamines.

b **False**. The catecholamines are released into the general circulation by exocytosis from the secretory granules. The intracellular microtubular network and an increase in the cytoplasmic free calcium ion concentration are involved in the exocytosis process.

c **False**. The catecholamines are lipophobic and cannot freely enter their target cells. Their receptors are on the target cell membranes and are members of a family of proteins which have seven intramembrane domains, and intra- and extracellular regions.

d **True**. There are two main classes of receptors for the catecholamines, these being α and β receptors. In general, adrenaline has a greater affinity for β receptors than noradrenaline, which has a greater affinity for α receptors. Various subtypes have been identified (e.g. α_1, α_2, β_1, and β_2) each type being associated with a different G protein. Different intracellular second messengers are associated with the different receptor subtypes.

e **True**. Some catecholaminergic effects occur following the intracellular generation of cyclic AMP. For example, the metabolic effects of adrenaline, initiated by binding to receptor subtype β_2, are mediated by activation of the adenyl cyclase–cyclic AMP system.

P.4 a **True**. This methylation of noradrenaline to adrenaline only occurs in chromaffin tissue which contains the relevant enzyme, phenylethanolamine-N-methyl transferase (*not* present in sympathetic postganglionic nerves).

b **True**. In humans approximately 80% of adrenomedullary catecholamine production is adrenaline, most of the remainder being noradrenaline.

c **False**. The plasma noradrenaline concentration is much greater than the adrenaline concentration because most of the noradrenaline enters the circulation from the sympathetic postganglionic nerve endings, with a relatively small contribution from the adrenal medulla. In contrast, the only important source of adrenaline is the adrenal medulla which normally has a total catecholamine output considerably lower than the noradrenergic discharge from the sympathetic terminals.

d **True**. This is an important metabolic effect of adrenaline, and it occurs mainly in liver *and* muscle, unlike glucagon which only stimulates hepatic glycogenolysis.

e **False**. The direct effects of catecholamines on cardiac muscle are on heart rate (chronotropic effect) and on the force of contraction of the heart (inotropic effect). Catecholamines increase heart rate (tachycardia) and force of contraction.

B. Adrenal cortex

P.5 a **True**. Each adrenal gland consists of an outer cortex (cortex means 'bark') surrounding the central medullary tissue. Functionally, the adrenal cortex and adrenal medulla operate relatively independently of each other and can be considered as two separate endocrine glands.

b **True**. These are (from outer to inner, respectively) the zona glomerulosa, the zona fasciculata, and the zona reticularis. Not only are these zones histologically different but the outer and two inner zones are also associated with the production of different hormones.

c **True**. The adrenal cortical hormones are all steroids, and they are called collectively, corticosteroid hormones.

d **True**. There is a well-developed sympathetic innervation to the chromaffin cells of the adrenal medulla (preganglionic fibres, see above) but the autonomic innervation of the adrenal cortical cells is scarce and its physiological significance unclear.

e **True**. Adrenal androgens form a significant part of circulating androgens in females (and can produce androgenic effects when produced in excess, as in Cushing's syndrome), but are a very small part of total circulating levels in males in whom the major source is the testes.

P.6 a **True**. Complete destruction or loss of the adrenal glands is not compatible with life, and aldosterone is believed to be the essential hormone. In its absence, there is a gradual loss of salt and fluid from the body which can, in extreme (fortunately rare) cases, result in severe dehydration, hypotension, coma, and death (cf. Addisonian crisis).

b **True**. The final part of the synthesis pathway is due to 18-hydroxylation, and the relevant enzyme (a $P-450_{c11}$ enzyme) is only found in the cells of the zona glomerulosa.

c **True**. Other steroids with mineralocorticoid activity are produced but only in small amounts (but see P.11 on cortisol).

d **True**. All steroids are derived from cholesterol which is either synthesized from acetate by the cells (a relatively minor source) or, more importantly, taken up from circulating lipoproteins.

e **False**. Steroids are lipophilic and can diffuse across all cell membranes. Very little steroid hormone is normally present in the adrenal cortical cells.

P.7 a **True**. Much of the aldosterone in the circulation is transported bound to plasma protein (over 50%) mostly associated with the albumin fraction, with the globulin transcortin binding a relatively small proportion.

b **True**. The first detectable sign of aldosterone action is an increase in mRNA approximately 20 minutes after addition of aldosterone. The hormone enters its target cell readily through the lipid membrane and binds to its intracellular receptor. The hormone–receptor complex enters the nucleus where it activates the transcription process (genomic action). Consequently, new protein molecules are synthesized. There is recent evidence that aldosterone may also have a much more rapid non-genomic action in certain cells (e.g. lymphocytes).

c **True**. The chief target tissues for aldosterone are the kidneys (by far the most important), the gastrointestinal tract, and the salivary glands.

d **False**. Aldosterone stimulates sodium reabsorption in the distal convoluted tubule and early cortical section of the collecting duct of the renal nephron. Aldosterone also stimulates potassium and hydrogen ion secretion into the tubular lumen of the distal nephron.

e **False**. Aldosterone has no established effect on the proximal tubule. Water reabsorption is passive along the proximal tubule, and follows the (very small) osmotic gradient established by the movement of sodium and other osmotically active particles across the epithelial cell layer. Since there is no evidence for a proximal tubular effect of aldosterone (e.g. on sodium reabsorption), the hormone will not influence water reabsorption across this early section of the nephron.

P.8 a **False**. Corticotrophin from the adenohypophysis is said to have a 'permissive' effect on aldosterone production, only. Its actions on adrenal cortical cells include the stimulation of early common precursor synthesis (e.g. of pregnenolone from cholesterol), which provides increased substrate available for aldosterone synthesis in response to other stimuli.

b **True**. The renin–angiotensin system is the most important influence on aldosterone production. A decapeptide, angiotensin I, is cleaved from a circulating precursor protein angiotensinogen which is synthesized in the liver. Angiotensin I loses two of its amino acids as a result of the action of an angiotensin-converting enzyme (ACE) system to form the octapeptide angiotensin II. This polypeptide is the most potent stimulus for aldosterone production from the zona glomerulosa cells.

c **False**. If the plasma sodium ion concentration *decreases* by more than 10 mmol/litre it has a direct stimulatory effect on aldosterone production.

d **True**. The juxtaglomerular cells of the renal afferent arteriole release the enzyme renin into the circulation. It acts on angiotensinogen to form the peptide angiotensin I, precursor of angiotensin II (see above). Thus, plasma renin activity (PRA) and aldosterone production are normally associated with each other such that if circulating PRA increases aldosterone production will increase. There is clear evidence that aldosterone and angiotensin II both exert negative feedback effects on renin release. If aldosterone production increases for some other reason (e.g. an adrenal adenoma), PRA levels are decreased.

e **True**. Salt appetite is stimulated as part of the normal physiological response to salt deficiency. A decrease in salt (i.e. sodium) in the plasma will stimulate aldosterone directly as part of the overall response to retain salt. In addition, salt deficiency might be associated with hypotension and increased sympathetic activity, which both stimulate renin release.

P.9 a **True**. This enzyme plays a key role in protecting the kidneys from excessive stimulation by cortisol by converting it to the relatively inactive molecule cortisone. This has the effect of removing cortisol from the vicinity of the mineralocorticoid receptors (MR) in the distal nephron. This is necessary because both cortisol and aldosterone have similar affinities for the MR, so the more prevalent glucocorticoid is removed in order to allow aldosterone to exert its renal effects. Licorice extracts contain chemicals (e.g. glycyrrhetinic acid) which inhibit the action of 11β-hydroxysteroid dehydrogenase; consequently, cortisol exerts an excessive mineralocorticoid effect with potential clinical problems.

b **True**. However, the expansion is self-limiting and a frank oedema does not develop.

c **True**. Sodium retention occurs when mineralocorticoid excess is present chronically and this is associated with a modest expansion of the extracellular fluid. It is believed that this, long term, is the cause for corticosteroid-induced hypertension.

d **True**. Atrial natriuretic hormone, as its name implies, produces an increased excretion of sodium in the urine so that its action tends to counteract the aldosterone-induced increase in sodium reabsorption.

e **False**. The renal actions of aldosterone occur mainly in the distal convoluted tubule and early part of the cortical collecting duct. The increase in sodium reabsorption (or the increase in potassium secretion) induced by aldosterone in this region of the nephron will not have any major effect on the maintenance of the medullary gradient.

P.10 a **True**. The relevant P-450 enzymes required for the synthesis of the glucocorticoids are present in these parts of the adrenal cortex. The principal glucocorticoid in humans is cortisol. The early stage in the synthesis pathway, from cholesterol to progesterone, can take place in all three zones of the adrenal cortex. However, the subsequent conversion of progesterone to 17α-hydroxyprogesterone can only take place in the two inner zones where the necessary enzyme ($P-450_{c17}$, also known as 17β-hydroxylase) is present.

b **False**. Aldosterone is not a precursor for cortisol; it is produced in the outer zona glomerulosa where the specific enzyme required for the final conversion stages from corticosterone to aldosterone (cytochrome $P-450_{c11}$, also known as 18-hydroxylase) is located. Cortisol requires certain specific enzymes located in the zonae fasciculata and reticularis (see above).

c **True**. All the steroid hormones are lipophilic and so can diffuse across cell membranes as soon as they are synthesized. For this reason steroid hormones are not stored to any extent in the endocrine cells.

d **True**. Between 0.1–0.4 μmol of aldosterone and 30–80 μmol cortisol are produced by the adrenal glands daily. The plasma concentrations of the two steroids are also markedly different, being of the order of 100–450 pmol/litre (recumbent) and 200–800 pmol/litre (ambulatory) for aldosterone compared with 200–700 nmol/litre (at 9 a.m.) and below 250 nmol/litre (at midnight) for cortisol.

e **True**. The release of cortisol by most (if not all) stressors is a key endocrine feature of the normal stress response. In the absence of normal amounts of circulating glucocorticoids, even a mild stress can be fatal (cf. Addison's disease).

P.11 a **True**. Other molecules with some glucocorticoid activity are produced (e.g. deoxycortisol, corticosterone) but these are of minor importance in humans.

b **True**. This plasma protein is a globulin which normally binds approximately 75% of the circulating cortisol, with a further 15% bound to albumin; the remainder is free (i.e. unbound). Transcortin also transports some aldosterone.

c **True**. Corticotrophin, also known as adrenocorticotrophic hormone (ACTH), is produced by the corticotroph cells of the adenohypophysis. This 39 amino acid polypeptide is the main controlling influence on adrenal cortisol production.

d **True**. When produced in excess (e.g. Cushing's syndrome) cortisol exerts a mineralocorticoid effect on sodium reabsorption. Also if the renal enzyme 11β-hydroxysteroid dehydrogenase is inhibited, cortisol is not converted to the relatively inactive molecule cortisone (see P.9a above) in which case it binds competitively to the mineralocorticoid receptors and produces an excessive aldosterone-like effect on salt and water balance.

e **True**. All steroid hormones have intracellular receptors to which they bind, cortisol binding to its glucocorticoid receptor (GR). The hormone–receptor complex then enters the nucleus where it exerts a genomic effect which results in increased protein synthesis. Cortisol, like other steroids, may have more rapid, non-genomic effects which may be mediated by other (perhaps membrane) receptors.

P.12 a **True**. This hepatic action removes biologically active cortisol from the circulation. A similar action, by renal 11β-hydroxysteroid dehydrogenase, allows aldosterone free access to its own receptor.

b **False**. Aldosterone, not cortisol, controls sodium reabsorption by the distal nephrons. Cortisol normally has a very minor role in this regard, although when produced in excessive amounts (i.e. in Cushing's syndrome) then it exerts a significant effect via the mineralocorticoid receptors in the distal convoluted tubules.

c **True**. The results of this effect are commonly observed when excessive amounts of circulating cortisol are present (i.e. in Cushing's syndrome). The wasting of arms and legs, and thinness of the skin which results in easy bruising, and the formation of purple striae are presenting features of the syndrome.

d **True**. This is at least partly a consequence of glucocorticoid-induced protein catabolism which provides suitable aminoacids for gluconeogenesis. In Cushing's syndrome chronic, excessive amounts of circulating cortisol can increase the blood glucose level such that diabetes mellitus ('adrenal diabetes') can result.

e **False**. Only protein/polypeptide hormones can be synthesized by non-endocrine tumours (i.e. ectopic production). Indeed, corticotrophin is one biologically active polypeptide which can be produced ectopically. Consequently, the adrenal glands are stimulated by this ectopic corticotrophin to produce cortisol, excessive quantities of which can result in Cushing's syndrome.

P.13 a **True**. The pulsatile release of cortisol occurs in response to the pulsatile release of its principal stimulus, the adenohypophysial hormone corticotrophin. Corticotrophin, in turn, is released in pulses because it is controlled by the pulses of corticotrophin releasing hormone (and vasopressin) from the hypothalamus.

b **False**. Cortisol levels in the blood are at their lowest around midnight and reach their peak usually around 8–9 a.m. This circadian rhythm is an important characteristic of normal cortisol production. Cortisol produced by an adrenal adenoma or in response to ectopic corticotrophin may not show a clear circadian variation.

c **False**. The only positive feedback effect on the hypothalamo–hypophysial axis is exerted by 17β-oestradiol during the late follicular phase of the menstrual cycle. Cortisol only has negative feedback effects on the hypothalamus and on the anterior pituitary.

d **True**. This is called an indirect negative feedback loop, operating at the level of the hypothalamus, and it involves the cortisol-induced inhibition of corticotrophin releasing hormone and vasopressin. Cortisol also has a direct negative feedback effect on the adenohypophysis, decreasing the production of corticotrophin.

e **False**. Cortisol has no clear effect on aldosterone production. (However, since cortisol has negative feedback effects on corticotrophin production, and corticotrophin has a 'permissive' action on aldosterone synthesis, it is feasible that cortisol *could* influence aldosterone.)

P.14 a **True**. They are actually synthesized in both inner zones of the adrenal cortex (zonae fasciculata and reticularis). The main stimulus for their production is corticotrophin from the adenohypophysis.

b **True**. Other more potent androgens, such as testosterone, are also produced in the adrenals, albeit in even smaller amounts. Androgens are also synthesized by the gonads in both sexes, particularly by the testes in males.

c **True**. Androgens are aromatized to oestrogens (by aromatase enzymes) in the gonads (testes or ovaries) and in peripheral and central tissues. A significant amount of oestrogen (the relatively weak oestrone) is synthesized from androgen precursors, mainly androstenedione, in adipose tissue and this becomes an important source of oestrogen in women after the menopause.

d **True**. Adrenarche occurs approximately 2 years before the pubertal increase in gonadal steroid production. It is associated with an increased production of adrenal androgens, the precise functions of which are still relatively obscure (but see below).

e **True**. The stimulation of pubic and axillary hair growth is the only known physiological effect of the adrenal androgens released at adrenarche.

SAQ Answers

P.15

The difference between the effects of noradrenaline and adrenaline is essentially their relative affinities for α and β receptors. Noradrenaline is a much more potent stimulator of α receptor-mediated actions, such as arteriolar vasoconstriction, then adrenaline which is particularly on β_2 receptors that mediate vasodilatation. In humans, noradrenaline administered intravenously will produce an initial tachycardia and a powerful vasoconstriction of arterioles, particularly in skeletal muscle, skin, and splanchnic bed. This vasoconstriction produces a large increase in total peripheral resistance, and the consequent rise in mean arterial blood pressure stimulates the baroreceptors in the carotid sinus and aortic arch, resulting in a reflex bradycardia (and a decrease in cardiac output). In contrast, adrenaline produces an increase in heart rate (tachycardia), some vasoconstriction via the α receptors but also a vasodilatation via β receptors. The mean arterial blood pressure does not increase very much, the baroreceptors are not stimulated and a reflex bradycardia is not elicited.

P.16

The principal mineralocorticoid in humans is aldosterone. In the distal nephron (distal convoluted tubule and cortical distal tubule) it stimulates sodium reabsorption and potassium/hydrogen ion secretion (see Fig. 5.1). Aldosterone binds to intracellular receptors, the hormone–receptor complex enters the nucleus and stimulates nuclear gene transcription resulting in new intracellular protein synthesis. Possible actions of these proteins include changes in luminal membrane

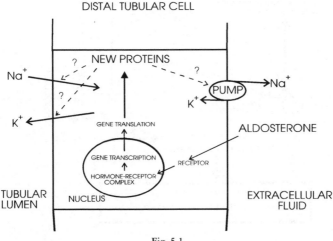

DISTAL TUBULAR CELL

Fig. 5.1

permeability to sodium and potassium ions (e.g. synthesis of new ion channels) and increased serosal membrane Na^+/K^+-ATPase pump activity.

P.17

The neurohypophysial hormone, vasopressin, is released into the general circulation when osmoreceptors in the hypothalamus are stimulated by an increase in extracellular fluid osmolality. Sodium chloride provides the chief solute constituents (approximately 95%) of the plasma (e.g. extracellular fluid) osmolality so any change in the sodium ion concentration will influence vasopressin release. The mineralocorticoid, aldosterone, from the zona glomerulosa of the adrenal cortex stimulates sodium reabsorption from the distal nephron and consequently the plasma osmolality will increase. This stimulates the release of vasopressin which acts on the renal collecting ducts to increase water reabsorption. Thus, aldosterone acts to increase the amount of sodium in the extracellular fluid while vasopressin acys to restore the sodium concentration by stimulating water reabsorption. (The osmoreceptors operate around a predetermined set point.) The same information is provided in Fig. 5.2.

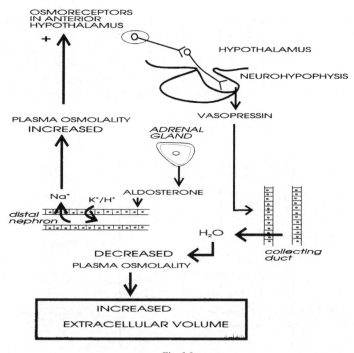

Fig. 5.2

P.18

The key words to mention in this answer are: the juxtaglomerular cells (or apparatus), renin, angiotensinogen (from liver), angiotensin I, angiotensin II (and even angiotensin III), angiotensin converting enzyme (ACE), adrenal cortex, zona glomrulosa, aldosterone, corticotrophin (or ACTH), plasma Na^+ and K^+ concentrations. (See Fig. 5.3.)

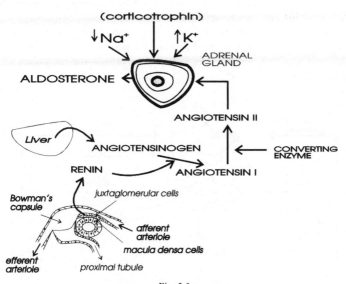

Fig. 5.3

P.19

The glucocorticoid cortisol has many effects on a variety of target tissues. The four actions required can be chosen from the following examples: (a) metabolic effects, which include stimulation of protein catabolism, hepatic gluconeogenesis, and lipolysis (and redistribution of fat to facial and truncal regions when excess cortisol is present); (b) mineralocorticoid activity (usually minor compared with aldosterone); (c) renal effect (e.g. required for excretion of water load); (d) cardiovascular influence (e.g. increases vascular sensitivity to catecholamines); (e) necessary for the normal stress response; (f) influence on immune system (important in endocrine–immune interactions); (g) growth.

In Cushing's syndrome, excessive metabolic effects of cortisol may be manifest as: (i) loss of muscle protein (muscle wasting, weakness) and thinning of skin tissue resulting in easy bruising and formation of purple striae; (ii) hyperglycaemia due to excessive gluconeogenesis, etc. (leading to 'adrenal diabetes', in approximately 10% of patients); (iii) redistribution of fat (e.g. characteristic moonface). Excessive mineralocorticoid activity may result in hypertension due to the sodium retention.

Excessive glucocorticoid effects on the immune system (immunosuppression) result in increased susceptibility to infection. In children there may be reduced linear growth.

P.20

Key features to be shown in a diagram illustrating the control of cortisol production are: corticotrophin releasing hormone (CRH, or corticoliberin), vasopressin (VP), hypothalamus, adenohypophysis (anterior pituitary), corticotrophin (or adrenocorticotrophic hormone, ACTH), adrenal cortex (perhaps specifying the inner zonae fasciculata and reticularis), direct and indirect negative feedback loops. Additional controlling factors can be included (e.g. bring in the interleukins which can be produced from cells of the immune system). (See Fig. 5.4.)

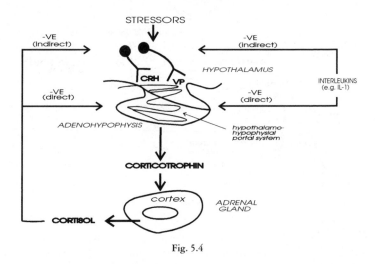

Fig. 5.4

The adrenals (Clinical)

Multiple Choice Questions

C.1

A 67-year-old female inpatient with a long history of well-controlled epilepsy is rehabilitating following a fractured femur. She is noted to have facial plethora and hypertension, raising the question of Cushing's syndrome. Urinary cortisol excretion was 300 and 285 nmol/24 hours on two successive days (N < 320).

Overnight dexamethasone suppression test (2.0 mg) results in an early morning serum cortisol of 220 nmol/litre (N < 100). Serum ACTH (9 a.m.) is 23 ng/litre (N < 25). Which of the following is/are true?

a Pituitary-dependent Cushing's syndrome has not been excluded
b The patient is likely to have an ectopic ACTH syndrome
c A two dose level dexamethasone suppression test should be performed
d Longstanding phenytoin therapy (for her grand mal epilepsy) could explain these findings
e It is likely that no endocrine disorder is present

C.2

A 35-year-old woman complains of weight gain and weakness, and is found to be hypertensive and diabetic. Pituitary-dependent Cushing's disease is suspected. Which of the following findings would support this diagnosis?

a Urinary cortisol excretion of 380 and 410 nmol/24 hours on 2 consecutive collections (N < 320), and undetectable serum ACTH levels by sensitive immunoradiometric assay
b Suppression of early morning cortisol to less than 50 nmol/litre 8 hours after oral dexamethasone 2 mg
c No identifiable abnormality on pituitary MRI scan
d Markedly raised plasma androgen levels
e Exaggerated ACTH response to CRH infusion

C.3

Which of the following strategies is/are appropriate for the treatment of pituitary-dependent Cushing's disease?

a Bilateral adrenalectomy
b Cyproheptadine
c Trans-sphenoidal removal of the pituitary adenoma
d External beam cobalt source radiotherapy
e Expectation of spontaneous remission

C.4

A 54-year-old woman with a blood pressure of 155/90 and a marked premenstrual 'tension' syndrome presents with weakness. She is found to have consistent hypokalaemia within the range 2.4–2.8 mmol/litre (NR 3.8–5.3). Urine potassium excretion is 58 mmol/24 hours. Serum aldosterone is 2350 pmol/litre (NR 80–450) and ambulant serum renin activity is 0.2 pmol/ml/hour (NR 0.5–3.0). Which of the following entities may be responsible?

a Primary hyperaldosteronism
b Potassium secreting villous adenoma of the bowel
c Liquorice ingestion

d Diuretic abuse
e Ectopic ACTH syndrome

C.5

Which of the following is/are true in the syndrome of primary hyperaldosteronism?

a It is responsible for approximately 5% of cases of newly diagnosed hypertension
b Most cases are due to a single adrenal adenoma
c Hypokalaemia developing during diuretic therapy is a clue to the presence of this disorder
d Spironolactone is capable of correcting the hypertension and hypokalaemia in almost all patients
e Hypomagnesaemia may be a contributory cause of the presenting muscular weakness

C.6

For which of the following complications of long-term, high-dose therapeutic corticosteroids is/are preventive strategies available?

a Growth retardation in children
b Peptic ulceration
c Osteoporosis
d Suppression of the pituitary–adrenal axis
e Diabetes mellitus

C.7

A 40-year-old man with fatigue and weight loss is suspected of having primary adrenocortical insufficiency (Addison's disease). Which of the following additional findings would support this diagnosis?

a A family history of autoimmune thyroid disease
b Patchy areas of skin depigmentation
c Postural hypotension
d A 9 a.m. serum ACTH level of 10 ng/litre (NR < 25 ng/litre)
e A serum cortisol of 230 nmol/litre before, and 260 nmol/litre 30 minutes after IV 250 μg tetracosactrin

C.8

In the treatment of adult primary adrenocortical deficiency, which of the following principles should be followed?

a Administration of cortisol once daily to avoid risk of steroid side-effects
b Suspension of cortisol replacement in the presence of vomiting
c Addition of mineralocorticoid only if hypotension is present
d Doubling or tripling the cortisol dose in the presence of severe emotional distress

e Wearing an identification bracelet or pendant indicating steroid replacement therapy

C.9

Which of the following is/are true in the disorder of congenital adrenal hyperplasia (CAH)?

a The prevalence of CAH is approximately 1 in 10 000 births
b Consanguinous marriages increase the risk of CAH
c The condition may be fatal if not diagnosed in the first two weeks of life
d Once a child with CAH is born to a couple, procedures are available for antenatal assessment of subsequent conceptions for the presence of CAH
e CAH occurs more frequently in females

C.10

In a 3-year-old child with ambiguous genitalia.

a The presence of hypertension makes the diagnosis of CAH unlikely
b If CAH is confirmed, steroid replacement can cause complete regression of abnormal sexual differentiation
c The dose of glucocorticoid replacement can best be monitored using plasma cortisol levels
d Final mature height may be above average if steroid doses at this age are inadequate
e With appropriate steroid replacement, fertility in adulthood is likely

C.11

In a 35-year-old woman, a calcified area overlying the right diaphragmatic shadow is noted on a routine chest X-ray. A subsequent abdominal MRI scan confirms that a gallstone is responsible. However, an incidental solid 8 mm diameter 'nodule' is also noted in the left adrenal. The patient is symptomatically well. Which of the following is/are true?

a 5–10% of healthy people harbour such lesions
b It is likely to be malignant
c Routine investigations are likely to identify a hypersecreting adrenal adenoma
d Removal of the adrenal lesion is mandatory
e Other endocrine glands should be evaluated for similar lesions

C.12

A 24-year-old man awaiting elective surgery for inguinal hernia repair is found to have a blood pressure of 170/105. On questioning, he has had recent episodes of sweating and faintness, so that the possibility of phaeochromocytoma is raised. Which of the following is/are true?

a The hypertension should be further investigated once his operation has been done b Three successive 24-hour urine collections for VNA (vanillyl mandelic acid) of 29, 31, and 28 μmol/24 hours (N $<$ 40) make this diagnosis untenable

c The blood pressure response to tyramine is a preferable test to biochemical screening

d A family history of hypertension makes the diagnosis less likely

e The presence of hypokalaemia makes a diagnosis of hyperaldosteronism more likely

Short Answer Questions

C.13

Name 5 symptoms and signs of pituitary-dependent Cushing's disease. In each case identify their pathophysiological basis.

C.14

A 25-year-old Caucasian male without a family history of hypertension is found to have a persistent blood pressure of 170/115 despite resting. Write short notes on diagnostic process required to identify a possible causative endocrinopathy?

MCQ Answers

C.1 a **True**. Although urinary cortisol excretion is normal, the cyclical nature of Cushing's disease is such that elevated levels are not always present. The other values quoted are entirely consistent with this diagnosis of hypercortisolism.

b **False**. Ectopic ACTH is almost invariably associated with marked elevations of urinary cortisol (and serum ACTH): see also Chapter 14, C.2.

c **True**. Suppression of urinary cortisol to $<$100 nmol/24 hours on 2 mg dexamethasone daily for 3 days would exclude the diagnosis. In patients with pituitary dependent Cushing's disease, such suppression only occurs with 8 mg daily for 3 days. The high–normal serum ACTH excludes the possibility of adrenal adenoma as a cause.

d **True**. Phenytoin induces P-450 microsomal enzyme activity, which increases the hepatic clearance of administered steroid. The negative feedback effect is accordingly diminished, and the value of the test negated. A number of other drugs share this effect.

e **True**. Elderly, hospitalized, anxious, or depressed patients often fail to suppress cortisol with conventional dexamethasone doses. Two out of three of these factors are operating in this case, so that the findings as presented are likely to represent 'normal' adrenal function.

C.2 a **False**. In pituitary-dependent Cushing's disease, serum ACTH is raised or at least detectable: the suppressed serum ACTH by negative feedback as in the quoted test profile would be consistent only with adrenal adenoma or carcinoma.

b **False**. Cortisol has been normally suppressed. A failure of cortisol suppression by exogenous steroid is consistent with *all* forms of Cushing's syndrome, but is found also in the elderly (especially institutionalized), the depressed, and those with either severe acute or chronic illness: conversely the quoted test result excludes Cushing's syndrome in all its forms.

c **True**. The pituitary microadenoma may be too small to identify even on MRI scan: hyperplasia of ACTH producing cells has also been described, presumably secondary to hypothalamic stimulation.

d **False**. High plasma androgen levels are more suggestive of adrenal adenoma or carcinoma.

e **True**. In pituitary dependent Cushing's disease, pituitary ACTH response to a variety of stimuli may be exaggerated. This includes insulin-induced hypoglycaemia, the negative feedback stimulus of metyrapone administration, and the exaggerated response to intravenous corticotrophin releasing hormone (CRH).

C.3 a **True**. This is a rapid means of correcting cortisol excess. However, because of consequent reduced feedback inhibition of ACTH release, the responsible pituitary adenoma may escalate in size in 10–25% of cases, infiltrating parasellar structures, and causing ACTH-mediated hyperpigmentation (Nelson's syndrome). Pituitary irradiation reduces but does not eliminate this risk.

b **True**. Mild cases may respond to this drug which inhibits serotonin-mediated ACTH release. Ketoconazole and metyrapone are two other occasionally useful drugs for temporary control, both of which act directly on the adrenal. They are useful prior to surgery. Metyrapone inhibits 11β-hydroxylase activity, but the sites of action of ketoconazole on steroid biosynthesis are still incompletely understood.

c **True**. This is the preferred approach, ideally after lateralizing studies using petrosal venous sinus sampling to identify the concentration gradient. The investigation is highly specialized, and is only carried out in a few centres.

d **True**. This approach is only occasionally used because of slow response rate, necessitating simultaneous and long-term administration of an adrenal biosynthetic blocking agent.

e **False**. Although there is small spontaneous remission rate due to presumed infarction of the tumour, definitive treatment is usually mandatory.

C.4 a **True**. Although most patients are hypertensive, this may not be a striking feature. Serum renin levels are low in primary hyperaldosteronism, due to aldosterone-induced volume expansion, and this confirms the diagnosis.

b **False**. Urinary potassium levels would be low in this condition, to compensate for enhanced gastrointestinal loss. Serum renin levels would be raised or normal.

c **False**. Glycirrizinic acid (found in liquorice) and the anti-ulcer drug carbenoxolone (now little used) inhibit 11β-hydroxysteroid dehydrogenase. This increases mineralocorticoid (corticosterone) production, and simulates the clinical picture of primary hyperaldosteronism. However, both serum aldosterone and renin are normal, or more usually suppressed.

d **False**. In addition to hypokalaemia, diuretic excess will induce volume depletion. Serum aldosterone (and renin) would accordingly be increased.

e **True**. Although physiologically, ACTH has little or no effect on the zona glomerulosa, the ectopic ACTH (or CRH) syndromes induce preferential mineralocorticoid excess because of very high blood ACTH levels encountered. The cushingoid clinical features often take longer to appear than the hypokalaemic symptoms. Serum renin levels are suppressed, but aldosterone levels are not necessarily markedly raised; the mineralocorticoid effects of aldosterone precursors are often dominant.

C.5 a **False**. At most, 1:500 (0.2%) newly identified hypertensives have primary hyperaldosteronism. Serum aldosterone is raised and serum renin suppressed. Secondary hyperaldosteronism (raised serum renin and aldosterone) is rather more frequently present, secondary to ischaemic renal lesions, particularly renal artery stenosis: the rare Bartter's syndrome has a similar profile and is due to hyperplasia of the juxta–glomerular apparatus.

b **False**. Better imaging and biochemical assays have allowed bilateral hyperplasia to be identified at least as (if not more) frequently than solitary adenoma: a characteristic postural rise in aldosterone is the hallmark of hyperplasia.

c **False**. Only very rarely is hypokalaemia in the course of diuretic therapy due to primary hyperaldosteronism: discontinuing the diuretic almost always restores normo-kalaemia. Hypokalaemia always should be corrected before investigating for hyperaldosteronism, since it directly inhibits aldosterone release, whatever its aetiology.

d **True**. Spironolactone (100–400 mg daily) is effective whether hyperplasia or adenoma is responsible. Long-term spironolactone therapy is also an acceptable alternative to surgery.

e **True**. Aldosterone also increases urinary magnesium excretion, and this may contribute both to musculoskeletal weakness as well as proneness to cardiac arrhythmias in older individuals.

C.6 a **False**. Alternate day steroid dosage and use of concurrent growth hormone therapy have been shown to be ineffective. IGF-I treatment may be shown to be of benefit, although most steroid effects on growth inhibition are mediated by a direct effect on growth hormone and IGF-I receptors on cartilage and bone.

b **True**. Both H2 receptor blockers and proton pump inhibitors are effective in preventing acid hypersecretion and consequent dyspepsia.

c **True**. Concurrent use of bisphosphonates has been shown to be effective in reducing steroid-induced bone loss, and should probably be employed in all patients requiring more than 7.5 mg prednisolone (or equivalent) for a period in excess of 4 months.

d **False**. Variable degree of temporary (rarely permanent) suppression of the pituitary–adrenal axis follows such courses of steroids irrespective of dose schedule or steroid type. ACTH has been used, in parallel with the steroids to 'protect' the adrenal. However, the major effect of steroid suppression is at the hypothalamic–pituitary level.

e **False**. There are no effective inhibitors of the multi-site hyperglycaemic effects of corticosteroids, which principally enhance hepatic gluco-neogenesis, suppress insulin release, and reduce insulin sensitivity in muscle and liver.

C.7 a **True**. Approximately 30% of patients with Addison's disease will either have a family history of autoimmune thyroid disease or will themselves have autoimmune thyroid dysfunction. The latter situation sometimes self-corrects after steroid replacement: the mechanism of this correction is unknown.

b **True**. Around 30% of patients have vitiligo, which may precede or follow the diagnosis of Addison's disease: this circumscribed patchy depigmentation is due to an antibody to a melanocyte antigen, probably the 69 kDa enzyme tyrosinase, which plays an important part in melanin synthesis. Sometimes the vitiligo is in striking contrast to the ACTH-mediated hyperpigmentation. Conversely, patients presenting with vitiligo alone should be assessed with antiadrenal and antithyroid antibodies as a guide to follow-up. The life-long cumulative prevalence of such organ-specific immune disorders in patients with vitiligo is not accurately known.

c **True**. Supine hypotension is due to hypovolaemia (sodium depletion): the additional postural drop is due to the lack of cortisol which in normal subjects potentiates the effect of catecholamines on vascular tone.

d **False**. In primary adrenocortical insufficiency, negative feedback stimulates very high ACTH levels, often exceeding 200 ng/litre. A low serum ACTH in the presence of low serum cortisol suggests adrenal insufficiency of hypothalamic–pituitary origin.

e **True**. Basal cortisol levels are often in the normal range in newly diagnosed patients with Addison's disease due to maximal stimulation from high endogenous ACTH levels. The failure to respond to synthetic ACTH is 'abnormal'. This phenomenon may also occur occasionally in normal subjects and more often in hypopituitarism. Therefore, an abnormal response should be followed either by multiple ACTH dose stimulation, intravenous tetracosactrin stimulation, or a serum ACTH measurement.

C.8 a **False**. Because of its short half-life, cortisol needs to be given twice or ideally 3 times daily, usually with the higher dose in the morning: a regime of 10 mg, 5 mg, 5 mg is common. Steroid side-effects are rare with cortisol replacement in correct dosages

b **False**. Such an action could precipitate adrenal 'crisis'. The steroid dose actually needs to be supplemented (*not reduced*) under these circumstances, ideally by the IM or IV route (100 mg stat), partly because of lack of absorption, and partly because of the increased steroid requirement with illness *of any type*.

c **False**. Mineralocorticoid replacement (usually fludrocortisone 50–150 μg daily) is *mandatory* in all cases. Mineralocorticoid needs can theoretically be met by using a higher dosage of cortisol, but glucocorticoid side-effects would then be a real risk. Serum renin levels can be used as a guide to adequacy of fludrocortisone replacement dose.

d **True**. Emotional stress is normally as large a stimulus to increased cortisol release as is physical disease. Hence, doses should be doubled or tripled during the acute stressful event.

e **True**. The major cause of death in Addison's disease is a failure to increase or parenterally administer steroid doses together with any additional stress. Easily visible identification with a pendant or bracelet lowers the risk of overlooking diagnoses in unconscious patients in 'crisis'.

C.9 a **True**. With a gene frequency of 1:50 for these collective enzyme defects, 1:2500 matings will be 'at risk'. Since these disorders are inherited as autosomal recessive traits, 1:4 offspring will be affected giving a prevalence of 1:10 000.

b **True**. As with all autosomally recessive disorders, this holds true.

c **True**. The severe salt-losing forms of 21-hydroxylase (and extremely rare 3β-hydroxysteroid dehydrogenase) deficiency result in collapse and vomiting from a combination of dehydration and cortisol deficiency, a fatal combination which can readily be misdiagnosed as infection.

d **True**. Samples taken by the procedure of chorionic villous sampling can be analysed for 'gene carrier status'. If positive, steroid therapy during pregnancy can prevent or minimize anomalous intrauterine genital development

e **False.** Prevalence is probably identical in males and females. However, androgen excess in pubertal or late developing forms in males is clinically inapparent, only presenting as infertility (which is sometimes correctable by steroid therapy).

C.10 a **False.** In one of the less common forms of congenital adrenal hyperplasia, 11β-hydroxylase deficiency, hypertension is almost the rule. This is due to accumulation of corticosterone derivatives with high mineralocorticoid activity. Hypertension resolves with physiological steroid replacement.

b **False.** At best, steroid replacement will halt further progression of abnormal genital changes. Surgery is very likely to be necessary.

c **False.** The only reliable method of monitoring is by regular checks of (serum) 17-hydroxyprogesterone or (urinary) pregnanetriol, which must be reduced into the normal range.

d **False.** Under-replacement with steroid allows continued androgenic hypersecretion. This will enhance growth rate initially (as part of precocious puberty), but androgen-mediated premature epiphyseal fusion will result in reduced final mature height.

e **True.** Allowing for correction of genital abnormalities (i.e. labiocrotal fusion), fertility is often achievable.

C.11 a **True.** Approximately 10% of the normal population are found to have so-called incidentalomas of the adrenal identified when scans are performed for other indications. They may similarly be identified first at autopsy.

b **False.** Almost invariably the lesion is benign, although metastases from primary tumours elsewhere commonly occur in the adrenal because of its vascularity.

c **False.** Although it is usual to screen for hyperaldosteronism, Cushing's syndrome, phaechromocytoma, and androgenic tumours, in more than 90% of cases the lesion is non-secreting.

d **False.** Surgery is not indicated on the basis of a–c above. However, it is safer to follow up with serial scans at 6–12-month intervals. In practice, up to 50% of cases come to surgery, usually because of concern regarding the tumour growth pattern as assessed by imaging techniques. Histology almost invariably confirms non-functioning (benign) adenomas. The number of cases coming to surgery may be reduced in future years with the wider use of percutaneous adrenal biopsy.

e **False.** Although functioning adrenal adenomas may form part of the polyendocrine familial MEN-1 syndrome, non-functioning adenomas are usually not part of this syndrome, so that more extensive screening is not justified.

C.12   a   **False**. A surgical operation (or any form of acute stress) in a patient harbouring a phaeochromocytoma can result in a potentially fatal adrenergic hypertensive crisis. Beta-adrenergic blocking drugs reduce, but do not eliminate this risk.

b   **False**. Normal VMA levels are found in about 25% of patients with proven phaeochromocytoma, even with serial urine collections. Measurement of adrenaline and noradrenaline increases diagnostic sensitivity to around 95%.

c   **False**. Stimulation tests are theoretically useful, but are dangerous. They are rarely if ever indicated.

d   **False**. Although 'essential' hypertension is often familial, phaeochromocytoma can also be familial when part of the MEN-2 syndrome, so that a positive family history should not deter from pursuing a diagnosis of phaeochromocytoma.

e   **False**. Although hypokalaemia is suggestive of hyperaldosteronism, it is also found in about 30% of patients with phaeochromocytoma. The mechanism is unclear.

SAQ Answers

C.13

Hypertension: sodium retention, increased arteriolar tone; *central obesity*: steroid-induced hyperphagia and lipogenesis; *hyperglycaemia/diabetes*: increased gluconeogenesis, down-regulation of insulin receptors; *back pain*: osteoporosis; *striae*: increased catabolism of protein/defective collagen structure; *pigmentation*: ACTH excess (MSH effect); *weakness*: steroid myopathy.

C.14

Hyperaldosteronism: check for hypokalaemia and inappropriately raised urine potassium, raised serum aldosterone, and suppressed renin, possibly proceeding to adrenal imaging (ultrasound, CT, or MRI.) *Cushing's syndrome*: check for associated clinical features, plus raised 24-hour urine cortisol or abnormal overnight dexamathasone suppression test in conjunction with serum ACTH (normal–high or low depending on whether pituitary or primary adrenal cause). Proceed to imaging or 'long' dexamethasone suppression test. *Phaeochromocytoma*: ask about 'adrenergic symptoms' (although many cases are asymptomatic), check for episodic hypertension, family history (MEN-2 syndromes), raised 24-hour catecholamines (dynamic tests uncertain and unsafe), proceeding to adrenal MRI or other areas for suspected extra-adrenal tumour. *Congenital adrenal hyperplasia (11-hydroxylase defect)*: raised serum 17-hydroxyprogesterone levels (and deoxy steroids), blood pressure suppressible by steroids (Note *hyperthyroidism* and *primary hyperparathyroidism* as occasional causes.)

References
Physiology
See Wehling (1994) (Chapter 2) on non-genomic actions of steroid hormones (focus on aldosterone)

Topic: Glucocorticoid receptors and tissue sensitivity to glucocorticoids.

Bamberger, C. M. *et al.* (1996). *Endocrine Reviews*, 17, 245–68.

Topic: Immune-neuro-endocrine interactions.

Besedovsky, H. O. *et al.* (1996). *Endocrine Reviews*, 17, 64–102.

Topic: Angiotensin, its receptors and their antagonists.

Goodfriend, T. L. *et al.* (1996). *New England Journal of Medicine*, 334, 1649–54.

Topic: Hypothalamic–pituitary adrenocortical regulation (and the effects of anti-depressants).

Holsboer, F. *et al.* (1996). *Endocrine Reviews*, 17, 187–205.

Clinical
Topic: Investigation of adrenal masses.

Cook, D. *et al.* (1996). *American Journal of Medicine*, 101, 88–94.

Topic: Mineralocorticoid hypertension.

Gordon, R. D. (1994). *Lancet*, 344, 240–3.

Topic: Diagnosis and management of Addison's disease.

Oelkers, W. *et al.* (1996). *New England Journal of Medicine*, 335, 1206–12.

Topic: Diagnosis and management of Cushing's syndrome.

Orth, D. N. (1995). *New England Journal of Medicine*, 332, 791–803.

Topic: Primary hyperaldosteronism.

Vallotton, M. B. (1996). *Clinical Endocrinology*, 45, 47–60.

6 Male reproductive endocrinology (physiology)

Multiple Choice Questions

See also Chapters 4 (Qs 4, 19, 20); Chapter 5 (Qs 5, 14)

P.1 In the male genotype

a the phenotype is determined by the presence of either X or Y chromosomes

b development of the indifferent gonads into testes is initiated by the activation of a 'sex-determining region of the Y chromosome' (sry) gene

c the primitive Mullerian ducts develop into the male reproductive tract

d the developing Sertoli cells are stimulated to produce testosterone

e the testes have normally descended into the scrotum at birth

P.2 The testes

a contain two cell types called Leydig and Sertoli cells

b are the only source of androgens in males

c are a source of oestrogen

d produce haploid gametes called spermatids

e cease to produce mature spermatozoa from the ages of 50–60 years (the male menopause)

P.3 The seminiferous tubules

a consist of ducts lined by Leydig cells

b contain a fluid that is secreted by the Sertoli cells

c are lined with smooth muscle fibres

d release an androgen-binding protein into the seminiferous fluid

e extend along the full length of the penis

P.4 The Sertoli cells

a are linked together by gap junctions

b provide a blood–testis barrier to the passage of various molecules

c synthesize androgen receptors

d synthesize the protein hormone, inhibin

e are intimately involved with the development of spermatocytes into spermatids

P.5 The Leydig cells

a lie in the interstitium between adjacent seminiferous tubules
b are innervated by myelinated nerve fibres
c release spermatogonia into the basal compartment fluid of the seminiferous tubules
d down-regulate their luteinizing hormone receptors acutely in response to luteinizing hormone
e synthesize receptors for follicle-stimulating hormone

P.6 Androgens

a are 21-carbon steroids
b are synthesized from the precursor cholesterol
c are only synthesized by the Sertoli cells in the testes
d are only synthesized in males
e are transported in the blood mainly bound to sex hormone binding globulin

P.7 Testosterone

a is converted to oestrogen in adipose tissue
b is the principal circulating androgen in males
c can be converted to the more potent dihydrotestosterone in many peripheral tissues
d is essential for the maintenance of spermatogenesis
e binds to receptors on its target cell membranes

P.8 Testosterone and other androgens

a stimulate the development of the male reproductive tract
b stimulate lipogenesis
c stimulate protein anabolism
d maintain the accessory sex glands such as the seminal vesicles
e synergize with the adenohypophysial hormone somatotrophin to stimulate linear growth at puberty

P.9 Testosterone production

a is increased by many stressors
b is directly stimulated by decreased circulating glucose concentrations
c only occurs in the male genotype
d is released in pulses into the circulation
e follows a diurnal variation in adult males

P.10 The release of testicular testosterone

a involves the hypothalamic gonadotrophin releasing hormone (GnRH)
b is stimulated by luteinizing hormone (LH) from the adenohypophysis

    c is influenced by its negative feedback effect on the hypothalamo–adenohypophysial axis

    d decreases when circulating inhibin levels increase

    e is decreased in conditions of calorific deprivation

Short Answer Questions

P.11

Identify the two principal functions of the testes, and *briefly* explain how the two are linked

P.12

List three physiological actions of testosterone and describe its mechanism of action.

P.13

By means of a clearly labelled diagram explain how testicular function is controlled.

MCQ Answers

P.1 a **False**. It is only the short arm of the Y chromosome which contains the 'sex-determining region' gene.

    b **True**. This gene is associated with the production of a DNA binding protein called SRY protein which converts the early indifferent gonads into testes. The major site of expression of this gene is the developing Sertoli cells.

    c **False**. The Mullerian ducts, if allowed to, would develop into *female* reproductive tract. The Wolffian ducts when stimulated by testosterone develop into the male reproductive tracts.

    d **False**. The developing Sertoli cells synthesize a glycoprotein hormone called Mullerian inhibitory factor (MIH) which stimulates regression of the Mullerian ducts.

    e **True**. Migration of the testes downwards through the abdominal cavity and over the pubic bone so that they end up in the scrotal sac usually takes place by 35–40 weeks *in utero*. The descent of the testes appears to be under the control of MIH. It appears that in humans the testes function better at a temperature approximately 5°C lower than that of body (abdominal) temperature. If the testes remain within the abdominal cavity (cryptorchism, i.e. 'hidden testes') spermatogenesis may be arrested despite normal endocrine function.

P.2 a **True**. The Leydig cells are involved in steroidogenesis, the principal synthesized steroids being androgens notably testosterone. The Sertoli cells are intimately concerned with spermatogenesis (i.e. the production of spermatozoa).

b **False**. The testes are by far the most important source of androgens in males but the adrenal glands also produce small quantities of them. The principal androgen produced by the testes is testosterone (total serum concentration in adult males: 10–35 nmol/l; in adult premenopausal women: 1–2.5 nmol/l) which can be converted to the even more potent dihydrotestosterone in peripheral tissues. The adrenal glands are a minor source of androgens in males, these consisting mainly of the weak androgens dehydroepiandrosterone (and its sulphate) and androstenedione, which can be converted to the more potent testosterone and dihydrotestosterone in peripheral tissues. The adrenals are a far more important source of circulating androgens in women.

c **True**. Some of the testicular androgen synthesized by the Leydig cells is converted to oestrogen by various tissues (including the testicular Leydig and Sertoli cells) in the presence of aromatase enzyme.

d **True**. This is an important function of the testes and is an essential element of the sexual reproductive process.

e **False**. In men, production of spermatozoa continues throughout life. With old age (e.g. over 70 years) there may be a decrease in the number of spermatozoa in seminal fluid, and an increase in the number of abnormal spermatozoa produced.

P.3 a **False**. The seminiferous tubules are lined by Sertoli cells, not Leydig cells which are found in the interstitium between seminiferous tubules.

b **True**. The active secretion results in a seminiferous fluid of quite different composition from the basal compartment fluid. For example, in comparison with either plasma or lymph, selective transport processes result in a seminiferous fluid which has lower Na^+ and higher K^+ concentrations, a lower total protein concentration (although some proteins are only found in the seminiferous fluid, e.g. androgen binding protein), a lower testosterone concentration but higher inositol concentration.

c **False**. The only part of the male reproductive tract lined by smooth muscle fibres is the final segment, the vas deferens, which serves as a reservoir for spermatozoa. The seminiferous tubules actively secrete fluid, much of which is reabsorbed in the epididymis prior to the vas deferens. Any impedence to flow in front of the epididymis results in accumulation of fluid and detrimental increase in back pressure in the seminiferous tubules. A vasectomy (ligature of the vas deferens) allows the seminiferous fluid (including spermatozoa) to be removed in the epididymis without it accumulating and damaging the tubules.

d **True**. This protein is synthesized by the Sertoli cells, is specific to the seminiferous fluid, and binds androgen (and oestrogen). It appears to play a similar role to sex hormone binding globulin in the blood.

e **False**. The seminiferous tubules lie within the testes. These tubules open into the rete testis in the hilum of the gland, and seminiferous fluid from this region drains into the vasa efferentia which then come together to form the epididymis. Finally, the seminiferous fluid enters the vas deferens which joins the urethra near the base of the penis. It is the urethra, the common duct for urine from the bladder (via the ureters) and seminiferous fluid from the testes, which passes along the full length of the penis opening at the tip of the glans.

P.4 a **True**. The Sertoli cells can intercommunicate through the gap junctions and this is probably important for their normal function. It may be relevant, for example, for the spermatogenic cycle which appears to link the stage of the developing spermatocyte to the section of seminiferous tubule.

b **True**. For this reason, the seminiferous fluid contains many molecules secreted by the Sertoli cells, and its composition differs from that of the basal compartment fluid (see answer to P.3b). In addition it provides a barrier to the movement of cells and other molecules (e.g. proteins) back into the blood where they could elicit an autoimmune response.

c **True**. The Sertoli cells synthesize androgen receptors and consequently respond to testosterone in various ways. For example, testosterone stimulates the Sertoli cells with regard to their support for the development of the secondary spermatocyte to spermatid stage of spermatogenesis.

d **True**. This protein hormone exerts a negative feedback control on the hypothalamo–hypophysial axis with particular reference to follicle-stimulating hormone.

e **True**. Secondary spermatocytes and spermatids can become completely enveloped by the Sertoli cells which appear to play an important role in their development. Testosterone is probably necessary for this developmental role of the Sertoli cells.

P.5 a **True**. The Leydig cells lie in the intersitium between the seminiferous tubules and were originally called interstitial cells. The hormone which stimulated them was originally called interstitial cell-stimulating hormone but is now known as luteinizing hormone

b **False**. There is no evidence for any direct innervation of these cells, whether myelinated or non-myelinated.

c **False**. The principal function of the Leydig cells is to produce androgens, principally testosterone which has many effects including the stimulation of spermatogenesis. However, they do not have anything to do with releasing spermatogonia into the basal compartment; these primary germ cells end up here during fetal development.

d **True.** The Leydig cells are stimulated and maintained by luteinizing hormone (LH) from the adenohypophysis. However, after LH administration there is a down-regulation of LH receptors within 24 hours which partly accounts for the subsequent desensitization to further LH.

e **True.** The Leydig cells mainly synthesize receptors for luteinizing hormone (LH) which is their principal stimulator. However they do also respond to follicle-stimulating hormone (FSH) which stimulates the synthesis of LH receptors. It must be presumed, therefore, that they respond to FSH by binding to FSH receptors which they synthesize.

P.6 a **False.** They are, indeed, steroid hormones but they have 19 carbon atoms, not 21 as in the precursor cholesterol and other steroid hormones such as cortisol, aldosterone, or progesterone.

b **True.** All testosterone is derived from the initial precursor steroid cholesterol. Most of the cholesterol enters the cells from the lipoprotein–cholesterol in the blood, but some cholesterol is synthesized from acetate.

c **False.** The Leydig cells are the principal source of androgens in testes. The Sertoli cells can convert testosterone to the more potent androgen dihydrotestosterone. (*Note:* see also next answer.)

d **False.** Androgens are produced by the adrenal glands in both sexes. Furthermore, androgens are also synthesized in the ovaries where they act as precursors for oestrogen synthesis. The follicular thecal cells synthesize androgens in response to luteinizing hormone (as do the Leydig cells in the male). The granulosa cells then convert the androgen to oestrogen in the presence of follicle-stimulating hormone (as do the Sertoli cells in the male).

e **True.** Over 60% of circulating androgens are transported in the blood bound to sex hormone binding globulin (SHBG), most of the remainder being bound to the albumin. Only 2% is present as free, unbound, hormone at any time. SHBG also transports a large proportion (more than 60%) of the oestrogen in the blood.

P.7 a **True.** Testosterone is aromatized to oestrogens (17β-oestradiol) in various peripheral tissues, particularly adipose tissue, which contain the aromataze enzyme complex necessary for the conversion. Of 5 mg/day of testosterone synthesized, approximately 0.02 mg/day of 17β-oestradiol is produced.

b **True.** Other androgens such as dihydrotestosterone, androstenedione, and dehydroepiandrosterone are present in the circulation, but testosterone is the main one.

c **True.** The more potent dihydrotestosterone is mainly synthesized from testosterone in target tissues which contain the 5α-reductase enzyme necessary for the conversion.

d **True**. Without testosterone (or its more potent derivative, dihydro-testosterone) the process of spermatogenesis is disrupted. This is mediated by the Sertoli cells which synthesize the necessary androgen receptors.

e **False**. Steroid hormones such as testosterone bind to intracellular receptors and, as hormone–receptor complexes, enter the target cell nucleus where they bind to specific hormone recognition elements along the target chromosome. Consequently, gene transcription takes place and the relevant new protein molecule mediating an action of testosterone is synthesized on ribosomes in the cytoplasm.

P.8 a **True**. This is the definition of an androgen. This action occurs first in the male fetus, but subsequent development and maintenance of the tract under androgen influence continues throughout life.

b **False**. Lipogenesis is not a physiological action of androgens.

c **True**. Androgens are protein anabolic agents, and have been used in many sports in order to stimulate muscular growth. (This practice is not accepted as legitimate by sporting authorities including the Olympic Committee.)

d **True**. This is an important physiological action of androgens. In the absence of circulating testosterone, the reproductive tract and the accessory sex glands such as the seminal vesicles may atrophy.

e **True**. The greatly increased androgen production which begins with puberty combines with the effects of somatotrophin to stimulate growth and development at this stage, including the linear *growth spurt*.

P.9 a **False**. Stressors generally inhibit the hypothalamo–adenohypophysial–gonadal axis, and in males the consequence is decreased stimulation of the Leydig cells resulting in reduced androgen synthesis.

b **False**. The principal stimulus for testosterone production is luteinizing hormone. Indeed, decreased caloric intake is associated with a *decreased* luteinizing hormone, and consequently testosterone, production (see also P.10).

c **False**. Testosterone is an androgen that is synthesized in both sexes, albeit in small amounts in females, and therefore occurs in both male and female genotypes. The adrenal glands synthesize androgens in both sexes, and in women some androgen is synthesized by the follicular thecal cells as a precursor for oestrogen production.

d **True**. There is a basal release of testosterone but it is mainly released in pulses determined by the pulsatile release of luteinizing hormone (LH) from the adenohypophysis. The pulsatile release of LH, in turn, is determined by the pulsatile release of gonadotrophin releasing hormone (GnRH) from the hypothalamus.

e **True**. There are larger pulses of testosterone released during the night than during the day. The diurnal variation is more pronounced at puberty.

P.10 a **True**. GnRH is the hypothalamic hormone which regulates the release of luteinizing hormone from the adenohypophysis.

b **True**. LH is the principal stimulus for testosterone production by the Leydig cells.

c **True**. The negative feedback influence of testosterone on both hypothalamus and adenohypophysis, to inhibit the release of GnRH and LH respectively, is an important physiological action of the hormone.

d **False**. Inhibin is a protein hormone produced by the testicular Sertoli cells in response to stimulation by the adenohypophysial hormone follicle-stimulating hormone (FSH). It has an important negative feedback effect on FSH but little regulatory effect on the production of adenohypophysial LH.

e **True**. This is probably due to a reduction in the pulses (probably in both frequency and amplitude) of GnRH from the hypothalamus with a consequent decrease in LH from the adenohypophysis.

SAQ Answers

P.11

The two principal functions of the testes are: (a) steroidogenesis and (b) spermatogenesis.

The first function is associated with the Leydig cells which synthesize the steroid hormones called androgens, the main one being testosterone. This hormone acts partly as a precursor molecule and its main derivative, the formation of which is catalysed by 5α-reductase in various target tissues including the Sertoli cells of the seminiferous tubules, is the more potent molecule dihydrotestosterone. The Sertoli cells are associated with the process of spermatogenesis which consists of various progressive stages of development of the spermatogonia in the basal compartment fluid, from primary (diploid) to secondary (haploid) spermatocytes, to spermatids, and finally to mature spermatozoa.

The two functions of the testes are linked together because spermatogenesis is regulated by hormones, specifically the androgens (steroidogenesis) as well as two adenohypophysial hormones, luteinizing hormone (via androgen production) and follicle-stimulating hormone.

P.12

Testosterone has various physiological actions, any three of which could be identified in answer to this question. They include: (a) stimulation of spermatogenesis, (b) development and maintenance of the male reproductive tract, (c) development and maintenance of the male secondary (or accessory) sex glands which include seminal vesicles, bulbo-urethral glands, and prostate, (d) stimulation of protein synthesis, (e) stimulation of sebaceous gland secretion, (f) growth spurt at puberty, (g) crucial developmental effects in the fetus, (h) behavioural effects (e.g. aggression, etc.), and (i) negative feedback regulation of hypothalamic and pituitary hormones GnRH and the gonadotrophins respectively.

All steroid hormones, including androgens such as testosterone, are lipophilic and can enter their target cells with ease. Their receptors are intracellular. Having bound to its receptor the hormone–receptor complex enters the nucleus and acts on a specific gene which it recognizes by means of a hormone recognition element on the activated receptor. It then acts as a transcription factor, resulting in the formation of specific mRNA which is translated into a new protein on ribosomes in the cytoplasm. The new proteins act within the cell and initiate the effects associated with androgen action.

P.13

Control of testicular function is associated chiefly with the control of Leydig and Sertoli cell activity by hormones of the hypothalamo–adenohypophysial–gonadal axis. Figure 6.1 illustrates the principal features of the stimulatory pathways and the negative feedback loops linking the endocrine glands which comprise this axis (GnRH, gonadotrophin releasing hormone; LH and FSH, luteinizing hormone and follicle-stimulating hormone, respectively).

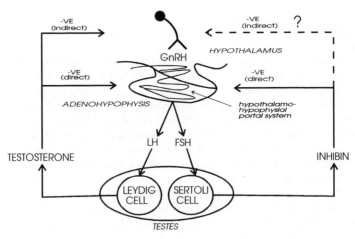

Fig. 6.1

Male reproductive endocrinology (Clinical)

Multiple Choice Questions

C.1

Which of the following statements is/are true in relation to the clinical features of male hypogonadism?

a If developing prepubertally, height often exceeds arm span by 5 cm or more

b Gynaecomastia is more commonly associated with primary gonadal (hyper-gonadotrophic) than with hypogonadotrophic hypogonadism

c The commonest cause of hypogonadism presenting at age 16 is simple delayed puberty (small-delay syndrome: constitutional delay in growth and development)

d Testicular size differentiates hypothalamic–pituitary (secondary) from gonadal (primary) causes of hypogonadism

e Reduced male sexual libido and potency are often due to hypogonadism

C.2

A 28-year-old male presents with gradually waning libido and potency and increasing fatigue. Serum testosterone is 5 nmol/litre (NR 10–26), serum LH 2.0 U/litre (NR 1–10) and serum FSH 1.0 U/litre (NR 1–8). He had mumps orchitis at the age of 20, his testes are small but there are otherwise no abnormal clinical findings. Which of the following is/are consistent with these findings?

a His hypogonadism may be secondary to mumps infection

b The abnormalities are consistent with the development of a pituitary tumour

c Stimulation with continuous, pulsed, or repeat daily GnRH injections is able to differentiate the underlying cause of his hypogonadism

d He may have a peripheral androgen-resistance syndrome

e The clinical and biochemical presentation is consistent with Kallman's syndrome

C.3

Which of the following statements is/are consistent with Klinefelter's syndrome?

a The prevalence is approximately 1:800 of the male population

b The definitive leucocyte karyotype is 47-XXY

c Hypogonadism and infertility are invariably present

d Diabetes is more common than in the general population
e Correction of hypogonadism increases the prospects of fertility

C.4

Which of the following mechanisms are known to be involved in the induction of gynaecomastia?

a Decreased hepatic elimination of endogenous oestrogen
b Ectopic production of oestrogen by malignant tumours
c Blocking of androgen receptors by drugs
d An increase in serum sex hormone binding globulin (SHBG)
e An increase in adipose tissue aromatase activity

C.5

'Cryptorchidism' is the term used to describe non-descent of the testes, which are normally expected to be bilaterally present in the scrotum by the age of 12. Which of the following statements is/are true in connection with this process, or its failure?

a Fertility is reduced in males with either current or previously undescended testes
b Gonadotrophin stimulation usually differentiates late-descending from anatomically ectopic testes
c Leydig cell function is unaffected in boys with undescended testes
d There is an increased rate of malignant change in cryptorchidism
e Hypothalamic–pituitary disease may be responsible for testicular non-descent

C.6

In relation to the causes of erectile impotence, which of the following statements is/are true?

a It is a rare complication of diabetic autonomic neuropathy
b Psychological factors are the main or a contributory component in 30% of cases
c A positive erectile response to intracavernosal injection of prostaglandin supports a structural arterial or venous abnormality
d Treatment of hypertension is an important cause of impotence
e Venous circulatory defects within the corpora cavernosa are as important as arterial factors in the aetiology of cases beyond the age of 50

C.7

Infertility is present in 5–10% of the male population. In regard to the causes and treatment of this disorder, which of the following statements is/are true?

a Almost 90% of infertile males are currently untreatable
b A raised serum FSH suggests potential responsiveness to treatment
c Varicocoele of the scrotum is a common cause
d Demonstration of azoospermia in a semen sample precludes successful therapy
e Immunological factors affecting sperm are rarely responsive to treatment

C.8

Lower serum androgen levels are frequently seen in ageing compared to younger men. In regard to this phenomenon, which of the following is/are true?

a A significant number of cases of biochemical hypogonadism in elderly men are secondary to systemic illness

b Primary testicular failure occurs in the ageing man in a manner which parallels ovarian failure in menopausal women

c Osteoporosis is a consequence of androgen deficiency in ageing men

d Adult male hypogonadism reduces the risk of coronary artery disease

e Normalization of serum androgen levels in ageing men is an important objective of geriatric care

C.9

In the treatment of hypogonadism, which of the following statements is/are true?

a Oral therapy represents a first-line approach to androgen replacement

b Treatment of hypogonadism in adolescence requires large doses for optimal androgenization

c Intramuscular injection of testosterone esters represents reliable and safe replacement in most patients

d Gonadotrophin therapy is a more appropriate treatment of hypogonadism in patients with hypothalamic or pituitary disease

e Adverse effects of long-term androgen replacement rarely need to be considered

MCQ Answers

C.1 a **False**. Hypogonadism allows continued growth of long bones due to failure or delay of epiphyseal fusion. Although the lower limbs participate in this process, the combined elongation of the two arms results in an arm span which often exceeds height by 5 cm. The sole–pubis measurement also usually exceeds the pubis–crown measurement by 3 cm or more in hypogonadism. These combined features identify the so-called eunuchoid body habitus characteristic of hypogonadism of prepubertal onset.

b **True**. Gynaecomastia is due to relative oestrogen/androgen excess. The high gonadotrophin levels resulting from the failing testis in primary hypogonadism is known to produce selectively higher oestrogen to androgen ratios. Hence, gynaecomastia is more frequently found in primary testicular disorders such as Klinefelter's syndrome.

c **True**. The physiological spectrum of pubertal onset is wide. Hypogonadism at age 15–16, especially if associated with delayed growth or reduced growth velocity, is likely to be due to the (physiological and self-correcting) small-delay syndrome. This is essentially a form of hypogonadotrophic hypogonadism, although the reduced growth component must signify simultaneous physiological delay in growth hormone secretion and/or action.

d **False**. Testicular size is not a guide as to cause. However, the testis in primary hypogonadism (best exemplified by Klinefelter's syndrome) tends to be firmer, due to hyalinization of the seminiferous tubules and peritubular fibrosis.

e **False**. Hypogonadism is the cause of reduced libido and potency in only around 10% of cases. Both libido and potency are mainly psychologically determined: even marked hypogonadism may occasionally be associated with retained libido and potency. One of the few organic causes of reduced libido in either sex is hyperprolactinaemia.

C.2 a **False**. Although mumps infection can affect Leydig cell function, the main damage is to seminiferous tubules. Furthermore, by inducing testicular damage, negative feedback would result in raised FSH (and perhaps LH) levels.

b **True**. The biochemical abnormalities are consistent with either a pituitary or a hypothalamic lesion, and a CT (or preferably) MRI scan is essential. Measurement of serum prolactin may identify a readily treatable prolactinoma, causing hypogonadotrophic hypogonadism either by compression of the normal pituitary, or by short loop negative feedback of prolactin on gonadotrophin release.

c **False**. Although on theoretical grounds, responsiveness of LH and FSH to GnRH should signify hypothalamic (rather than pituitary) disease, these stimulation tests are unreliable. MRI scanning is a more sensitive method of identifying important structural changes in this clinical setting.

d **False**. Peripheral androgen resistance rarely presents as hypogonadism, but rather as varying degrees of feminization. Furthermore, since these are genetic syndromes, the dynamic process represented by this case presentation would not be consistent.

e **False**. Although the biochemical profile in this case is consistent with Kallman's syndrome, this is a genetic syndrome almost always resulting in a much earlier presentation with failed pubertal development and associated features such as anosmia, cleft palate, neurosensory deafness, renal tract dysgenesis, and facial asymmetry.

C.3 a **True**. Most studies show a prevalence of 1:500 to 1:1000. The prevalence is higher in populations suffering from chronic psychiatric syndromes, including personality disorder and schizophrenia (approximately 1:100).

b **False**. Although 47-XXY is the commonest genotype revealed by leucocyte culture in patients with this clinical syndrome, this is not invariable. Leucocytes may carry XY, or reveal mosaics such as XY/XXY: the 47-XXY karyotype may only be found in fibroblasts. Mosaic forms usually have less striking clinical features (i.e. absence of gynaecomastia and less severe hypogonadism).

c **False**. Varying degrees of hypogonadism occur: 10–20% have normal serum testosterone and secondary sexual characteristics, and are only diagnosed when they present with infertility. Even infertility is not invariable in the mosaic variants.

d **True**. Diabetes occurs with approximately 2–4 times the prevalence of the general population. No sex chromosome-linked determinants of insulin release or action have so far been clearly identified to explain this phenomenon.

e **False**. If azoospermia is present (which is almost invariably the case), androgen replacement carries no benefit.

C.4 a **True**. This occurs typically in hepatic cirrhosis, where hepatocyte dysfunction causes decreased elimination of various steroid hormones, including cortisol and oestrogens. Persistent hypercortisolaemia is usually prevented by negative feedback, whereas this mechanism appears not to be operative with hyperoestrogenaemia.

b **False**. Oestrogens (as indeed all steroids) are rarely produced ectopically by tumours. However, Leydig cell testicular tumours (usually benign) produce oestrogen and associated gynaecomastia. Many tumours, including germ cell tumours of the testis and ovary and particularly bronchogenic carcinoma produce hCG, which in turn induces gynaecomastia via hyperoestrogenaemia.

c **True**. A variety of drugs including spironolactone, flutamide, and cimetidine have androgen receptor blocking activity, increasing (tissue) oestrogen/androgen ratios. In the various forms of congenital androgen resistance, anything from mild gynaecomastia to normal female-type breasts are seen, depending on the extent of the androgen receptor defect.

d **True**. SHBG preferentially binds androgen when compared to oestrogen. Any condition which increases SHBG will accordingly result in a raised *free* oestrogen/androgen ratio. This is seen in hyperthyroidism, and with spironolactone (which produces marked gynaecomastia because of additional suppression of androgen production and peripheral androgen blocking effects).

e **True**. Aromatase activity (converting androgen to oestrogen) is present in adipose tissue: the larger quantum of breast tissue of obese males is in part due to this phenomenon, rather than a simple pectoral fat accumulation.

C.5 a **True**. The absolute or relative infertility which is found in about 70% of patients with undescended testes is due in part to the higher intra-abdominal temperature which inhibits spermatogenesis. In addition, the truly ectopic testis is more likely to be morphologically abnormal to begin with. Accordingly, even surgical placement and tethering of the testes into the scrotum (orchidopexy) does not reduce the likelihood of infertility below 20%.

b **True**. 'Physiologically' delayed descent of the testes is correctable either by giving gonadotrophin by injection over a 6-week period, or by using pulsed subcutaneous or intermittent intranasal GnRH. This is an important diagnostic/therapeutic test before resorting to abdominal exploration. However, simple retractile testes (due to anxiety or environmental cold) can be identified by showing spontaneous appearance in the scrotum during immersion in a hot bath. In this event, no other treatment is required.

c **False**. Varying degrees of Leydig cell hypofunction (hypogonadism) may be seen in the longer-term follow-up of patients with treated or untreated cryptorchism. This is more likely to be due to fundamental abnormality of the gonad rather than the result of exposure to raised intra-abdominal temperature.

d **True**. The cryptorchid testis has a prevalence of malignancy of 8%, around 40 times higher than that of a control population. Restoring the testis to the scrotal location reduces but does not completely abolish this relative risk.

e **True**. Testicular descent is partially under control of pituitary gonadotrophins. Later or absent descent is seen particularly in boys with congenital forms of hypogonadotrophic hypogonadism (Kallman's syndrome) and to a lesser extent in small-delay syndrome (delayed puberty).

C.6 a **False**. Impotence is present in approximately 20–30% of diabetic men, where it is due to autonomic neuropathy in about 50% of cases. Ejaculatory impotence is additionally present in about one-quarter of cases, and may be responsible for infertility due to retrograde ejaculation.

b **True**. Sudden onset, variable severity, and retained nocturnal erections are the hallmarks. Many cases respond to explanation, reassurance, or psychotherapy, but some require additional treatment using vacuum methods, intracavernosal prostaglandin/papaverine, or phentolamine.

c **False**. Intracavernosal prostaglandin is only successful if both the arterial blood supply and the veno-occlusive mechanisms are intact. Neuropathic, psychological, and hypoandrogenic states do not impair this response.

d **True**. Many of the drugs used in the treatment of hypertension may induce impotence. Thiazide diuretics, methyl-dopa, beta-adrenergic, and calcium channel blocking drugs may all cause impotence. Furthermore, lowering blood pressure may reduce penile arterial perfusion in the presence of arteriosclerotic and narrowed penile feeder vessels. Other drugs which can cause impotence include tricyclic antidepressants and other drugs with anticholinergic activity, and cimetidine (due to its antiandrogenic effects).

e **True.** If intracavernosal prostaglandin fails to elicit an erection, more than 75% of such patients will have venous lesions as a major or minor contributory factor. Abnormal or ectopic veins and abnormal venous shunts can be displayed by cavernosal venography, and are sometimes amenable to surgical correction. However, arterial insufficiency remains a common cause of impotence in older age groups.

C.7 a **True.** Treatment is often unsuccessful. Adverse predictive factors include testicular biopsy findings of maturation arrest and tubular hyalinization. Chromosomal disorders and testicular atrophy resulting from cytotoxic drugs, radiotherapy, testicular torsion, and (previous) undescent all present uncorrectable lesions. Sperm concentration/donor insemination represents a possible way forward in some cases. Either idiopathic or acquired (e.g. pituitary tumour) gonadotrophin deficiency is rarely identified in the investigation of the infertile male, but treatment is often successful using combined LH and FSH preparations.

b **False.** Seminiferous tubule/spermatogenic failure is associated with reduced inhibin production which by negative feedback raises serum FSH. If serum FSH is raised to more than twice the upper normal range, further investigation and therapeutic intervention is probably not worthwhile.

c **False.** Minor varicocoeles are quite a common finding in the general population. Larger ones raise scrotal temperature and thus to some extent impair fertility, possibly where an additional defect pre-exists. Response to surgical correction of varicocoele is not as common as previously assumed.

d **False.** Total absence of sperm calls for testicular biopsy. Normal biopsy findings dictate a need to identify obstruction at various levels either at the epididymal or vasal level. Surgical correction is often not possible. In this instance, sperms can be harvested by microepididymal sperm aspiration (MESA). Artificial insemination can be carried out, or more successfully intracytoplasmic sperm injection directly into an oocyte and thus fertilized *in vitro* (IVF).

e **False.** Sperm autoimmunity is a potentially treatable cause of infertility. The semen profile may vary from complete azoospermia to apparent normality. The sperm-mucus penetration test and measurement of surface immunoglobulins on sperm are the screening tests. High-dose corticosteroid therapy results in an approximate 25% success rate over 6 months.

C.8 a **True**. Inhibition of the hypothalamic–pituitary–gonadal axis results from both acute severe illness and chronic disease, most strikingly following burns, trauma, and systemic infection, as well as in chronic respiratory and renal disease and advanced malignancy. The mediators of hypothalamic inhibition are unknown, and the process is further complicated by a rise in SHBG levels (and hence a fall in the free androgen fraction). This occurs particularly where the underlying disease process affects hepatic function. All these effects increase with age.

b **False**. Oocyte depletion and failure underlie the female menopause, causing hypergonadotrophic hypogonadism. In contrast, in males, although there is an element of reduced Leydig cell function, LH pulse frequency and amplitude decline with age: raised gonadotrophin levels are unusual even with very low total or free testosterone levels.

c **True**. Muscle and bone are affected by waning androgen levels, superimposed on age-related, hormone-independent bone loss. Fracture rates double with each decade above 60. Spinal vertebral compression can also be identified in 25% of men between the ages of 55 and 75 years.

d **True**. On the available data, hypogonadism does appear to be protective against coronary artery disease. This is partly based on higher serum HDL cholesterol levels, but may involve non-lipid mechanisms affecting endothelial cell function.

e **False**. On current evidence, androgen replacement may benefit bone density and muscle tone (and hence reduce fracture risk). Appropriately randomized studies are not yet complete. The potentially deleterious effects on lipids (and hence vascular disease) and on benign prostatic hypertrophy and latent prostatic carcinoma may outweigh the potential benefits. Only the results of prospective studies will resolve this issue and perhaps help to define subgroups of the elderly who may benefit from androgen replacement.

C.9 a **False**. Unmodified testosterone orally has too short a half-life to be practical. Alkylation at the 17-alpha position results in weak androgens which resist hepatic metabolism. It is difficult to achieve satisfactory therapeutic levels either with these or with beta-esters, such as testosterone undecanoate, and their use is indicated only in the mildest cases.

b **False**. Treatment is rarely indicated before age 14. Large doses are not required, and if employed risk psychological distress from rapid androgenization, and premature epiphyseal fusion. For these reasons, in delayed puberty 6-week courses of gonadotrophin to 'trigger' puberty are preferable to depot testosterone. In primary (testicular) hypogonadism, smaller doses of testosterone oenanthate (50 mg 2–3 weekly) are suggested starting doses.

c **True**. Esterification of the 17β-hydroxy group increases fat solubility, and results in slow release of testosterone following hydrolysis. Testosterone oenanthate provides the most constant serum testosterone levels at a dosage range of 250 mg every 2–4 weeks, with greater variability using preparations of mixed esters. Testosterone patches and implantable pellets can also be used.

d **False**. For long-term replacement, the use of the necessary frequently injectable LH preparations (usually chorionic gonadotrophin) is not needed. Treatment as in c above suffices. Long-term use of testosterone replacement does not impair the later responsiveness to gonadotrophin when induction of spermatogenesis may be required.

e **False**. Androgen replacement is absolutely contra-indicated in known carcinoma of the male breast or prostate. Acne and psychological instability may occur when androgens are first introduced, especially in higher dosage. Because of their anabolic action polycythamia may occur, while use of the 17-alkyl substituted androgens can result in cholestatic jaundice and hepatic adenoma or rarely angiosarcoma.

References

Physiology

Topic: Uses (and abuses) of androgens in men.
Bagatell, C. J. *et al.* (1996). *New England Journal of Medicine*, **334**, 707–14.
Topic: Malnutrition and reproductive function in the male.
Bergendahl, M. *et al.* (1995). *Trends in Endocrinology and Metabolism*, **6**, 145–59.
Topic: Hormonal control of spermatogenesis.
McLachlan, R. I. *et al.* (1995). *Trends in Endocrinology and Metabolism*, **6**, 95–100.

Clinical

Topic: Gynaecomastia.
Braunstein, G. D. (1993). *New England Journal of Medicine*, **328**, 490–5.
Topic: Male infertility.
Howards, S. S. (1995). *New England Journal of Medicine*, **332**, 312–17.
Topic: Erectile dysfunction.
Korenman, S. J. (1995). *Journal of Clinical Endocrinology and Metabolism*, **80**, 1985–8.
Topic: Treatment of hypogonadism.
Nieschlag, S. (1996). *Clinical Endocrinology*, **45**, 261–2.
Topic: Investigation of hypogonadism.
Plymate, S. (1994). *Endocrinology and Metabolism Clinics of North America*, **23**, 749–72.
Topic: Treatment of cryptorchidism.
Polascik, T. J., (1996). *Journal of Urology*, **156**, 804–6.

7 Female reproductive endocrinology (physiology)

Multiple Choice Questions

See also Chapters 4 (Qs 4, 15–17, 19, 20, 29–31); Chapter 12 (Qs 2, 3)

P.1 *In the female fetus*

a phenotype is determined by a pair of X chromosomes
b the indifferent gonads develop into ovaries
c The number of potential ova reaches a maximum just prior to parturition
d the Wolffian ducts fail to develop into the male internal reproductive tract because of the secretion of an ovarian Wolffian inhibitory hormone
e subsequent male-type behaviour (e.g. 'tomboyism') in childhood may be associated with the *in utero* presence of large amounts of androgens

P.2 *In girls the pubertal growth spurt*

a coincides with adrenarche (the time when adrenal androgen production is increased)
b is associated with the beginning of menstrual cyclicity
c usually occurs approximately two years earlier than in boys
d is initiated by the increasing quantities of circulating gonadal steroids
e is retarded when blindness has been present from birth

P.3 *The menstrual cycle*

a with rare exceptions is 28 days long
b initially involves the development of a group of ova and their follicles
c consists of hypotensive and hypertensive phases in arterial blood pressure
d is comprised of ovarian and endometrial cycles
e is associated with cyclic changes in ovarian steroid production

P.4 *The cyclic changes which take place in the ovaries*

a are concerned with the ripening and release of mature ova
b begin at parturition
c take place throughout life
d are associated with the growth and development of a Graafian follicle
e can be divided into follicular and luteal phases

P.5   *The process of ovulation*

a   generally occurs at the end of each cycle
b   is induced by the surge of luteinizing hormone
c   only occurs in the presence of mature spermatozoa
d   is associated with the termination of the first meiotic division
e   generally coincides with the full moon

P.6   *The follicular phase of the ovarian cycle*

a   begins with the shedding of the endometrial lining (menstruation)
b   is induced by decreasing levels of adenohypophysial gonadotrophins
c   is associated with various follicles undergoing atresia
d   normally coincides with increasing concentrations of 17β-pestradiol in the blood
e   is absent in women following hysterectomy (removal of the uterus)

P.7   *The developing follicles*

a   consist of outer thecal and inner granulosa cells
b   each contain an ovum
c   may number as many as 15 at the beginning of each cycle
d   are stimulated by the gonadotrophins in the circulation
e   release increasingly large quantities of progesterone into the general circulation

P.8   *The production of oestrogen during the follicular phase*

a   is mainly by the ripening ova
b   is proportional to the number of developing follicles
c   occurs chiefly by collaboration between thecal and granulosa cells
d   involves the initial synthesis of androgens by the granulosa cells
e   depends on appropriate stimulation by adenohypophysial gonadotrophins

P.9   *The luteal phase of the ovarian cycle*

a   follows the process of ovulation
b   involves the transformation of remaining granulosa and thecal cells into luteal cells
c   is initiated by the LH surge
d   is associated with rising concentrations of oestrogen and progesterone
e   coincides with the secretory phase of the endometrial cycle

P.10   *The endometrial cycle*

a   comprises proliferative and secretory phases
b   prepares the endometrium for the possible implantation of a fertilized ovum

c is associated with a progesterone-stimulated initial increase in endometrial growth

d is controlled by the adrenal glucocorticoid hormone cortisol

e is terminated by the withdrawal of ovarian hormonal support

P.11 17β-oestradiol

a is the principal oestrogen produced during the menstrual cycle

b is synthesized from androgenic precursors

c is a 21-carbon steroid

d is less potent than oestriol on a molecular basis

e binds to intracellular receptors

P.12 The oestrogens

a maintain the functions of the oviducts (Fallopian tubes) and uterus

b contribute to breast development

c stimulate the production of a cervical mucus that is easily penetrated by
spermatozoa

d exert a negative feedback on the production of adenohypophysial
gonadotrophins

e can induce some degree of salt and water retention

P.13 17β-oestradiol

a induces the LH surge

b stimulates protein synthesis

c elevates the basal body temperature

d plays a protective role against hypertension during the menstrual
cycle

e decreases the circulating cholesterol concentration

P.14 Progesterone

a is mainly synthesized during the ovarian follicular phase

b is the principal progestogen produced during the menstrual cycle

c is a polypeptide hormone

d is synthesized by luteal cells

e is partly transported in the blood bound to the plasma globulin transcortin

P.15 The progestogens

a stimulate protein anabolism

b contribute to breast development

c stimulate endometrial secretory activity

d inhibit oestrogen synthesis during the luteal phase

e exert a negative feedback on the hypothalamo–adenohypophysial axis
during the follicular phase

P.16 *Fertilization of the ovum*

a usually takes place within the Graafian follicle
b can often take as long as 6 days
c involves the collaborative action of at least two spermatozoa
d necessitates the presence of oestrogen and progestogen in order for it to occur
e is associated with the expulsion of the second polar body

P.17 *Implantation*

a occurs after the first cell divisions have taken place
b involves the process of decidualization
c usually occurs within 24 hours of fertilization
d initiates the formation of the syncytiotrophoblast
e in humans is interstitial

P.18 *Pregnancy*

a starts with the successful implantation of the developing blastocyst
b requires the cyclic production of oestrogens and progesterone
c usually lasts approximately 60 weeks in humans
d is dependent on ovarian steroid hormones throughout
e is associated with the decreased production of adenohypophysial gonadotrophins

P.19 *Oestrogen production during pregnancy*

a is mainly from the ovarian corpus luteum
b is chiefly oestriol
c increases so that high plasma concentrations are present prior to parturition
d is stimulated by human placental lactogen
e is dependent on the feto-placental unit after the first 6 weeks

P.20 *Parturition*

a involves relaxation of the cervical ligaments
b arises following contractions of the myometrium
c is associated with spontaneous milk ejection
d can be induced by oxytocin
e is inhibited by prostaglandin $PGF_{2\alpha}$

P.21 *Lactation*

a is initiated by stimulation of tactile receptors around the nipples
b is stimulated by prolactin
c is inhibited during pregnancy by the maintained very high levels of oestrogens and progesterone

    d involves an oxytocin-stimulated milk ejection reflex
    e can occur in males under appropriate hormonal stimulation

Short Answer Questions

P.22
Briefly describe the menstrual cycle identifying the principal ovarian and endometrial events.

P.23
Identify the principal oestrogens produced: (a) during the menstrual cycle, and (b) during pregnancy. List three physiological actions of oestrogens and briefly explain the chief features of their mechanism of action.

P.24
Draw simple graphs illustrating the principal changes in adenohypophysial and ovarian hormone concentrations during a typical menstrual cycle.

P.25
Explain by means of a diagram how the ovarian hormones influence gonadotrophin production from the adenohypophysis during the menstrual cycle, including the hypothalamus in your answer.

P.26
List the principal features of the fertilization and implantation processes.

P.27
Explain with the aid of a diagram how contraction of the myometrial muscle is stimulated at parturition.

P.28
Briefly explain the term neuroendocrine reflex arc using either prolactin or oxytocin as your example.

P.29
Briefly explain how oestrogens and progestogens can have contraceptive effects when administered as 'the pill'.

MCQ Answers

P.1 a **True.** The development, and hence appearance, of the female is determined by a pair of XX chromosomes while the male phenotype is determined by X and Y chromosomes.

b **True.** In the absence of the sry (sex-determining region of the Y chromosome) gene and the SRY protein which activate the Sertoli cells in the male, the indifferent gonads develop into ovaries.

c **False** The maximum number of potential ova, usually around 6–8 million, is reached by the 20th week *in utero*. This number then begins to diminish as they undergo atresia. Just prior to parturition the number of potential ova is already down to about 2 million.

d **False.** The reverse is true, i.e. the female Mullerian ducts develop into the female internal reproductive tract because of the absence of a testicular Mullerian inhibitory hormone.

e **True.** There does seem to be an increased likelihood that the presence of an increased androgenic influence on a female fetus is associated with a more 'boyish' behaviour in early life. Note that in later life these girls appear to develop perfectly naturally and have no special problems in rearing their families.

P.2 a **False.** Adrenarche (the time of increased adrenal androgen output) occurs approximately two years before the pubertal growth spurt. It occurs in both sexes, the androgens stimulating axillary and pubic hair growth (and perhaps having other, so far unclear, effects).

b **False.** The beginning of menstrual cyclicity (menarche) is the first obvious sign that reproductive development has begun in girls, often coinciding with the pubertal growth spurt.

c **True.** Females enter the pubertal growth and development phase on average some two years earlier than boys i.e. usually beginning between the ages of 12 and 14 years in girls and 14 to 16 years in boys.

d **True.** The increasing ovarian steroid hormone output at the beginning of puberty, in the presence of sufficient concentrations of circulating somatotrophin, initiates the pubertal growth spurt.

e **False.** Blind girls do not seem to have a retarded menarche or pubertal growth spurt, indicating that in humans the retinal–pineal gland influence on sexual maturation is not a key determinant.

P.3 a **False.** There is actually quite a lot of variability in the length of the menstrual cycle so that while it is appropriate to consider the average length to be 28 days it can vary from 20 to 40 days between women, and can also vary from cycle to cycle in the same woman.

b **True.** At the beginning of each cycle a small group of ova within their pre-antral follicles (often between 12 and 15) enter the development process.

c **False.** The arterial blood pressure may vary throughout the cycle, as indeed it does during each 24 hours, but it certainly does not vary so much as to go from hypotensive to hypertensive phases.

d **True.** The changes in ovarian and uterine structure and function which determine the ovarian and endometrial cycles are linked together by the hormones produced by the ovaries during each menstrual cycle.

e **True.** The cyclic changes in ovarian steroid production are essential in determining the different phases of the menstrual cycle. The ovarian cycle consists of pre- and post-ovulatory follicular and luteal phases respectively, while the endometrial cycle consists of proliferative and secretory phases.

P.4 a **True.** The ripening and release of a mature ovum (oocyte) is the central event of each menstrual cycle. The preparation of the uterus, for the successful implantation of the dividing blastocyst should fertilization of the ovum have occurred, is linked to the ovulatory process by the production of ovarian hormones.

b **False.** The regular changes of each menstrual cycle begin at puberty. The age at onset of the first menstrual cycle is called menarche.

c **False.** Menstrual cycles begin at menarche and end at the menopause, which usually occurs between the ages of 50 and 60 years.

d **True.** The most advanced (i.e. Graafian) follicle which survives to the end of the follicular phase is intimately associated with the ripening ovum released at ovulation.

e **True.** The follicular phase is the first part of the cycle and is associated with the growth and development of follicles, and the luteal phase follows the mid cycle event of ovulation.

P.5 a **False.** Each menstrual cycle is associated with ovarian changes which are considered in two phases: the follicular and luteal phases. Ovulation occurs mid cycle, between these two phases.

b **True.** The surge of the adenohypophysial gonadotrophin luteinizing hormone (LH) is the main determinant of the final maturation of the ovum and the critical changes in follicular cell development which culminate in the process of ovulation. The smaller surge in follicle-stimulating hormone (FSH) release from the adenohypophysis, which occurs simultaneously, may also have some role in initiating the ovulatory process

c **False.** The process of ovulation is determined by the pre-ovulatory LH (and FSH) surge; mature spermatozoa are not involved. Interestingly, the act of copulation may trigger the process in other animals, but there is little evidence for this occurring in humans.

d **True.** The first of the polar bodies is expelled from the ripe ovum at ovulation.

e **False.** A poetic idea that has no relation to the truth!

P.6 a **True.** This is the endometrial lining grown during the previous cycle.

b **False.** It is induced by *increasing* levels of gonadotrophins (LH and FSH) at the beginning of the cycle

c **True.** Of the 15–20 follicles entering the developmental process at the beginning of the follicular phase most (indeed usually all but one) undergo atresia.

d **True.** As the follicles grow they produce increasing amounts of oestrogen in response to the gonadotrophins.

e **False.** A hysterectomy would have no effect on the ovarian cycle (i.e. the follicular and luteal phases, and the ovulatory process). Removal of the uterus will simply mean that one of the target tissues for the ovarian steroids will be missing, and pregnancy becomes impossible.

P.7 a **True.** Each follicle consists of cells which differentiate into an outer layer of thecal cells and an inner layer of granulosa cells. It is the collaboration between these two cell types that produces the oestrogens released during the follicular phase of the ovarian cycle

b **True.** Within each developing follicle the inner layer of granulosa cells surrounds an ovum. As the granulosa cells secrete oestrogen-rich fluid during the follicular phase of the ovarian cycle, an antrum filled with fluid forms. In the final, surviving follicle in each cycle, the granulosa cells have proliferated into an outer layer in contact with the thecal cells and an inner layer surrounding the ovum

c **True.** The number of follicles entering each cycle can be as high as 20. Usually, only one of those follicles (called the Graafian follicle) will survive to the end of the follicular phase and release its ovum from the ovary. The pre-ovulatory follicle diameter is usually between 20 and 25 mm. By this late stage, all the other follicles have degenerated and been absorbed into the ovarian stroma (a process called atresia).

d **True.** The gonadotrophins from the adenohypophysis stimulate the cells of the developing follicle. LH stimulates the thecal cells to synthesize androgens while FSH stimulates the granulosa cells to convert these androgens (by aromatization) to oestrogens (mainly 17β-oestradiol).

e **False.** Large amounts of progesterone are only produced and released into the general circulation) during the luteal phase of the ovarian cycle, not during the follicular phase when basal amounts are released. There is a small increase in progestogen (mainly 17α-hydroxyprogesterone) produced by the follicle cells just prior to ovulation.

P.8 a **False.** The ripening ova do not synthesize the enzymes necessary for the production of steroid hormones. Oestrogens, mainly 17β-oestradiol, are synthesized as a consequence of the collaboration occurring between the thecal and granulosa cells of the follicle.

b **False.** As the follicular phase progresses the increasing production of oestrogen is associated with *decreasing* numbers of follicles since many of them undergo atresia. The increased production of oestrogen is associated more with the increased growth (proliferation) and development of the thecal and granulosa cells of the growing dominant follicle. Increased synthesis (i.e. numbers) of LH and FSH (and oestrogen) receptors by the different cells will be associated with a greater stimulation of steroid synthesis.

c **True.** As described above, oestrogen production by the growing follicles is mainly the result of collaboration between the two layers of follicle cells, the outer thecal and the inner granulosa cells. The thecal cells produce androgens which are aromatized to oestrogen by the granulosa cells which contain the necessary aromatase enzymes.

d **False.** The thecal cells synthesize androgens. While the thecal cells may produce small amounts 17β-oestradiol by direct aromatization of androgen, by far the greater amounts of oestrogen are produced as a consequence of the collaboration between thecal and granulosa cells. (The granulosa cells do not appear to synthesize androgens themselves.)

e **True.** The thecal cell production of androgens is stimulated by LH while the aromatization of androgen to oestrogen in the granulosa cells is stimulated by FSH, *and* by oestrogen (mainly 17β-oestradiol), an example of autocrine regulation which follows a positive feedback loop (i.e. the more oestrogen produced, the greater the stimulation of oestrogen production).

P.9 a **True.** The ovarian cycle is divided by the process of ovulation into follicular and luteal phases, the latter occurring after release of the ripened ovum.

b **True.** After ovulation the granulosa (and probably some of the thecal) cells become transformed into luteal cells, so called because they contain a yellowish carotenoid pigment called lutein.

c **True.** The LH surge induces the final maturation of the ovum and also stimulates the growth and development of the follicle cells which results in the release of the ovum into the peritoneal cavity (ovulation). LH does not penetrate the follicle cell layers, and does not bind to the ovum. Consequently, effects by LH on the ovum must be indirect, mediated by some mechanism stimulated within the follicle cells.

d **True.** The LH (and probably the FSH) stimulates the luteal cells to synthesize progesterone (and 17α-hydroxyprogesterone) in steadily increasing amounts, *and* 17β-oestradiol (in humans). Small amounts of androgens are also released.

e **True.** The progesterone, in the presence of 17β-oestradiol in humans, stimulates the secretions of the developed endometrium.

P.10 a **True.** The changes which take place in the uterine wall (the endometrial cycle) during the menstrual cycle are first proliferative (the proliferative, i.e. growth, phase) and then, after ovulation, secretory (the secretory phase). The proliferative phase occurs under the influence of oestrogens, the circulating (and local) levels of which are steadily increasing in the presence of basal amounts of progesterone only (i.e. corresponding to the follicular phase of the ovarian cycle). After ovulation the follicular remnants form the corpus luteum, which secretes oestrogen (17β-oestradiol) and increasing amounts of progesterone. In the presence of oestrogen (in humans), progesterone stimulates the endometrium to secrete a nutrient-rich fluid.

b **True.** The secretions of the endometrium which are released in the second half of the menstrual cycle will support the initial growth and development of the blastocyst in the uterus, should fertilization have occurred. This is the whole purpose of developing the endometrium and then stimulating it to secrete appropriately.

c **False.** The initial proliferative (growth) phase of the endometrial cycle is stimulated by 17β-oestradiol in the *absence* of progesterone.

d **False.** Cortisol has many effects but these do *not* include control of the endometrial cycle.

e **True.** This does indeed follow from withdrawal of ovarian hormonal support, as occurs towards the end of each cycle if implantation has not occurred.

P.11 a **True.** Other oestrogens (e.g. oestrone and oestriol) are produced but are of minor importance during the menstrual cycle. In contrast, feto-placental oestrogen production during pregnancy is mainly of the less potent oestriol.

b **True.** All oestrogens are derived from androgenic precursors. During the menstrual cycle these are mainly androstenedione and testosterone which are synthesized by the thecal cells.

c **False.** The precursor cholesterol is a 21-carbon steroid, as are later precursors in the synthesis pathway (e.g. progesterone and 17α-hydroxy-progesterone). The principal adrenal steroids, aldosterone and cortisol, which are derived from these precursors, are also 21-carbon molecules. In contrast, androgen derivatives are 19-carbon molecules and oestrogens which themselves are derived from androgens, are 18-carbon steroids.

d **False.** 17β-Oestradiol is the most potent of the naturally occurring oestrogens; it is more, not less, potent than oestriol (and oestrone).

e **True.** All steroid hormones are lipophilic, enter cells and bind to intra-cellular receptors. Subsequently, oestrogens exert genomic effects which result in the synthesis of new protein molecules.

P.12 a **True.** The oestrogens have important developmental and maintenance effects on various tissues which include the reproductive tract (e.g. oviducts and uterus).

b **True.** Various hormones are probably necessary for the normal development and maintenance of the breasts, and these certainly include oestrogens.

c **True.** Oestrogens, in the absence of progesterone as occurs in the proliferative phase of the endometrial cycle, stimulate the secretion of a watery cervical mucus which is easily penetrated by spermatoxoa.

d **True.** The negative feedback effect of oestrogen on gonadotrophin production is the normal state of affairs. This is particularly true for LH production (the protein inhibin probably playing the dominant regulatory role for FSH). However, under certain specific conditions which arise towards the end of the follicular phase the oestrogen exerts a *positive* feedback effect on LH (and FSH) production, resulting in the pre-ovulatory surge.

e **True.** The precise nature of the involvement of oestrogens in salt and water balance is unclear; however, it does stimulate hepatic protein synthesis and one such protein is angiotensinogen which is a precursor for angiotensin II, a molecule involved in salt and water balance. An interaction between oestrogens and the antidiuretic hormone, vasopressin, is also of potential physiological significance.

P.13 a **True.** High circulating concentrations of 17β-oestradiol, if present for a minimum period of 36 hours *in the absence of high circulating concentrations of progestogen*, have a positive feedback effect on the hypothalamo–hypophysial axis resulting in the pre-ovulatory LH (and FSH) surge.

b **True.** Oestrogens are mild protein anabolic agents, and at least part of their growth-promoting effects are associated with the stimulation of protein synthesis.

c **False.** This is an effect associated with the progesterone produced during the luteal phase. A rise in basal body temperature is a useful clinical indicator that ovulation has taken place, and that the luteal phase (and its associated production of progesterone) has begun.

d **True.** Oestrogens produced cyclically are associated with a protective effect on the cardiovascular system, menstruating women being less prone to pathological hypertension than men, for example. This protective effect in women is lost after the menopause. However, this effect is reversed if oestrogens are present at high concentrations chronically (and hypertension has been associated with oestrogenic contraceptive pills).

e **True.** This is another protective effect of oestrogens which is lost at the menopause, and which is probably associated with the lower incidence of cardiovascular disease (e.g. thrombosis) recorded in menstruating women.

P.14 a **False.** Progesterone is mainly synthesized during the luteal phase of the ovarian cycle. Basal amounts are produced during the follicular phase, with a small increase occurring just before ovulation.

  b **True.** Another progestogen, 17α-hydroxyprogesterone, is also synthesized, particularly before ovulation has occurred, but progesterone is far more important being produced in high concentrations during the luteal phase.

  c **False.** Progesterone is one of the first steroids produced from the 21-carbon precursor, cholesterol; this steroid hormone also has 21 carbon atoms.

  d **True.** Progesterone is mainly synthesized by, and released from, the luteal cells of the corpus luteum in response to stimulation by LH. This is the principal source of progesterone during the menstrual cycle.

  e **True.** Transcortin is a plasma binding protein particularly associated with the transport of other 21-carbon steroids such as the adrenal corticosteroids cortisol and aldosterone. However, it does also bind and transport progesterone in the circulation.

P.15 a **False.** Progestogens are generally mildly catabolic with respect to protein, as well as on carbohydrate and lipid metabolism.

  b **True.** Along with oestrogens (and other hormones) progestogens play a role in breast development. Oestrogens are probably the main stimulators of breast development (e.g. of the ducts, lobules, and alveoli). However, the hypertrophy of the breasts which occurs during pregnancy is a consequence of increased circulating levels of oestrogens and progesterone, as well as of other hormones such as insulin and prolactin.

  c **True.** The endometrium thickens and develops during the proliferative phase, and the secretory glands have enlarged and become coiled within the endometrium. During the luteal phase, in the presence of circulating oestrogens, progesterone stimulates the glands to secrete a nutrient-rich fluid into the uterus.

  d **False.** Progesterone and 17β-oestradiol are both produced during the luteal phase. Together they exert a negative feedback effect on the hypothalamo–hypophysial system resulting in an inhibition of gonadotrophin release from the adenohypophysis. Consequently, this major gonadotrophin stimulus on steroid production by the corpus luteum decreases, and progesterone and 17β-oestradiol production decreases.

  e **False.** The circulating concentration of progesterone does not increase above basal levels during most of the follicular phase. There is a small pre-ovulatory increase in progestogen production which, it has been suggested, may potentiate the positive feedback effect of the 17β-oestradiol at this stage.

P.16 a **False.** Fertilization takes place after the egg has been expelled from the ovary (i.e. at ovulation). The spermatozoa deposited within the vagina swim into the uterus and move up the Fallopian tube, their passage here being assisted by the wafting movements of the cilia lining the walls. Fertilization of the ovum (or oocyte) usually occurs within the Fallopian tubes.

b **False.** The actual process of fertilization, involving the fusion of spermatozoon and ovum, normally takes place within hours of the spermatozoon reaches the egg.

c **False.** It only takes one spermatozoon to fertilize an ovum. Indeed, it is more likely that spermatozoa will inhibit each other: certainly, once one spermatozoon has penetrated the outer zona pellucids surrounding the oocyte, various enzyme-induced effects occur which greatly reduce the likelihood of other spermatozoa binding to the oocyte.

d **False.** Both oestrogen and progesterone are required for implantation of the blastocyst should a successful fertilization occur, but not for the fertilization process itself.

e **True.** The second polar body is expelled at the time of fertilization, so that a truly haploid ovum can fuse with a haploid spermatozoon. The first polar body was expelled from the ovum at the time of ovulation.

P.17 a **True.** The fertilized ovum has already undergone the first few cell divisions to form a morula as it travels down the Fallopian tube and reaches the uterus. By the time of implantation, two distinct groups of cells are already distinguishable: the inner cell mass (which will develop into the conceptus) and an outer trophectoderm cell layer.

b **True.** When the implanting blastocyst (specifically the outer trophectoderm layer) makes contact with the endometrium, changes are initiated in the underlying maternal stroma. These regional changes in cell structure and function produce a tissue which will provide the necessary nutrients for subsequent development of the implanting embryo. This process occurs rapidly (within hours), and is called *decidualization*. The signal which initiates it is still uncertain, although prostaglandins and/or histamine have been proposed.

c **False.** Implantation usually takes place at least 4–5 days after fertilization, by which time many cell divisions have already taken place. Nutrients and other necessary molecules secreted by the endometrium reach the growing cell mass within the uterine cavity by simple diffusion. By the time the blastocyst stage has been reached it is unlikely that sufficient provision of nutrients can reach all the cells by simple diffusion alone. The need to develop a more efficient delivery system becomes of paramount importance, hence the necessity for implantation.

d **True.** The formation of the synctiotrophoblast occurs after implantation and when decidualization of underlying endometrial tissue has occurred. It is an early stage in the development of the feto-placental unit.

e **True.** In humans, the endometrial tissue fuses over the implanted blastocyst. This type of implantation is called 'interstitial'.

P.18 a **True.** While fertilization and early cell divisions have already occurred before implantation, the true beginning of pregnancy, involving the development of the special relationship between mother and fetus and the formation of the feto-placental unit, must be implantation.

b **False.** Once the blastocyst is implanted, the production of oestrogens and progesterone will increase steadily throughout pregnancy (i.e. it is no longer cyclic). The signal for the maintained production of these steroid hormones is the production of maternal chorionic gonadotrophin (hCG) which is released into the maternal circulation as soon as the blastocyst has implanted. This hormone stimulates the corpus luteum to produce oestrogen and progesterone, thereby taking over the role of the adenohypophysial LH which is inhibited by the rising ovarian steroid concentration. By week 10 the feto-placental unit is producing the necessary oestrogens and progesterone and the corpus luteum is no longer necessary for the continued maintenance of pregnancy.

c **False.** It normally lasts approximately 40 weeks when measured from the date of the last menstruation in humans, this being the last clear event the woman will usually know (dates for ovulation, fertilization, or implantation not usually being known). The pregnancy itself is usually considered to consist of three trimesters.

d **True.** The steroid hormones oestrogens and progesterone are necessary throughout pregnancy. While at first maintenance of the ovarian corpus luteum is necessary for the production of these steroids in ever-increasing quantities, the feto-placental unit gradually takes over this function.

e **True.** The raised levels of oestrogens and progesterone ensure the maintained negative feedback effect on adenohypophysial gonado-trophin production throughout pregnancy. Consequently LH and FSH production are inhibited.

P.19 a **False.** The corpus luteum is vital for oestrogen (and progesterone) production during the first few weeks of pregnancy but not later on, when the placenta has taken over this role.

b **True.** While 17β-oestradiol is the main oestrogen produced during the normal menstrual cycle, oestriol is the main oestrogen produced during pregnancy. During the late stage of pregnancy the plasma oestriol concentration is of the order of 400 nmol/litre and the 17β-oestradiol concentration is approximately 50 nmol/litre.

c **True.** Both oestrogen and progesterone plasma concentrations increase steadily throughout pregnancy, reaching high levels prior to parturition. In order to account for the initiation of contractions of the myometrium at term, an oestrogen-dominated uterus is believed to be necessary.

d **False.** Human placental lactogen (hPL) is not believed to have any effect on oestrogen production during pregnancy. It is a protein of approximately 190 amino acids with a structure very similar to that of somatotrophin (growth hormone), and with structural similarities to prolactin. It is detectable in the maternal blood from about week 5, and rises steadily in direct proportion to placental weight. However, while it does not appear to have growth-promoting effects it does stimulate an increase in blood glucose concentration and it has some lactogenic activity. Reportedly, normal pregnancy can develop in its absence, so its precise physiological role is still controversial.

e **True.** After 5–6 weeks the ovaries can be removed and yet pregnancy can continue successfully until term. This is because by then the feto-placental unit has taken over the production of oestrogen and progesterone.

P.20 a **True.** One essential component of parturition is the relaxation of the cervix and the pelvic ligaments, an effect which is associated with the polypeptide hormone, relaxin. This hormone is synthesized by the ovarian corpus luteum, the uterus, and (particularly relevant to pregnancy) the placenta. Its structure is similar to that of insulin and the insulin-like growth factors IGF-I and IGF-II, i.e. it consists of two chains of amino acids linked by disulphide bonds (although the amino acid sequences are different). Intriguingly, circulating plasma levels appear to be higher at week 10 than later on in pregnancy.

b **True.** In addition to the relaxation of the pelvic ligaments, successful delivery of the baby requires regular contractions of the uterus. The uterine smooth muscle (myometrium) contracts at term with an increasing frequency. Usually, regular contractions every 2 to 5 minutes become established, and delivery of the baby normally follows within 24 hours.

c **False.** The milk ejection reflex is brought about by the pulsatile release of oxytocin, but only once milk production has been stimulated. Therefore, this only occurs after delivery of the baby even though quite large pulses of oxytocin are released prior to, and during, parturition. The reason for this is that milk production is stimulated by prolactin (and the collaborative action of other hormones), but only after removal of the inhibitory influence of the high concentrations of placental steroids (mainly oestrogen) present at parturition.

d **True.** One of the functions of oxytocin is to stimulate appropriately primed (e.g. by oestrogen) myometrial smooth muscle, and it is used clinically to induce labour. However, it is clear that oxytocin is not the prime inducer of parturition, since this can occur in the absence of the hormone. Rather, it seems that oxytocin plays a supportive role, probably enhancing the stimulatory effect of certain prostaglandins.

e **False.** Various prostaglandins, including $PGF_{2\alpha}$, actually stimulate myometrial contraction by increasing the cytoplasmic Ca^{2+} concentration of the smooth muscle cells.

P.21 a **True.** Tactile receptors around the nipple are stimulated by suckling during lactation. Consequently, increased activity along the afferent nerve pathway to the hypothalamus is associated with the stimulation of prolactin (involved in milk production) and oxytocin (milk ejection) release. The hormones provide the endocrine efferent limbs of the neuro-endocrine reflexes.

b **True.** Prolactin is the principal stimulator of milk synthesis (galacto-poeisis) by the alveolar cells of the breasts. Other hormones contribute to the milk synthesis process, including somatotrophin, the iodothyronines, and insulin.

c **True.** The high circulating levels of oestrogen (and androgen) during pregnancy block the action of prolactin on milk synthesis. This is why milk is not produced during pregnancy despite the increasingly high concentrations of circulating prolactin and placental lactogen. After delivery of the baby, steroid levels fall and prolactin can exert its powerful effect on galactopoeisis unchecked.

d **True.** The milk ejection reflex is one of the principal (known) physiological effects of oxytocin. The oxytocin stimulates contraction of the myoepithelial cells surrounding the mammary ducts; milk secreted by the alveolar cells into the ducts, following the action of prolactin, is then released in spurts from the pores in the nipple.

e **True.** Hyperprolactinaemia, arising as a consequence of a pituitary adenoma, is sometimes associated with milk flow (galactorrhoea) in men, and more commonly in women. Milk expression may be transient or intermittent, and presumably requires a certain level of circulating gonadal hormones for the prolactin to exert its physiological action.

SAQ Answers

P.22

The menstrual cycle is a regular series of events linking the ripening of an ovum and its release from its follicle with the preparation of the endometrium (and other tissues) should fertilization of that ovum occur, and implantation be imminent.

The menstrual cycle consists of two principal components: (a) the ovarian cycle and (b) the endometrial cycle linked together by the ovarian steroids (see Fig. 7.1).

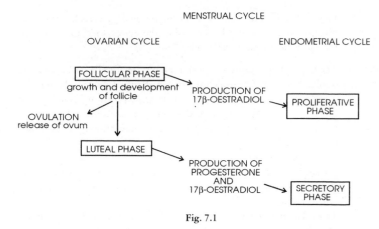

Fig. 7.1

P.23

The principal oestrogen produced during the menstrual cycle is 17β-oestradiol. During pregnancy, this oestrogen is also produced but far greater quantities of oestriol are synthesized by the feto-placental unit. The oestrogens have many physiological actions, some of the main ones being listed below. Any three of these actions could be given in your answer.

1. Growth and maintenance of female reproductive tract (including oviducts, uterus, cervix, vagina).

2. Growth and maintenance of breast tissue.

3. Stimulation of protein anabolism.

4. Effects on lipid metabolism (e.g. decreases plasma cholesterol concentration)

5. Effects on salt and water metabolism (e.g. via stimulation of hepatic angiotensinogen synthesis).

6. Negative *and positive* feedback effects on hypothalamo–adenohypophysial axis

7. Behavioural effects.

The mechanism of action of oestrogens involves: (i) binding to its intracellular receptor, (ii) the hormone–receptor complex linking to a specific section of nuclear DNA, (iii) acting as a transcription factor to activate a gene, (iv) the mRNA formed then being translated to a correct sequence of amino acids on ribosomes in the cytosol, and (v) the specific protein formed then mediating the physiological effect of the oestrogen.

P.24

The principal changes in adenohypophysial and ovarian hormone levels in the blood during a typical menstrual cycle are illustrated in Fig. 7.2. It is appreciated

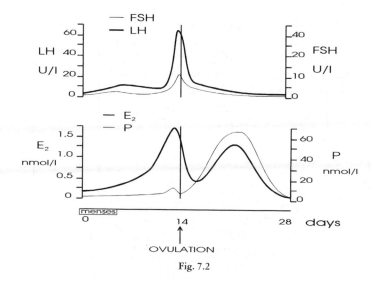

Fig. 7.2

that precise scales for the different hormones may not be known, but an attempt to obtain the orders of magnitude for the different hormones should be made (e.g. to show the much greater concentrations of progesterone than of oestrogen during the luteal phase). The important points to appreciate are: initial increases in plasma follicle-stimulating hormone (FSH) and luteinizing hormone (LH) concentrations at beginning of the cycle; FSH then decreases before rising just before ovulation (surge); LH does not decrease but does have a large surge just before ovulation; both LH and FSH then decrease during the luteal phase, being increasingly inhibited by the rising steroid levels. Oestrogen (17β-oestradiol, E_2) increases from beginning of the cycle, rising quite sharply during the late part of the follicular phase; then E_2 falls at start of the luteal phase and then rises to second peak mid luteal phase before falling towards the end of the cycle. Progestogen (P) is not produced above basal levels during the follicular phase until just before ovulation (increase here is mainly due to 17α-hydroxyprogesterone); after ovulation there is a large rise due to increased production of progesterone which reaches peak in mid luteal phase before decreasing towards the end of the cycle.

P.25

This question examines the negative and positive feedback effects of the ovarian steroids on the hypothalamo–adenohypophysial axis. It is possible that when progestogen is present in the circulation at a low concentration (i.e. before ovulation) it may potentiate the positive feedback effect exerted by the high circulating concentrations of oestradiol on LH (and FSH) at that stage. (This is not shown in Fig. 7.3.)

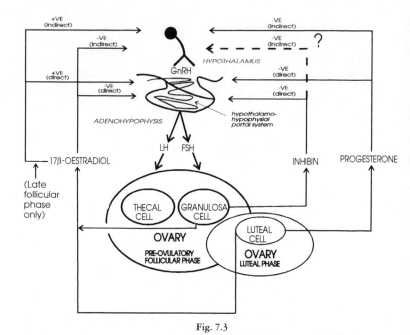

Fig. 7.3

P.26

The principal features of fertilization are:

1. Spermatozoa are deposited within vagina and uterus.

2. They swim up the oviducts (Fallopian tubes) where they encounter an ovum (oocyte) which has been released from an ovary at ovulation.

3. One spermatozoon (usually) fuses with the ovum to produce new diploid cell (i.e. full chromosome number of 23 pairs).

The principal features of implantation are:

1. Following the fusion of a spermatozoon and the oocyte within the Fallopian tube, cell division begins and by 4–5 days in the uterus the blastocyst stage is reached, with outer trophectoderm cells and inner cell mass. At this stage it is still unattached and receiving all its nutrients from the endometrial secretions.

2. On approaching the uterine wall, the blastocyst implants into the endometrium. This process involves the outer trophectoderm cells which somehow stimulate the underlying endometrium to undergo profound changes which are necessary for the establishment of a fetal-maternal link. The signal from the trophectoderm cells may simply be non-specific (e.g. tactile). Whatever the nature of this initial stimulus, it releases histamine and/or prostaglandins which cause a rapid disintegration of the underlying endometrium.

3. This effect on the underlying endometrium is called decidualization, and it involves the increased vascular permeability in the stroma of the area resulting in a local oedema, the breakdown of the intercellular matrix, and a growth of capillaries into the area.

4. The endometrial tissue gradually grows over the implanting blastocyst (in humans, called invasive implantation).

P.27

Contractions of the uterus involve the myometrial cells underlying the endometrium–placenta. Like all muscle cells, actin-myosin filaments link up by cross-bridges and as they pull together the muscle fibres shorten. The key event that allows actin and myosin to combine is the intracellular calcium ion concentration. The hormonal control of the Ca^{2+} concentration is shown in Fig. 7.4. The calcium binds to troponin protein allowing the actin and myosin to link together with the formation of cross-bridges necessary for muscle contraction. The effects of oestrogen (17β-oestradiol) and progesterone oppose each other, and are directed to increasing or decreasing intracellular calcium ions, respectively, via effects on oxytocin (more precisely on oxytocin receptor synthesis) and on prostaglandin synthesis ($PGF_{2\alpha}$ increasing movement of calcium into cytoplasm from intracellular storage sites).

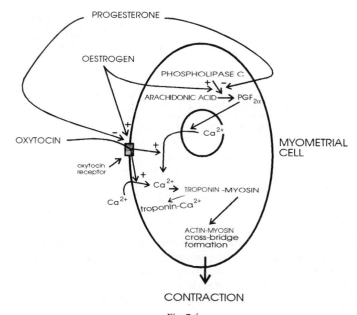

Fig. 7.4

P.28

A neuroendocrine reflex is a reflex which has an afferent neural pathway and an efferent endocrine (hormonal) pathway. Both prolactin and oxytocin are hormones released reflexly following stimulation of sensory receptors around the nipples (e.g. during suckling) and increased nerve activity in a polyneuronal afferent pathway which terminates in the hypothalamus. When this neural pathway is stimulated prolactin and oxytocin are released, from the adenohypophysis and the neuro-hypophysis respectively. Taking oxytocin as an example, the afferent pathway terminates on oxytocinergic neurones in the supraoptic and paraventricular nuclei (SON and PVN) in the hypothalamus. Oxytocin is released into the systemic circulation, and as the efferent pathway it reaches the myoepithelial cells lining the ducts in the breasts causing their contraction. Milk in the ducts is then ejected from the nipple—the milk ejection reflex. Figure 7.4 illustrates the basic elements of this pathway.

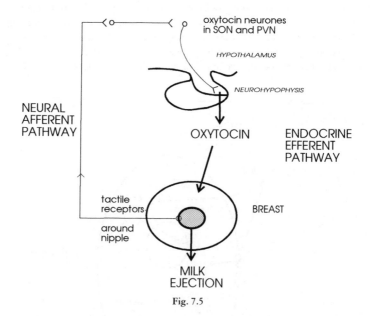

Fig. 7.5

P.29

There are various contraceptive pills available nowadays, and they contain various oestrogenic and progestogenic preparations. The essential contraceptive feature of the combined oestrogen and progestagen pill taken for a 21-day period is the negative feedback effect of the combined steroids on the hypothalamo–adenohypophysial axis. Biphasic or triphasic oral contraceptives involve the use of varying amounts of both oestrogen and progestogen during the cycle. The main contraceptive feature of these pills is the progestogen during the first half of the cycle which blocks the LH surge. Required doses are lower with less side-effects than the simple combined pill. Progestogens also stimulate a cervical secretion that is less penetratable by (and is a more hostile environment for) spermatozoa, and make the uterus less receptive to implantation.

Female reproductive endocrinology (Clinical)

Multiple Choice Questions

C.1

Which of the following are reliable indicators of the occurrence of ovulation?

a Mittelschmerz
b A fall of central body temperature during the second half of the menstrual cycle
c A rise of serum progesterone to greater than 20 nmol/litre during the second half (presumed luteal phase) of the menstrual cycle (normal follicular phase progesterone levels: 1–4 nmol/l).
d A change in the characteristics of cervical mucus
e Ultrasound evaluation of follicular size

C.2

In relation to causes of amenorrhoea, which of the following statements is/are true?

a Low or normal serum gonadotrophin levels suggest a primary gonadal cause
b Prolactin excess induces amenorrhoea mainly by impairing ovarian responsiveness to gonadotrophin stimulation
c Stress-mediated amenorrhoea is essentially a temporary form of hypogonadotrophic hypogonadism
d The amenorrhoea of hyperthyroidism is due to increased sex hormone binding globulin
e With the exception of pregnancy and the menopause, polycystic ovarian syndrome (PCOS) is the commonest cause of amenorrhoea.

C.3

In the assessment of amenorrhoea, which of the following statements is/are true?

a Adequacy of oestrogen production can be clinically confirmed by attempted induction of withdrawal bleeding by progestogen administration b GnRH stimulation tests are capable of differentiating pituitary from hypothalamic causes of hypogonadotrophic hypogonadism

c In the absence of drug effects, a serum prolactin of 950 mU/Litre (NR 200–450 nmol/l) strongly suggests a prolactinoma as the cause of amenorrhoea

d Clomiphene administration can be used to assess ovarian function by its direct stimulating effect on ovarian oestradiol production

e Persistently raised serum gonadotrophin (LH and FSH) levels in association with low oestradiol level (<100 pmol/l) is strongly indicative of an irreversible gonadal lesion

C.4

Polycystic ovarian disease/syndrome (PCOS) is present in 15–20% of females. Which of the following statements concerning clinical presentation is/are true?

a Oligo- or a-menorrhoea may alone be indicative of PCOS

b The presence or absence of menstrual abnormality is closely linked to the presence or absence of obesity, respectively

c In the absence of menstrual irregularity, it is unlikely that acne and seborrhoea are secondary to PCOS

d The distribution of abnormal hair growth and balding reflects the severity of androgen excess

e The clinical features of PCOS can be precisely simulated by congenital adrenal hyperplasia, masculinizing ovarian and adrenal tumours, and Cushing's syndrome

C.5**

In regard to the metabolic syndrome which often accompanies the polycystic ovarian syndrome, which of the following statements is/are correct?

a The hyperinsulinaemia which is frequently present is due entirely due to the frequently associated obesity

b The hyperlipidaemia of PCOS is only partly due to coexistent obesity

c Diabetes is more frequent than in the general population

d There is strong supportive evidence for increased coronary artery disease risk in PCOS

e Reduction of hyperinsulinaemia reduces serum androgen levels

C.6

In relation to the differential diagnosis of PCOS, which of the following statements is/are correct?

a Serum total testosterone is often normal in PCOS

b In patients presenting with hirsutism, raised levels of dehydroepiandrosterone sulphate (DHEAS) suggest an adrenal cause

c A basal serum 17-hydroxyprogesterone (17-OHP) above 12 nmol/litre suggests the possibility of late-onset (presumed heterozygous) congenital adrenal hyperplasia

d Patients with a serum total testosterone level above 5 nmol/litre have a greater than 80% chance of having an adrenal aetiology for their androgenic clinical features
e Low serum oestradiol with raised serum LH is the hallmark of PCOS

C.7

In the treatment of the androgenic manifestations of PCOS, which of the following approaches may be expected to be helpful?

a Electrolysis-based removal of affected hair
b Oestrogen supplementation
c Weight reduction
d Corticosteroid administration
e Antiandrogens

C.8**

In relation to management of the reproductive elements of PCOS, which of the following statements is/are true?

a In the absence of immediate desire for fertility, amenorrhoea alone does not constitute an indication for hormonal intervention
b Weight reduction improves fertility rate in PCOS
c Clomiphene citrate induces ovulation in more than 50% of infertile patients with PCOS
d The 80% pregnancy rate following ovarian diathermy justifies its use as a first-line treatment modality
e Combined GnRH agonist-gonadotrophin therapy is a logical treatment choice in the presence of clomiphene failure

C.9

Variation in age at menarche and periods of amenorrhoea are common. In regard to these phenomena, which of the following statements is/are true?

a Late menarche is partly familial
b Age at menarche does not influence bone density at maturity (peak bone mass)
c It is not known whether the amenorrhoea occurring as a result of intense protracted physical exercise (e.g. athletes), low body weight/calorie deprivation (anorexia nervosa), or both (ballet dancers) should be prophylactically treated with oestrogen replacement
d Amenorrhoea occurring during the treatment of certain psychiatric conditions is more likely to be due to the drugs employed, rather than to the disorder itself
e Amenorrhoea following discontinued administration of the contraceptive pill does not usually reflect any underlying disorder

C.10

In regard to the syndrome of gonadal dysgenesis (Turner's syndrome), which of the following statements is/are true?

a Absence of both webbing of the neck and a wide carrying angle (cubitus valgus) makes the diagnosis unlikely

b There is a high prevalence of coexistent congenital cardiovascular and renal anomalies

c Fibrous 'streak gonads' are a prerequisite for making the diagnosis

d Normal growth can be restored by appropriate oestrogen replacement

e Conception is feasible using egg donation and *in vitro* fertilization procedures (IVF)

C.11**

In the syndrome of testicular feminization, which of the following statements is/are correct.

a The karyotype is invariably 46 XY

b Serum testosterone levels are reduced compared to normal males

c Partial forms are more commonly assigned to a male gender

d Gonadectomy is not indicated

e The condition is inherited as autosomal dominant

C.12

Which of the following phenomena is/are known to be due to the reduction of circulating oestrogen which occurs at the menopause?

a Increased vaginal secretions

b A fall in serum LDL cholesterol

c Vasomotor symptoms of flushing

d An increased tendency to depression

e Bone loss due to reduced bone formation (osteoblastic activity)

C.13

In regard to premature menopause or ovarian failure (hypergonadotrophic hypogonadism), which of the following statements is/are true?

a It is partly familial

b By age 60, there is an increased risk of osteoporosis when compared with age-matched women with normal-age menopause

c The risk of cerebrovascular and coronary occlusive events (stroke and heart attack) is increased compared with women having a normal-age menopause

d Autoimmune ovarian destruction is the major cause

e Once amenorrhoea has been established for 3 months in biochemically confirmed cases, infertility can be assumed

C.14

Which of the following statements is/are correct in assessing the indications for and advantages of oestrogen replacement in the menopause?

a Oestrogen replacement reduces bone fracture rate when introduced at any stage following the menopause

b The absolute benefits of oestrogen replacement on the incidence of heart attack and stroke are not known

c Vasomotor flushing and vaginal dryness are absolute indications for oestrogen replacement

d Oral oestrogens are superior to transdermal oestrogen patches in terms of effects on hepatic lipid production

e Urinary frequency and proneness to urinary tract infection may respond to oestrogen replacement

C.15

Which of the following statements is/are correct in assessing the contra-indications to and disadvantages of oestrogen replacement in the menopause?

a Unopposed oestrogen (i.e. without progestogen) should not be used in the presence of an intact uterus

b Breast cancer risk is increased by the use of hormone replacement therapy (HRT) in women with a positive family history

c There is an increased risk of venous thromboembolism in women receiving postmenopausal oestrogen

d Previous myocardial infarction is a contra-indication to oestrogen replacement

e Cyclical withdrawal bleeding is an inevitable consequence of safe oestrogen replacement regimens

MCQ Answers

C.1 a **False.** The iliac fossa or lower central abdominal pain which occurs as a result of follicular rupture (ovulation) is well recognized by some patients, but in sufficiently specific and consistent to be used as a reliable indicator of ovulation.

b **False.** Basal body temperature (BBT) begins a rise of at least 0.2 °C synchronously with the LH surge associated with ovulation, with maximum rise of about 0.4 °C, 48 hours later. The early morning at resting criteria are all important if the test is to have value. The ris BBT is secondary to the elevated progesterone, which in turn stim release of thermogenic norepinephrine.

c **True.** Co-incident with the LH surge of ovulation, serum prog rises, reaching a maximum about 8 days later with maturing of the corpus luteum. A luteal phase value of 20 nmol is highly suggestive and 40 nmol/litre confirmatory of ovulation. Urinary pregnanediol, the metabolite of progesterone can also be used.

d **False.** Women may notice an increase of cervical mucus at ovulation. Various chemical changes in the mucus are suggestive, but not confirmatory of ovulation. For several days after ovulation, mucus quality alters (spinnbarkheit) so that the ability to sustain a thread of cervical mucus between glass slides is impaired.

e **True.** Transvaginal ultrasound can 'track' the progressive growth (to between 18 and 25 mm), rupture, and regression of a dominant follicle which comprise the process of ovulation. It is the gold standard against which other methods are measured, possibly paralleled only by diurnal measurement of serum or urinary LH.

C.2 a **False.** Ovarian causes of amenorrhoea result in a primary reduction of oestrogen secretion, and a corresponding *increase* in pituitary gonadotrophin release. Included in these causes are gonadal dysgenesis (Turner's syndrome), premature ovarian failure, ovarian damage from radiotherapy or chemotherapy, and rarely, oocyte failure associated with myotonia dystrophica and galactosaemia.

b **False.** Prolactin receptors have been identified on granulosa cells. Both *in vivo* and *in vitro*, hyperprolactinaemia inhibits ovarian oestrogen response to gonadotrophin stimulation. However, the major effect of prolactin excess is mediated by gonadotrophin inhibition: both serum oestradiol and gonadotrophins are low in the presence of significant hyperprolactinaemia.

c **True.** Probably acting exclusively via dopaminergic stimulation, gonadotrophin secretion is inhibited by stress. Exercise amenorrhoea occurs through similar pathways. It is contentious whether the hypogonadotrophic hypogonadism of anorexia nervosa is mediated by calorie deficiency, low body weight, the primary psychological state which is associated with this condition or a combination of these factors.

d **True.** Thyroid hormones directly stimulate hepatic SHBG production, with increased oestradiol and a consequent reduction in free oestradiol. This may represent one factor contributing to amenorrhoea in this condition, although other currently unidentified factors are probably also responsible.

e **True.** Amenorrhoea, and even more frequently oligomenorrhoea is very common in PCOS, a condition affecting 15–20% of the female population, based on large-scale population screening with pelvic ultrasound.

a **True.** Medroxyprogesterone, 5–10 mg daily for 5 days normally causes withdrawal bleeding if sufficient oestrogen is present to induce prior endometrial build up. However, there is a significant incidence of false positive responses. A negative response is nevertheless indicative of hypooestrogenaemia. A better marker of 'adequate' oestrogen activity is follicular-phase endometrial thickness, which should exceed 5 mm on ultrasound measurement.

b **True.** The behaviour of serum LH and FSH following a single bolus GnRH injection may be expected to differentiate hypothalamic causes (response present) from pituitary causes (response absent). However, in long-standing hypothalamic disorders, this is unreliable because of pituitary gonadotroph involution. 'Priming' the pituitary with daily GnRH infusion for 5 days, followed by single bolus GnRH stimulation restores pituitary responsiveness, if it is otherwise normal (the Snyder test protocol).

c **False.** Rises of serum prolactin to 1000 mU/litre (or sometimes higher) are seen in stressed or depressed patients, who may also have amenorrhoea (although this is primarily due to hypothalamic anovulation mediated directly by stress).

d **False.** Although clomiphene does have a minor direct effect on the ovary, its major effect is induced by blocking hypothalamic oestrogen receptors. A doubling of LH pulse frequency has been demonstrated and serum LH (and oestradiol) rises. It therefore represents a useful test of intactness of the hypothalamic–pituitary–ovarian axis.

e **True.** Ideally, this biochemical combination should be demonstrated on two or more occasions before presuming that ovarian failure is present.

C.4 a **True.** There is marked variability in androgen production in PCOS. Furthermore, despite high androgen levels, target organ (e.g. skin) effects are dependent on 5α-reductase activity (and consequent active dihydrotestosterone synthesis) in the skin, which is also highly variable.

b **True.** Obesity reduces serum SHBG, increasing free androgen levels. In addition, obesity induces hyperinsulinaemia, which it itself responsible for enhancing ovarian androgen synthesis. Menstrual irregularity is strongly related to obesity, although the precise nature of this relationship is not understood: androgen excess alone is not sufficient to cause it.

c **False.** Postadolescent 'common' acne vulgaris and seborrhoea may alone be manifestations of PCOS. Both the biochemical and ultrasound features may be indistinguishable from more typical PCOS patients.

d **False.** The pattern of hirsutism is highly variable, and this may be partly dependent on distribution of 5α-reductase enzyme activity or on other currently indefinable genetic factors. Androgen-dependent balding, dominated by frontal hair recession may occur in the absence of hirsutism.

e **True.** Late-onset (heterozygous) congenital adrenal hyperplasia is diagnosed in around 2% of patients presenting with clinical androgen excess without true virilization: indeed, polycystic ovaries commonly coexist, for reasons which are not clear. True virilism (voice deepening, breast atrophy, muscle hypertrophy, clitoromegaly) may be seen in patients with rare androgenizing tumours of the adrenal or ovary (hilus cell tumours, arrhenoblastoma). Cushing's syndrome may also masquerade as PCOS.

C.5 a **False.** As mentioned in C.4b, hyperinsulinaemia relates to obesity. However, serum insulin in PCOS is about double that of non-PCOS cases for a given weight. Its mechanism is not understood. Extreme hyperinsulinaemia is seen in the HAIR-AN (hyperandrogenaemia insulin-resistance acanthosis nigricans) syndrome, in which the underlying insulin resistance is due to mutations in, or autoantibodies to the insulin receptor. The characteristic furrowed hyperpigmentation is often seen (and more frequently identified on biopsy) in axillary and neck skinfolds.

b **True.** High serum LDL and triglyceride, and low HDL cholesterol are seen in PCOS, even when corrected/adjusted for body weight.

c **True.** Diabetes prevalence is 2–7 times more frequent in PCOS. It is not clear whether this association represents diabetes developing as a consequence of insulin resistance/obesity, or whether the insulin resistance and relative hyperinsulinaemia, which is a feature of type 2 (non-insulin-dependent) diabetes results in enhanced androgen synthesis.

d **False.** Although the above constellation of findings suggests a strongly atherogenic profile, this has not yet been confirmed on the basis of adequate epidemiological studies.

e **True.** Reduction of hyperinsulinism by weight reduction, or experimentally using the drugs metformin or diazoxide secondarily reduces serum androgen levels. It also results in regression of acanthosis nigricans, which represents the cutaneous response to chronic marked hyperinsulinaemia.

C.6 a **True.** *Total* serum testosterone is raised in only 30–50% of ultrasound proven cases of PCOS. However, the coexistent reduced SHBG level renders the *free* testosterone level (usually calculated as total testosterone divided by SHBG multiplied by 100: NR 1.5–4.5) elevated in more than 90% of cases.

b **False.** Although DHEAS is an adrenal androgen, exogenous oestrogen suppresses the moderately raised levels sometimes found in PCOS, suggesting abnormal intraovarian pathways.

c **True.** This is a realistic threshold, above which the likelihood of CAH increases. Values of 17-OHP at this level justify a short synacthen stimulation test (250 μg IV): 30-minute 17-OHP maxima above 30 nmol/litre support a diagnosis of late onset CAH.

d **True.** Irrespective of the presence of true virilism (as defined in C.4e above), such levels of total testosterone justify adrenal imaging and dynamic tests of adrenal cortisol and androgenic function (stimulation and suppression).

e **False.** Unless there is coexistent pathology, serum oestradiol (and other oestrogens) are normal in PCOS. This is responsible for the endometrial build up, which represents a risk of malignant change in amenorrhoeic PCOS patients. Serum LH is however often raised, although the mechanism of this is not understood.

C.7 a **True.** This is probably the most effective method of dealing with coarse facial hair, and is also applicable to other body regions. Individual approaches to other cosmetic treatment modes such as shaving, waxing, and chemical hair removal require exploration with the patient, for whom they may not be acceptable.

b **True.** Although adequate oestrogen production exists in PCOS, supplemental oestrogen, given cyclically with a non-androgenic progestogen suppresses serum LH (which reduces ovarian androgen production). Exogenous oestrogen also down-regulates peripheral tissue androgen receptors. Its benefits are usually modest.

c **True.** As indicated above, obesity not only leads to higher rates of anovulation, but also causes hyperandrogenaemia via obesity-related hyperinsulinaemia and by reducing serum SHBG levels. Although a highly desirable goal, weight reduction is no more easily achieved than in obese women without PCOS.

d **False.** This was postulated in the past to be a useful approach. However, there is no demonstrated benefit except in the uncommon subgroup with late onset CAH. Even here, other forms of therapy may be preferable long term, given the side-effect profile of even low corticosteroid doses.

e **True.** Spironolactone has androgen blocking as well as mineralocorticoid blocking effects. It is usually well tolerated. Its progestational effects sometimes cause irregular bleeding. Cyproterone acetate, given either continuously with the contraceptive pill, or cyclically with oestrogen alone has shown inhibitory effects on hair diameter and growth rate. Finasteride, an inhibitor of 5α-reductase has shown early promise of benefit in some cases.

C.8** a **False.** In amenorrhoeic women with PCOS, the continued effect of normal circulating oestrogen results in endometrial hyperplasia, believed to be a premalignant process. Accordingly, regular withdrawal bleeding should be induced with progestogen alone, or more conveniently with oestrogen–progestogen combination.

b **True.** A 5% reduction in weight has been shown to significantly improve fertility rate, even in the absence of additional therapy. As indicated above, the reduction of serum androgen is probably irrelevant: the mechanism of the fertility benefit resulting from reducing serum insulin levels has not yet been adequately explained.

c **True.** Clomiphene is safe, and correctly used has a low incidence of multiple pregnancy. Ovulation is achieved in about 75% of treated cases. However, successful fertilization occurs in only 50% of cases. The persisting and even enhanced serum LH levels associated with clomiphene are thought to impair oocyte development and thereby explain this discrepancy: miscarriage and multiple pregnancy rates are also higher.

d **False.** Ovarian diathermy is a recent laparoscopic variation of the ovarian wedge resection procedure first used empirically in 1935. The means by which this focal trauma achieves about a 70% ovulation and fertility rate is unknown. In contrast to clomiphene, LH levels fall post-operatively: hence higher fertility/ovulation ratios and lower miscarriage rates. Androgen levels also decrease for a variable period. Postoperative adhesions may occur. Most centres regard the procedure as second- or third-line therapy.

e **True.** Theoretically, this is optimal therapy. High-dose GnRH agonist therapy down-regulates and hence suppresses LH release. Subsequent pulsed GnRH or more commonly combined FSH/LH induces ovulation. Being a more complex procedure, and despite a 60–65% fertility rate in the best centres, it usually represents a second-line approach, to follow a failed clomiphene protocol.

C.9 a **True.** Age at menarche has a familial component. Nutritional, physical health, and psychological factors are important modifiers.

b **False.** The older the age at menarche, the lower the peak bone mass. Similar relationships have been noted in males: delayed puberty is associated with reduced bone mass in later life.

c **True.** Osteoporosis has been noted in all the stated groups. The adverse bone effects of oestrogen deficiency are clearly not reversed or counteracted by the muscular activity associated with exercise. The possible benefits of oestrogen replacement are not yet known.

d **True.** Many drugs used in the treatment of depression and schizophrenia, including phenothiazines, neuroleptics, and antipsychotics as well as other drugs (metoclopramide, cimetidine) have dopaminergic activity. They stimulate prolactin release and accordingly variably suppress gonadotrophin release. The longer-term consequences of the resulting oestrogen deficiency are still unknown. Psychiatric disorders themselves may, in some instances, cause amenorrhoea directly, presumably based on associated stress and nutritional factors.

e **False.** Investigation of 'post-pill amenorrhoea' usually identifies clearcut pathology. Stress-induced amenorrhoea, prolactinoma, and poly-cystic ovarian syndrome are together responsible for 95% of cases. However, investigation should only be initiated after amenorrhoea has been present for 6 months.

C.10 a **False.** Although these two clinical features are common in the classical 45 XO karyotype, they may be absent in chromosomal mosaics, which may account for up to 30% of cases. Patients may present only with minor short stature and primary amenorrhoea.

b **True.** Coarctation of the aorta and horseshoe kidney are the commonest associated anomalies, but other congenital heart defects are also well recognized.

c **False.** Streak gonads are found in most patients and require no surgical intervention. However, XO/XX mosaics may have a unilateral dysfunctional gonad, while in XO/XY mosaics, a unilateral ovo-testis may be associated with clinical hyperandrogenism: such gonads are predisposed to undergo malignant change (gonadoblastoma) and should ideally be removed prophylactically.

d **False.** Short stature is not due to oestrogen deficiency, but to defective growth hormone and somatomedin receptors in the dysplastic bone of these patients. Oestrogen replacement may induce a minor temporary increase in growth velocity. Growth hormone similarly produces a growth rate increment, but final mature height is only improved by 2–3 cm at best.

e **True.** With oestrogen replacement, uterine maturation occurs rapidly. IVF procedures have succeeded in many cases. Cephalopelvic dispro-portion makes Caesarean section a safer approach for delivering the baby.

C.11 a **True.** Genetically, all cases are male 46 XY: the defect lies in defective androgen receptors in all tissues. All complete forms are phenotypically female, and may sometimes not e diagnosed until presenting with infertility!

b **False.** Serum testosterone (and all other androgen levels) are those found in unaffected males. Serum LH is commonly raised, probably com-pensating for increased androgen to oestrogen conversion by tissue aromatase activity.

c **False.** Partial androgen insensitivity results in variable degrees of gynaecomastia, a variable uro-genital sinus and clitoral enlargement. Despite some voice deepening, sexual orientation is usually female, and this is a more acceptable phenotype. Apart from reconstructive surgery, oestrogen supplementation is the usual strategy.

d **False.** The gonads (testes) are usually undescended, or at best labial in position in incomplete forms of testicular feminization. They are accordingly more prone to malignant change and are ideally removed as soon as possible, followed by oestrogen supplementation.

e **False.** Since all cases are infertile, autosomal dominant inheritance cannot apply.

C.12 a **False.** Vaginal secretions diminish in proportion to the reduction in circulating oestrogen. The consequent vaginal dryness may result in dyspareunia and also increases the risks of vaginal infection.

b **False.** Compared to men, women are relatively protected from atherosclerotic vaso-occlusive events until the menopause. Serum LDL rises and HDL falls as a consequence of oestrogen deficiency, partly accounting for the escalating vascular risk of the intermediate and late postmenopausal period of life (see also Chapter 13, C 7a).

c **True.** Although the mechanism of the menopausal flush is not clear, it appears to be directly due to oestrogen deficiency. Although it was considered that the raised gonadotrophin level of the menopause may play a part in flush causation, perhaps through diminished pulse frequency, flushes are also seen in hypopituitarism, albeit less frequently. Prostaglandins may also be involved: some cases respond to prostaglandin inhibitors.

d **False.** Although there is an increased occurrence of depression in the perimenopausal period, psychosocial rather than biological factors are responsible. Trials reveal that any benefits of oestrogen are due to alleviation of disabling flushes, and that there is no direct connection between depression and oestrogen deficiency.

e **False.** Oestrogens primarily inhibit *osteoclastic* bone resorption by opposing parathormone action on bone receptors, and possibly stimulating calcitonin secretion. They may also impair differentiation of mature osteoclasts from marrow precursors. A subsidiary action of oestrogen on osteoblasts may be mediated by oestrogen-sensitive growth factors such as IGF-I and transforming growth factors.

C.13 a **True.** A family history of early menopause is encountered in approximately 25% of cases in which there is no apparent additional pathology.

b **True.** With menopause (whether spontaneous or artificial) occurring before age 40, the risk of bone density falling below an arbitrary 'fracture threshold' is three times greater than with a normal menopause (see also Chapter 9, C.10d).

c **True.** The risk represents a reversal of the protection afforded to women through physiological oestrogen exposure. This risk is partly linked to adverse changes in the serum profile (see C.10b above), but also may be due to a demonstrated abnormality of blood flow and effects on vascular endothelial and haemorheological characteristics.

d **False.** In approximately 20% of cases, premature ovarian failure coexists with other organ-specific autoimmune disorders such as Hashimoto's disease, insulin-dependent diabetes, and Addison's disease. Lymphocytic infiltrates similar to that seen in the thyroid in Hashimoto's disease are also found in the ovary in affected cases: antibodies directed against both the corpus luteum as well as granulosa cells have been identified in no more than 25% of patients in whom no other pathology is present. Other causes to be considered are (congenital) galactosaemia (where excess galactose has been shown experimentally to reduce germ cell migration to the genital ridges), the neurological disorder, myotonia dystrophica, and damage from either radiotherapy or cancer chemotherapy (alkylating agents).

e **False.** Ovarian biopsy of patients with apparently idiopathic premature ovarian failure shows apparently viable oocytes in about 20% of cases. In accord with this, 25% of cases resume ovulation spontaneously at least in the short term. Pregnancy has been occasionally reported during oestrogen replacement.

C.14 a **False.** Current evidence only supports a benefit on fracture rate if oestrogens are introduced within 3 years and possibly 6 years of the menopause. However, at any time point following the menopause, the decline of bone density is slowed by oestrogen. There is no evidence that concurrent progestogen reduces these benefits.

b **True.** At present, all prospective studies on protective effects of oestrogen are of non-randomized subjects: confounding lifestyle factors may be partly responsible for the observed 30–50% reduction in myocardial infarction, and a lesser benefit on cerebrovascular accidents (stroke). The effect of progestogens of different types is not yet known: they may diminish benefits.

c **False.** Vasomotor flushing usually resolves spontaneously and also may respond to cimetidine: the use of oral oestrogens may delay the process of spontaneous resolution. Vaginal dryness can be treated by topical dienoestrol cream, although transvaginal absorption occurs with excessive use.

d **False.** Notwithstanding the 'first pass' hepatic effects of orally administered oestrogen, transdermal oestrogen has similar beneficial effects on total and LDL–cholesterol. The rise of HDL–cholesterol is higher with oral oestrogen, but may be offset by the induction of hypertriglyceridaemia related to hepatic production of increased VLDL. Only controlled prospective studies are capable of resolving significant differences.

e **True.** The external urethral epithelium shares oestrogen responsiveness with vaginal epithelium. Notwithstanding reports of symptomatic benefit with oral and vaginal oestrogen, there are no controlled studies on which to place any firm reliance.

C.15 a **True.** In different studies, unopposed oestrogen increased the risk of endometrial carcinoma by 3–7 times. It should therefore only be sued in hysterectomized women. There is no evidence of increased cancer risk in the ovary or any other tissue.

b **True.** The life risk of breast carcinoma increases from 1:13 to about 1:7 with a family history of breast carcinoma before age 50. Most estimates attribute a 1.1–1.4 risk ratio to the effect of postmenopausal oestrogen, whether or not there is a positive family history.

c **True.** An increased venous thromboembolic risk ratio of 1.1–1.5 has been attributed to oestrogen therapy. Current methods of predicting prothrombotic tendency by measurement of coagulation proneness (Leiden and other protein factors) are unsatisfactory.

d **False.** Data on secondary prevention (following a first myocardial infarction episode) reveal a probable 50% *reduction* in re-infarction risk. It is likely that this benefit is mediated by non-lipid factors involving vascular endothelium and blood flow characteristics, presently unspecified.

e **False.** Continuous combined oestrogen–progestogen combinations appear to provide relative protection against bone and vascular consequences of the menopause, and without the complication of withdrawal bleeding. The results of long-term studies are still awaited. Other steroids with mixed oestrogenic/androgenic potency (tibolone) are probably equally bone-protective: their effect on vascular prognosis is currently unknown.

References

Physiology

Topic: Relaxins.
Bryant-Greenwood, G.D. *et al.* (1994). *Endocrine Reviews*, 15, 5–26.
Topic: Oestrogen receptors in tissues not generally recognised as target sites.
Ciocca, D.R. *et al.* (1995). *Endocrine Reviews*, 16, 35–62.
Topic: The pre-ovulatory LH surge.
Clarke, I.J. (1996). *Trends in Endocrinology and Metabolism*, 6, 241–7.
Topic: Possible roles of growth factors in female reproduction (including developing embryo–maternal interactions).
Giudice, L.C. *et al.* (1995). *Trends in Endocrinology and Metabolism*, 6, 60–9.
Topic: Regulation of ovarian follicle development.
Gougeon, A. (1996). *Endocrine Reviews*, 17, 121–55.
Topic: The mechanism of action of progesterone.
McDonnell, D.P. (1995). *Trends in Endocrinology and Metabolism*, 6, 133–8.
Topic: Oestrogen and progesterone effects on vascular sensitivity.
White, M.M. *et al.* (1995). *Endocrine Reviews*, 16, 739–51.

(Clinical)

Topic: Hormonal treatment of the menopause.
Belchetz, P.E. (1994). *Lancet*, 330, 1062–71.

Topic: The polycystic ovary syndrome.

Franks, S. (1995). *New England Journal of Medicine*, **335**, 617–23.

Topic: Female infertility.

Healy, D.L. (1994). *Lancet*, **343**, 1539–44.

Topic: Psychological and sexual aspects of the menopause.

Pearce, J. *et al.* (1995). *British Journal of Psychiatry*, **167**, 163–73.

Topic: Testicular feminization.

Quigley, C.A. (1995). *Endocrine Reviews*, **16**, 217–32.

Topic: Androgens and hair growth.

Randall, V.A. (1994). *Clinical Endocrinology*, **40**, 439–58.

Topic: Turner's syndrome.

Saenger, P. (1996). *New England Journal of Medicine*, **335**, 1749–54.

Topic: Evaluation of secondary amenorrhoea.

Warren, M. (1996). *Journal of Clinical Endocrinology and Metabolism*, **81**, 337–42.

8 The thyroid (Physiology)

Multiple Choice Questions

See also Chapter 4 (Qs 3, 18); Chapter 12 (Q 5)

P.1 The normal thyroid gland

a is situated in the chest
b consists of two linked lobes of tissue
c requires a direct neural link with the brain in order to function
d is composed mainly of follicles filled with a protein-rich gel
e produces iodinated molecules derived from the amino acid tyrosine

P.2 The iodinated thyroid hormones

a are synthesized in the follicular cells
b are tri- and tetra-iodinated thyronine molecules
c are formed as a result of coupling reactions which link mono- and di-iodinated tyrosyl groups on a thyroidal globulin protein
d are stored as follicular colloid
e include the calcium-regulating hormone calcitonin

P.3 Iodide

a is a necessary component of the diet
b is present as iodide in the extracellular fluid
c diffuses into the thyroid follicular cells
d if chronically deficient, results in the development of a goitre
e is essential for normal iodothyronine synthesis

P.4 Tri-iodothyronine

a is the main iodothyronine synthesized by the normal thyroid gland
b is the principal active iodothyronine
c is produced by the monodeiodination of tetra-iodothyronine (thyroxine) in target tissues
d is transported in the blood mostly bound to the thyroglobulin
e binds to intracellular receptors in its target tissues

P.5 *Thyroxine (tetra-iodothyronine)*

    a is merely a precursor prohormone

    b can be deiodinated to the biologically inactive tri-iodothyronine known as 'reverse T_3'

    c has a longer biological half-life than tri-iodothyronine

    d stimulates the nuclear transcription process in many target cells

    e stimulates the removal of cholesterol from the blood

P.6 *The iodothyronines*

    a have short latencies of 6–12 minutes

    b stimulate basal metabolism in all target cells

    c increase protein synthesis and degradation

    d have catecholaminergic effects partly by stimulating β-receptor synthesis

    e are important for normal growth and development of the fetus and infant

P.7 *The actions of the iodothyronines*

    a are dependent on their activation of G proteins in the plasma membrane

    b may be associated with the intracellular activation of cyclic AMP

    c often involve the intracellular synthesis of mRNA

    d are mediated by the intracellular generation of prostaglandins

    e may be inhibited by the hormone, calcitonin

P.8 *Regulation of iodothyronine production*

    a is an important function of the adenohypophysis (anterior pituitary)

    b is primarily due to the actions of thyrotrophin (thyroid-stimulating hormone)

    c is mainly under the inhibitory control of circulating iodide in the blood

    d involves negative feedback loops to the hypothalamus and pituitary

    e is influenced by the autonomic innervation of the follicular cells

Short Answer Questions

P.9

Draw a labelled diagram clearly illustrating the principal features of iodothyronine synthesis, storage, and release.

P.10

Briefly describe how the iodothyronines are transported in the blood. Identify the biologically active component and indicate how changes in hepatic proteogenesis might affect thyroid function.

P.11

Briefly describe the physiological role of the iodothyronines using the condition of hypothyroidism to illustrate your answer.

P.12

List *three* important effects of iodothyronines on metabolic processes, and explain how each of these processes would be affected in hyperthyroidism.

P.13

Briefly describe three possible mechanisms of action of the iodothyronines in their target cells, specifying which is likely to be the principal one.

P.14

Draw a labelled diagram illustrating the main regulatory influences on the thyroid follicular cells, indicating clearly the feedback loops involved.

MCQ answers

P.1 a **False.** The thyroid gland is situated in the neck, anterior to the trachea. However, if enlarged it can extend into the upper mediastinum.

      b **True.** The two lobes of the thyroid are joined by a thin strand of tissue called the isthmus.

      c **False.** There is good evidence for an autonomic innervation of the follicular cells (and thyroid blood vessels), and the brain (specifically the hypothalamus) is very important for thyroid regulation (see P.8 below), but a *direct* neural link with the brain does not exist.

      d **True.** The gel is composed mainly of iodinated thyroglobulin protein (i.e. the storage form of the iodothyronines).

      e **True.** The starting point for iodothyronine hormone synthesis is the iodination of tyrosine amino acids present as tyrosyl residues incorporated in the thyroglobulin protein synthesized by the follicular cells. The peroxidase enzyme responsible for catalysing the iodination is located in the apical membrane and the reaction probably takes place along this membrane.

P.2 a **True.** The iodinated thyroid hormones, or iodothyronines, are synthesized in the follicular cells of the thyroid. The other cell type in the thyroid is the parafollicular cell which produces the polypeptide hormone, calcitonin. (For more information about this hormone see Chapter 9).

      b **True.** initial iodination of the tyrosyl residues on the thyrogulin molecules produces either mono- or di-iodotyrosyls. A coupling reaction, which involves a configurational change in the structure of the protein molecule, results in mono- and di-iodotyrosyl groups linking together to form the tri- and tetra-iodothyronines which remain incorporated in the thyroglobilin protein.

c **True.** As explained in the previous answer, the iodinated tyrosyls link together to form tri- and tetra-iodothyronines which are still incorporated in the thyroglobulin protein molecule. Actual production of the iodothyronine hormones involves the proteolysis of the thyroglobulin molecule which ultimately results in the release of tri- and tetra-iodothyronines into the circulation.

d **True.** The thyroglobulin (containing the iodinated thyronines) is secreted into the follicular space by exocytosis where it is stored. Sufficient of these thyroid hormones is stored here for up to 6 months' normal requirement.

e **False.** Calcitonin is a polypeptide hormone synthesized by the parafollicular cells; it is *not* iodinated.

P.3 a **True.** Iodine is present as iodides in the water (the main source) and the soil—hence present in small amounts in various vegetables. The daily dietary requirement (and urinary excretion) of iodine is 50–150 μg. Nowadays, it is often added to table salt and bread. Seaweed is a particularly good source. It is important to be aware that various medicines and other dietary components may contain iodinated products.

b **True.** While some iodide is found in erythrocytes, most is to be found in the extracellular fluid. Organically bound iodide (as iodinated tyrosines and thyronines in thyroglobulin) is present in particularly high concentration in the thyroid gland.

c **False.** Iodide is actively transported from the extracellular fluid into the follicular cell by the iodide pump in the basal membrane. As a consequence of the activity of the iodide pump, iodide is 'trapped' within the follicular cells where it is greatly concentrated (25–50fold).

d **True.** Consequent on the deficiency of iodide there is a decrease in production of iodothyronines and a subsequent reduction in negative feedback on the hypothalamo–adenohypophysial axis. This results in the increased production of thyrotrophin (thyroid-stimulating hormone, TSH) which stimulates increased thyroid activity (including growth of gland and production of increased quantities of follicular colloid). This is manifest as a goitre.

e **True.** Without sufficient iodide the quantity of iodothyronines produced falls and consequently the signs and symptoms of hypothyroidism become evident.

P.4 a **False.** The main iodothyronine synthesized by the thyroid follicular cells is tetra-iodothyonine, also called thyroxine. However, in hyperthyroidism proportionately larger quantities of tri-ioodothyronine are synthesized and released by the thyroid gland; actual production of tri-iodothyronine remains smaller than that of thyroxine.

b **True.** Thyroxine (T_4) acts mainly as a precursor for the more active tri-iodothyronine (T_3) in many peripheral tissues.

c **True.** In addition to small amounts of tri-iodothyronine being produced by the thyroid follicular cells directly, thyroxine can be mono-deiodinated to the more active tri-iodothyronine (T_3) by peripheral tissues.

d **False.** Thyroglobulin is the storage protein found in the colloid and follicular cells. In the blood, the iodothyronines are transported mostly bound to a specific globulin protein called thyronine binding globulin (TBG) and also to the albumin and (for thyroxine) the prealbulin fractions.

e **True.** Intracellular (and perhaps intranuclear) receptors for the iodothyronines have been identified.

P.5 a **False.** Thyroxine can also bind to intracellular iodothyronine receptors, although with lesser affinity than T_3, and therefore it is a hormone in its own right—as well as being a precursor prohormone for T_3.

b **True.** Thyroxine can be mono-deiodinated in either one of two positions, to produce the biologically active T_3 (3,5,3'-tri-iodothyronine) or the biologically inactive 'reverse T_3' (3,3',5'-tri-iodothyronine).

c **True.** The half-life ($T_{1/2}$) of thyroxine is approximately 7 days compared with a much shorter $T_{1/2}$ of 1–2 days for T_3. In addition to the shorter half-life, T_3 also has a shorter latency of 12 hours compared with that of T_4 (approximately 72 hours).

d **True.** Both iodothyronines probably exert their main physiological effects by stimulating the nuclear transcription process resulting in the synthesis of new proteins. Other mechanisms of action are also in contention, including a direct action on membrane transport processes and an action directly on the mitochondria perhaps working directly on the enzymes located in this intracellular structure.

e **True.** Both iodothyronines stimulate the removal and degradation of plasma cholesterol to a greater extent than they stimulate cholesterol synthesis. Consequently, hypothyroidism is associated with hyper-cholesterolaemia.

P.6 a **False.** The iodothyronines have long latencies (i.e. length of time elapsed before there is any evidence of any action) of approximately 12 and 72 hours for tri- and tetra-iodothyronine, respectively. These latencies are much longer than those for most other hormones, whether proteins/polypeptides or steroids.

b **False.** While the stimulation of basal metabolic rate is a fundamental effect of the iodothyronines, and it occurs in most cells of the body, there are nevertheless important exceptions. The principal exceptions are the cells of the brain, spleen, and testes. (*Note* that this does *not* mean that the iodothyronines have no effects on the cells of the central nervous system, however; merely that the basal metabolic rate is not increased in them.)

c **True.** Iodothyronines stimulate both protein synthesis and degradation processes. Normally, protein synthesis is influenced more than degradation, so the iodothyronines are considered to be protein-anabolic and hence growth-promoting. However, when iodothyronines are deficient there is an accumulation of 'old' protein and other molecules (e.g. mucopolysaccharides, hyaluronic acid, etc.) in the tissues which then retain water (hence the *oedema* of myxoedema).

d **True.** A stimulation of catecholamine β receptor synthesis by the iodothyronines may be one way in which the iodothyronines and the catecholamines interact. This could account, at least partly, for the partial correction of some of the defects of hyperthyroidism with β-adrenergic blockers such as propranolol.

e **True.** The growth-promoting effects of iodothyronines on the fetus are vital for normal development. If an iodothyronine deficiency is not corrected within weeks or months of birth, normal mental and physical development may not occur, resulting in a condition historically called 'cretinism'.

P.7 a **False.** While it is possible that iodothyronines have membrane effects (e.g. on ion channel activation) there is no evidence so far for either membrane receptors or G proteins being involved in their mechanism of action.

b **True.** It is still unclear exactly how the iodothyronines and the catecholamines interact, but their is some evidence to suggest an increase in catecholamine receptor synthesis by the iodothyronines and some evidence for an enhanced cyclic AMP synthesis by catecholamines in iodothyronine-primed tissues. Whether these effects are species-specific, tissue-specific, or of any physiological significance requires further study.

c **True.** This is generally believed to be the principal mechanism by which the iodothyronines influence cell activity.

d **False.** There is no evidence for any major involvement of prostaglandins in mediating actions of the iodothyronines.

e **False.** Calcitonin has no known effect on iodothyronine activity.

P.8 a **True.** The adenohypophysis produces a glycoprotein hormone which stimulates the production of the iodothyronines by the thyroid. This hormone is a molecule consisting of an α and a β chain, the 92 amino acid α chain being identical to the α chains of two other adenohypo-physial glycoprotein hormones, the gonadotrophins luteinizing hormone and follicle stimulating hormone. The specificities of the three molecules reside in their individual β chains which, for thyrotrophin is 110 amino acids long.

b **True.** The adenohypophysial hormone which stimulates iodothyronine production is called thyrotrophin (also known as thyroid-stimulating hormone).

c **False.** Iodide can inhibit 'organification' within the thyroid (an effect known as the Wolff–Chaikoff effect), but this is probably of minor importance under normal physiological conditions, the dominant controlling influence being thyrotrophin from the anterior pituitary.

d **True.** Iodothyronines have an important negative feedback influence on the hypothalamic production of thyrotrophin releasing hormone (TRH) and the adenohypophysial production of thyrotrophin (thyroid-stimulating hormone, TSH), by indirect and direct negative feedback loops respectively. Thyroxine is believed to be deiodinated to tri-iodothyronine in the thyrotroph cells of the adenohypophysis, and probably in the specific TRH producing neurones of the hypothalamus.

e **True.** The autonomic innervation (sympathetic fibres) to the thyroid gland terminate mostly on the blood vessels, but some innervation of follicular cells has also been detected. Therefore, autonomic activity may influence iodothyronine production indirectly, by altering blood flow through the gland, and/or directly by the innervation of the follicular cells.

SAQ Answers

P.9

The diagram required to answer this question is essentially the one shown as Fig. 8.1. The main features to include are: (a) the iodide pump in the plasma membrane, (b) the activation (oxidation in the presence of hydrogen peroxide) of iodide to a reactive form of iodine—perhaps the iodine radical, (c) the organic iodination reaction, i.e. iodination in position 3 alone or with position 5 of the tyrosyl groups on the thyroglobulin molecule forming mono- and di-iodotyrosines T_1 and T_2, (d) the coupling reaction to form tri- and tetra-iodothyronines T_3 and T_4, (e) the exocytosis of iodinated thyroglobulin into the follicle, (f) the uptake by endocytosis of follicular colloid containing iodinated thyroglobulin, (g) migration of lysosomes containing enzymes including deiodinases, (h) breakdown of thyroglobulin to release T_3 and T_4, and (i) movement of T_3 and T_4 into the circulation (by diffusion or carrier-mediated transport across the cell membrane).

P.10

The iodothyronines (T_3 and T_4) are almost entirely bound to plasma proteins in the circulation so that the 'free' (i.e. unbound) component of total T_4 is 0.05%, while

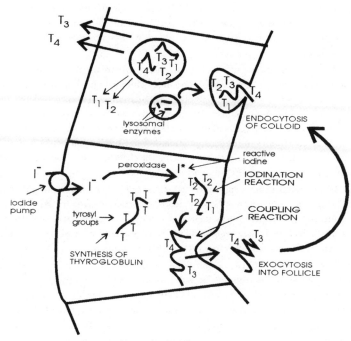

Fig. 8.1

for T_3 this component is some 10 times greater at 0.5%. Most (approximately 80%) of the T_3 and T_4 is bound to the specific (high affinity) globulin called thyronine binding globulin (TBG). Most of the remaining T_4 is bound to a prealbulin (approximately 15%) with a very small component bound to the low affinity (but high capacity) albumin. In contrast, the remainder of the bound T_3 is associated with the albumin fraction only. A dynamic equilibrium exists between the free and bound hormone components and the plasma protein fractions.

Only the free hormone component is biologically active. Any alteration in the amount of the thyronine binding plasma proteins in the blood can influence thyroid function. Thus, for example, oestrogens (and oestrogen-containing contraceptive pills) stimulate hepatic TBG synthesis and this is associated with raised total T_4 (and to a lesser extent T_3) concentrations while androgens have the opposite effect. Usually, the free T_4 and T_3 components, which are active in the feedback control of the thyroid gland, are kept within their normal ranges.

P.11

Included in your answer should be the following points:

(a) The iodothyronines generally increase basal metabolic rate (BMR) and are caligenic (main exception: in brain). In hypothyroidism the BMR can be reduced by as much as 40%; the decreased caligenesis (there may be a small drop in basal body temperature) is associated with a cold skin, and the patient has a poor tolerance of cold.

(b) T_3 and T_4 promote protein synthesis, hence are important for growth and development. They are particularly important in childhood (and *in utero*) for both physical and mental development. Protein degradation is also increased by the iodothyronines. In hypothyroidism, decreased protein synthesis and protein catabolism results in retarded replacement of tissues (e.g. brittle nails, hair loss, poor wound healing) and contributes to the accumulation of water-binding molecules (e.g. the glycoprotein mucins) under the skin producing the characteristic tissue puffiness of the condition (gives rise to its clinical name of myxoedema).

(c) Lipid metabolism is influenced by T_3 and T_4 such that although both anabolic and catabolic pathways are stimulated the main effect is on degradation. Consequently in hypothyroidism there is a gradual increase in fat accumulation resulting in increased body weight (often despite a reduced appetite) and the plasma cholesterol level tends to rise (hypercholesterolaemia).

(d) T_3 and T_4 also stimulate carbohydrate metabolism, and again both glycogen synthesis, gluconeogenesis, glycogenolysis, glycolysis, and even glucose absorption by the small intestine are all increased. In hypothyroidism, the main manifestation on carbohydrate metabolism may be the reduced intestinal absorption of glucose.

(e) Another consequence of hypothroidism is the possible development of a yellowish tinge to the skin (due to increased build-up of carotenes normally used in vitamin A synthesis, which is reduced in this condition).

(f) Effects on the central nervous system are apparent in hypothyroidism. Indeed the slowness of thought and speech, memory impairment, and general lethargy are very common symptoms.

(g) Effects on the musculoskeletal, renal, and alimentary systems are also manifest in thyroid disease states. For example, general weakness and aching muscles are common presenting features.

(h) Interactions with other hormones, particularly catecholamines; they probably account for some of the effects of iodothyronines on certain metabolic pathways, the cardiovascular and nervous systems.

The effects of the iodothyronines are necessary for normal physiology, but are not vital for life itself.

P.12

In addition to the more general iodothyronine-stimulated increase in basal metabolic rate (BMR) and caligenesis, three more specific effects would be their actions on protein, carbohydrate, and lipid metabolism. Anabolic and catabolic processes are affected. The essential features of these effects can be exemplified by considering the condition of hyperthyroidism (thyrotoxicosis).

(a) BMR and calorigenesis would be associated with slightly raised basal body temperature, warm skin, vasodilatation, increased sweating, and poor tolerance of heat. Although appetite is often increased, body weight is generally reduced.

(b) Increased protein synthesis and degradation both occur but degradation is stimulated to a greater extent; the consequent net decrease in muscle mass contributes to the loss of body weight.

(c) The effects of iodothyronines on lipid metabolism are similar to those on protein, so that again lipid degradation is the net effect also contributing to the loss of body weight. Consequently, circulating levels of free fatty acids and glycerol increase, but the plasma cholesterol concentration decreases.

(d) Carbohydrate metabolism is also increased, with both anabolic and catabolic pathways stimulated. The oral glucose tolerance test is often abnormal (being prolonged and often similar to that seen in diabetics).

It may be appropriate to mention that interactions between the iodothyronines and other hormones (e.g. catecholamines, insulin) may also play a part in producing the metabolic effects described above.

P.13

The iodothyronines enter their target cells readily, possibly by passive diffusion although assisted transport involving carriers is also likely. Certainly, the iodo-thyronine receptors (of which there are at least two types) are intracellular and can be detected within the nucleus of target cells. Receptors have also been located in the mitochondria. The principal mechanisms of action being considered at present are: first and foremost, stimulation of protein transcription in the nucleus; second, direct stimulation of the mitochondria; and third (least likely) is the possibility that there is a direct effect on the plasma cell membrane.

The nuclear transcription mechanism involves the hormone–receptor complex binding to a specific site (the hormone response element) on the chromosome by means of the receptor DNA binding domains. Subsequently, specific transcription activation occurs and the resulting mRNA produced is translated into new protein on the ribosomes. A direct effect on mitochondrial DNA resulting in new protein synthesis (e.g. enzymes of the respiratory chain) has also been proposed. Effects of iodothyronines on the cell membrane are unlikely to be direct; rather, increases in membrane ATPase activity and or concentration may be brought about indirectly, as a consequence of other intracellular messenger systems. One such is cyclic AMP, the synthesis of which may be influenced by iodothyronines in certain specific target cell types.

P.14

Figure 8.2 illustrates the key features of the control of iodothyronine production. These include the production of thyrotophin releasing hormone (TRH) from the hypothalamus, thyrotrophin (thyroid-stimulating hormone, TSH) from the adenohypophysis (anterior pituitary), and the negative feedback loops involving

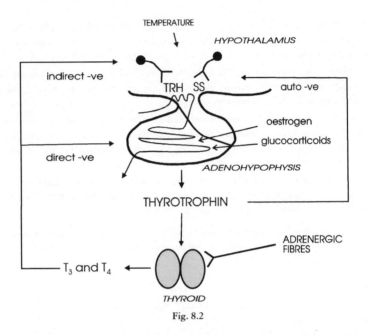

Fig. 8.2

iodothyronines acting at hypothalamic and pituitary levels to inhibit production of TRH and thyrotrophin respectively. In addition, the influence of the autonomic fibres to the thyroid could be indicated, as could the influence of other hormones such as the oestrogens (which may act by increasing the number of TRH receptors on the thyrotroph cells of the adenohypophysis). Glucocorticoids suppress TSH production but only when present in pharmacological amounts. The minor inhibitory influence on thyrotrophin production exerted by the hypothalamic neurosecretion somatostatin (SS) is shown.

The thyroid (Clinical)

Multiple Choice Questions

C.1

Most patients with thyroid dysfunction have an underlying disorder of thyroid autoimmunity. In this connection, which of the following statements is/are true?

a Raised serum levels of thyroglobulin (TGA) and microsomal (thyroid peroxidase: TPA) antibodies are found in approximately 2% of the adult population

b The diagnostic sensitivity of TPA for autoimmune thyroid disease exceeds 90%
c One or both of these antibodies are responsible for antibody-mediated thyroid follicular cell destruction
d Graves' hyperthyroidism is due to a stimulating thyrotrophin–receptor antibody
e The serum level of this stimulating antibody accurately predicts remission-proneness in hyperthyroidism

C.2

A 25-year-old woman presents with palpitations, weight loss, and heat intolerance. Hyperthyroid Graves' disease is suspected. Which of the following would *exclude* this diagnosis?

a Inability to feel a goitre
b A serum TSH of 1.3 mU/litre (NR 0.5–3.5)
c A serum *total* thyroxine of 130 nmol/l (NR 60–145)
d a thyroidal isotope (technetium) uptake of 1.1% 0f N < 5%)
e A serum-*free* thyroxine of 20 pmol/l (NR 12–24)

C.3

Three months postpartum, a 21-year-old woman presents with mood swings and a goitre. She is found to have raised serum-free T_3 and free T_4 levels, and suppressed serum TSH. Postpartum thyroiditis (PPTD) is considered as a possible diagnosis. Which of the following is/are consistent with this diagnosis?

a Coexistent thyroid ophthalmopathy
b Normal thyroid function tests 3 months later, without therapy
c Positive (1:1600) thyroid peroxidase (microsomal) antibody titre
d Tender thyroid enlargement
e Raised thyroidal uptake of technetium or radioidine

C.4

Which of the following is/are true in relation to the use of antithyroid (thiocarbamide) drugs?

a They are effective in the treatment of the hyperthyroidism of subacute (de Quervain's) thyroiditis
b Skin rash, arthralgia, and agranulocytosis are all common complications
c They act by blocking thyroidal hormone (T_4 and T_3) release
d They are regularly effective when given once daily
e Their action is inhibited by simultaneous iodide administration

C.5

Which of the following is/are true in relation to the use of beta-adrenergic blocking drugs in hyperthyroid Graves' disease?

a They can be used for definitive treatment
b They can be used in low dosage in the presence of asthma

c Cardio-selective beta blockers (e.g. atenolol) are preferable
d They are contra-indicated in the presence of thyrotoxic cardiomyopathy
e They have significant benefits on thyroid eye disease

C.6

Which of the following statements would you associate with the syndrome of thyrotoxic crisis (thyroid storm)?

a It is almost exclusively seen in the (biochemically) severest thyrotoxic states
b It is a significant complication of radioiodine therapy
c Hyperpyrexia and confusion are common clinical features
d Mortality (untreated) is about 20%
e Therapy with beta-adrenergic blockade and iodine administration are more important than antithyroid drugs

C.7

A 40-year-old man with confirmed hyperthyroidism is offered symptomatic therapy with beta-adrenergic blocking drugs, pending a decision about definitive treatment. Which of the following symptoms or signs would you expect to respond to this group of drugs?

a Weight loss
b Diarrhoea
c Palpitations
d Heat intolerance
e Tremor

C.8**

A 24-year-old woman with recently diagnosed with Graves' hyperthyroidism has been commenced on treatment with antithyroid drugs. Some weeks later, she is found to be pregnant. Which of the following statements is/are correct?

a Pregnancy usually enables women to maintain euthyroidism with lower doses of antithyroid drugs
b Incompletely controlled hyperthyroidism risks miscarriage
c Concurrent thyroxine therapy (block-replace therapy) is an appropriate method of preventing hypothyroidism in both mother and fetus
d Subtotal thyroidectomy is the only suitable alternative treatment of antithyroid drug hypersensitivity reactions occur
e Breast-feeding should be avoided if antithyroid drugs are used postpartum

C.9**

A new-born (5-day-old) baby girl is found to have a sinus tachycardia and possible lid retraction. Neonatal thyrotoxicosis is suspected. Which of the following is/are consistent with this diagnosis?

a Her mother was biochemically euthyroid (normal serum-free T4, free T3, and TSH) throughout pregnancy, and on no therapy
b The baby is likely to have thyroid microsomal (antiperoxidase) antibodies
c The presence of a large goitre in the baby suggests that the hyperthyroid state will require long-term antithyroid drug therapy
d Most cases do not require treatment because of a negligible mortality rate
e Late development of hypothyroidism is unlikely

C.10

A 60-year-old woman complaining of tiredness and dry skin is suspected of having hypothyroidism due to Hashimoto's disease. Which of the following investigations would *exclude* this diagnosis?

a Normal serum cholesterol
b A serum total thyroxine level of 85 nmol/litre (NR 60–145)
c A serum thyrotrophin (TSH) of 2.1 mU/litre (NR 0.5–3.5)
d Negative thyroid microsomal (peroxidase) antibodies
e A serum free T_3 of 5.5 nmol/litre (NR 4.8–8.5)

C.11

A 55-year-old woman with metastatic carcinoma of the breast and severe fatigue is found to have a serum total thyroxine of 40 nmol/litre (NR 60–145) and free thyroxine of 8.0 pmol/litre (NR 12–24). Serum TSH was normal (1.6 mU/litre). Which of the following differential diagnoses would be supported by these findings?

a Hashimoto's disease
b Sick euthyroid syndrome
c A tumour metastasis in the hypothalamic–pituitary axis
d Congenitally low thyronine binding proteins
e A side-effect of concurrent drug therapy

C.12

In the treatment of a 60-year-old man with primary hypothyroidism, which of the following statements apply?

a Coexistent ischaemic heart disease is a contra-indication to treatment
b It is desirable to use T_3 as well as T_4 to achieve "physiological' replacement
c Achievement of a normal serum TSH is the most reliable indicator of optimum thyroid hormone replacement
d Thyroid hormones can be omitted for 1–2 days without deleterious effect
e Biochemical monitoring is required every 2–3 months to ensure optimum dosage of thyroxine replacement

C.13

Which of the following is/are true in neonatal hypothyroidism?

a Prevalence is approximately 1:4000 births in most countries
b Neonatal screening programmes are not considered to be cost-effective
c Central nervous system development is impaired if treatment is delayed
d Multiplex families (more than one family member affected) are common
e Autoimmune thyroid destruction is the commonest cause

C.14

A 10-year-old girl with poor growth is found to be hypothyroid. Which of the following findings and statements is/are consistent with this diagnosis and its management?

a Thyroid microsomal (antiperoxidase) antibodies negative
b A bone age of 7.5 years (Greulich and Pyle)
c TSH-suppressive doses of thyroxine are desirable to allow 'catch-up growth' to occur
d Family screening for thyroid disorder is worthwhile
e She will be able to be weaned off thyroxine once growth is complete

C.15

An 82-year-old woman is admitted to hospital unconscious and hypothermic (rectal temperature 30°C). The differential diagnosis includes hypothyroid coma.

a Treatment with thyroid hormone(s) should be delayed until biochemical confirmation is available
b Hyponatraemia and hypercapnia are common biochemical accompaniments of this diagnosis
c Prompt rewarming with an electric blanket is desirable
d Corticosteroid administration is advisable
e The recovery rate is about 80%

C.16

In a 24-year-old woman, a solitary palpable nodule can be felt in the left lobe of the thyroid gland. Which of the following is/are associated with a high risk of malignancy of the thyroid?

a Hoarseness and dysphagia
b A family history of hyperparathyroidism
c Regional lymphadenopathy
d Increased isotope uptake in the nodule
e Multiple nodules seen either with ultrasound or isotope scanning

C.17**

A 35-year-old woman presenting with irregular tachycardia and a small goitre is being investigated for possible hyperthyroidism. Investigations reveal a free T_3 level of 12.8 pmol/litre (NR 4.8–8.5) and a serum TSH of 5.9 mU/litre (N 0.5–3.5). Which of the following diagnoses would be consistent with these biochemical findings?

a Hyperthyroid Graves' disease
b TSH producing pituitary tumour
c Thyroid hormone resistance syndrome
d Increased levels of thyronine binding proteins due to administration of an oestrogen-containing contraceptive
e Amiodarone administration for treatment of her cardiac arrythmia

C.18

Iodine and iodide are widely distributed in pharmaceutical drugs (e.g. multi-vitamin preparations, amiodarone, proprietary cough remedies), as contaminants of milk (udder and can sterilization), and in radiological contrast media. Which of the following conditions might such iodide excess cause?

a Graves' hyperthyroidism
b Hypothyroidism
c Hyperthyroidism in endemic goitrous areas
d Reduced efficacy of antithyroid (thiocarbamide) drugs
e Interference with the assay of serum thyroid hormones

Short Answer Questions

C.19

Hyperthyroidism may present with many different signs and symptoms. Identify one symptom and one sign for each of 5 of the body's systems. For each of your 10 items, identify the pathophysiology.

C.20

Hypothyroidism may present with many different signs and symptoms. Identify one symptom and one sign for each of 5 of the body's systems. For each of your 10 items, identify the pathophysiology.

C.21

Discuss *briefly* the ways by which vision may be compromised by thyroid eye disease (infiltrative ophthalmopathy).

C.22**

Write *brief* notes on the management of different stages of severity of thyroid eye disease (infiltrative ophthalmopathy).

C.23

A 25-year-old woman has low anterior neck pain and hyperthyroid symptoms and signs. Investigations have identified this as subacute (de Quervain's) thyroiditis on the basis of a raised erythrocyte sedimentation rate (ESR), raised serum free T_3 and a suppressed thyroid image on isotope scan. Write *short* notes on treatment and follow-up.

C.24**

'Recurrent/persistent hyperthyroidism following subtotal thyroidectomy for Graves' disease raises complex issues in management.' Discuss the basis for this statement.

C.25**

'The relapse rate of Graves' disease following a course of antithyroid drugs is high and unpredictable.' Write *short* notes on this statement.

C.26

'Endemic goitre is the world's commonest thyroid disorder, and goitrous cretinism its most serious consequence.' Write *short* notes on the prevention and treatment of this disorder.

MCQ Answers

C.1 a **False.** The prevalence of thyroid antibodies rises with each decade age group, and is 50–100% higher in females at any age. During the reproductive years, 5–10% of women are antibody-positive to TGA, and 12–15% to TPA, rising to 15% and 25%, respectively, by age 70.

b **True.** Earlier assays were less specific. Current enzyme-linked and radio-immunoassay techniques identify TPA excess in well over 90% of cases of autoimmune thyroid disease, although not necessarily consistently. However, some cases of histologically proven Hashimoto's thyroiditis, the archetypal autoimmune disease, are nevertheless associated with undetectable antibody levels.

c **False.** Neither antibody is cytotoxic, and their presence in the serum of patients with hypothyroidism represents an epiphenomenon of follicular cell damage induced by cell-mediated immune destructive processes: the ratio of CD4 to CD8 T lymphocytes is altered in autoimmune thyroid disorders. Some cases of hypothyroidism have intact follicular cells, the hypothyroidism representing the effect of blocking TSH receptor antibodies: some cases prove to be reversible.

d **True.** In more than 90% of cases of Graves' hyperthyroidism, an IgG antibody to TSH receptor known to stimulate thyroid cells *in vitro* is present in patient's serum. The placenta is permeable to this antibody, whose presence in the fetus of a currently or previously hyperthyroid mother probably accounts for all cases of neonatal hyperthyroidism.

e **False.** Although falling levels of stimulating antibody broadly relate to remission rates, it cannot be used in individual cases. A coexistent TSH receptor blocking antibody, detection of which is technically difficult, may be responsible for this lack of correlation and predictability.

C.2 a **False.** A goitre can only be palpated in 50–75% of patients with Graves' disease. Even with ultrasound, 5–10% of patients have a normal size thyroid. A better functional impression can be gained by performing an isotope scan, in which increased uptake is present in well over 90% of patients with Graves' disease.

b **True.** Serum TSH is suppressed to <0.1 mU/litre in all forms of hyperthyroidism except the rate conditions of TSH-producing pituitary tumours and thyroid hormone resistance (abnormal receptor function) syndromes. Serum TSH is accordingly a good screening test for hyperthyroidism (but see also Chapter 9, C.16e for an exception to this rule).

c **False.** Because thyroxine is 99.95% protein-bound, reduction in serum proteins, either hereditary (TBPA or TBG deficiency) or acquired (hypoproteinaemia of any cause) may result in a normal *total* serum T_4, even though serum-*free* T_4 and *free* T_3 levels are raised.

d **False.** Concurrent or previous iodide excess (e.g. resulting from previous contrast radiography, the taking of multivitamin pills containing iodine or cough medicines) expands the total body iodine pool and accordingly reduces thyroidal percentage uptake.

e **False.** Free T_3 alone is raised (T_3 toxicosis) in early/mild cases or if total body iodine is depleted as a result of a previous treatment course of antithyroid drugs. T_3 is preferentially synthesized in the iodine-depleted state. A rise of free T_4 may not occur for weeks or months.

C.3 a **False.** Although postpartum thyroiditis (or thyroid dysfunction: PPTD) is an autoimmune disorder, occurring in 5–10% of all pregnancies (usually asymptomatically), presence of ophthalmopathy almost invariably indicates Graves' disease. Graves' disease also frequently presents or relapses in the postpartum period, due to waning of the characteristic immune tolerance associated with pregnancy.

b **True.** The hyperthyroidism of PPTD is self-limiting, followed by euthyroidism. However, hypothyroidism occurs within 6 months in 5–10% of cases and in as many as 50% during long-term follow-up.

Such (biochemical) follow-up is accordingly very important, since symptoms may be very insidious in onset.

c **True.** PPTD is an autoimmune disorder: 12% of women are antibody-positive antenatally and approximately 50% of these will develop PPTD.

d **False.** In contrast to subacute (de Quervain's) thyroiditis, tenderness and soreness of the thyroid is rare in PPTD.

e **False.** Uptake of isotope will be suppressed (the test should only be performed in women who are not breast-feeding because of radiation dosage).

C.4 a **False.** In subacute thyroiditis, thyroid hormone discharge is induced by inflammation of the thyroid, not by increased synthesis. Beta-adrenergic blocking drugs will inhibit the major adrenergic features of tachycardia (palpitations), tremor and sweating.

b **False.** Skin rash and arthralgia are seen in as many as 3–5% of patients treated; agranulocytosis in only 0.1%. If rash or arthralgia occur, changing to an alternative drug of this group is successful in about 25–30% of cases. Although antihistamines have been (successfully) used for these milder side-effects, there is then a risk of developing the much more serious (and occasionally fatal) agranulocytosis.

c **False.** Thiocarbamides inhibit organification of iodide. Iodide itself in high concentrations is the only agent capable of inhibiting hormone release, hence its value in the treatment of thyroid storm.

d **False.** Hypermetabolism of the thyrotoxic state requires multiple daily dosage for *consistent* early control: once euthyroid, control by single daily dosage is almost invariably possible.

e **True.** Iodide competes with thiocarbamide drugs in their action on thyroidal peroxidase inhibition. Sudden loss of control during maintenance treatment with antithyroid drugs should raise the possibility of unsuspected iodine intake, usually from drugs.

C.5 a **False.** Although there is some evidence to support inhibited peripheral tissue T_4 to T_3 conversion, these drugs only reduce the adrenergic symptoms. They do not influence thyroid hyperfunction or the natural history of the disorder.

b **False.** A history of asthma is an absolute contra-indication to beta-adrenergic blockers, which can induce a severe and even fatal attack of asthma.

c **False.** Non-selective beta-adrenergic blockers benefit a wider range of adrenergically mediated clinical features. They should only be continued until the patient is euthyroid.

d **False.** They are only contra-indicated if there is a major additional primary cardiac problem (e.g. ischaemic heart disease). In this instance the negative inotropic effect resulting from reducing adrenergic tone might precipitate or worsen cardiac failure.

e **False.** Only the comparatively insignificant lid lag and retraction may be reduced: important infiltrative changes are unaffected by bets-adrenergic blockers.

C.6 a **False.** Even biochemically 'mild' hyperthyroidism can be complicated by thyroid storm, triggered by episodes such as an accident, intercurrent surgery for another condition, or severe infection.

b **True.** Radiation thyroiditis complicates some radioidine treatment episodes, usually 1–2 weeks after administration. It is not clear why some patients develop this complication, which may indeed lead to thyroid storm.

c **True.** These are the cardinal features, potentially confused with severe infection or septicaemia (which may of course coexist and be the cause of the condition). Cardiac arrythmias, sometimes leading to ventricular tachycardia or fibrillation are the potentially life-limiting events.

d **False.** Mortality (untreated) is considerably higher than this, approaching 100%: it rarely resolves spontaneously (mortality (treated) should be less than 10%.

e **True.** Mortality is directly related to adrenergic excess, and iodine administration is the only method of blocking thyroidal release of (preformed) T_4 and T_3. The onset of useful action of antithyroid drugs is slow by comparison, even when used in high doses.

C.7 a **False.** This symptom/sign is due to hypermetabolism, to which increased adrenergic activity contributes very little.

b **True.** Bowel hypermotility is adrenergically mediated.

c **True.** Palpitations in hyperthyroidism may be due to sinus tachycardia or to the irregularity associated with the development of atrial fibrillation. The slowing of ventricular rate by adrenergic blockade will produce symptomatic improvement in both situations.

d **False.** Heat intolerance is due to hypermetabolism and will be unaffected: sweating, however, is often reduced by beta-adrenergic blockers.

e **True.** This is often one of the most dramatic responses.

C.8** a **True.** This sensitivity to the action of antithyroid drugs becomes apparent early in the second trimester, as the immuno-tolerant state of pregnancy develops: occasionally, antithyroid drugs can even be discontinued altogether in the third trimester, although this risks rebound hyperthyroidism postnatally.

b **True.** Recurrent miscarriage may even be a presenting symptom of hyperthyroidism. There is also a risk of premature labour in untreated or incompletely treated cases, which may be linked to adrenergic effects.

c **False.** The placenta is only minimally permeable to thyroxine and trioiodothyronine, but is freely permeable to antithyroid drugs. A block-replace regimen would therefore maintain euthyroidism in the mother, but risk hypothyroidism in the fetus.

d **True.** Radioiodine is absolutely contra-indicated in pregnancy because of high fetal irradiation. Subtotal thyroidectomy in the second or early third trimester is safe. *Short-term* preparation with beta-adrenergic blockers and iodine is required unless the patient is biochemically euthyroid.

e **False.** Although all antithyroid drugs are excreted through breast milk, daily maternal doses of 10–15 mg carbimazole or 100–150 mg propylthiouracil are safe in terms of neonatal goitre induction. If a goitre does occur, it will regress after weaning, and does not predispose to thyroid dysfunction later in life.

C.9** a **True.** Neonatal hyperthyroidism is not due to transplacental passage of thyroid hormones (very low permeability factor). However, the placenta is permeable to thyroid-stimulating antibodies, which may continue to be present in the maternal circulation for years following previously treated (or unrecognized, self-limiting) Graves' disease.

b **False.** Only rare cases of neonatal hyperthyroidism are due to a Graves' process in the baby: most cases have no immunological abnormality of their thyroid.

c **False.** A goitre is often palpable, and has no prognostic significance.

d **False.** Mortality rate is as high as 60% in some series. Treatment by beta-adrenergic blockade, antithyroid drugs (and iodide in severe cases) is indicated in most affected babies, even though all cases completely remit within 6–8 weeks.

e **True.** Hyperthyroidism is self-limiting with no hypothyroid phase: the baby's thyroid resumes function spontaneously. However, the separate entity of transient noeonatal *hypothyroidism* does occur due to transplacental passage of thyroid blocking antibodies.

C.10 a **False.** Although a raised serum cholesterol is common in hypothyroidism (always reducing and often normalizing with treatment), a normal value does not exclude the diagnosis.

b **False.** The patient could be receiving oestrogen as menopausal hormone replacement therapy: this would falsely elevate an otherwise low *total* thyroxine level by increasing thyronine-binding proteins (especially TBG). A normal serum *free* thyroxine level would, however, make hypothyroidism unlikely as a course of her symptoms.

c **True.** A normal serum TSH excludes hypothyroidism due to primary thyroid disease (e.g. Hashimoto's). In pituitary hypothyroidism, however, serum TSH may be either low or normal.

d **False.** Thyroid antibodies are mostly present in high titre in auto-immune thyroid disease: however, about 10% of cases (with cytologically or histologically confirmed lymphocytic infiltrate) are indeed microsomal antibody (TPO) negative.

e **False.** Serum free T_3 is only low in severe hypothyroidism, serum levels being presumably maintained due to an adaptive enhanced peripheral deiodination of T_4.

C.11 a **False.** Serum TSH would be raised in this disorder, by the negative feedback effects of reduced free hormone levels.

b **True.** Low thyronine-binding proteins coupled to hypothalamic–pituitary 'turn-off' (both processes secondary to cachexia/catabolism) are responsible for this combination of findings in the so-called sick-euthyroid syndrome, which occurs in advanced malignancy, malnutrition, and other acute and chronic disease states.

c **True.** Malignant breast (and other) tumours quite commonly metastasize to the very vascular hypothalamic–pituitary region producing hypopituitarism. Serum TSH is often normal rather than low in this condition, for reasons which have not been elucidated.

d **False.** Low thyronine binding proteins (alone) would not account for low *free* serum thyroxine: total thyroxine levels would, however, be low.

e **False.** There are no drugs which suppress free thyroxine in serum (except exogenously administered T_3).

C.12 a **False.** Coexisting ischaemic heart disease is an indication for very gradual dose increases of thyroid hormones, ideally beginning at 25 μg daily: biochemical euthyroidism may not be safely achievable. Only rarely do such patients need to be left totally untreated.

b **False.** Thyroxine is peripherally metabolized to triodothyronine: with optimal replacement doses, both serum free T_3 and free T_4 will be within the normal range: T_3 does not need to be given.

c **True.** Almost invariably, a normal serum TSH is found to be accompanied by normal serum free T_4 and free T_3 levels. However, in this clinical setting, ischaemic cardiac symptoms may be precipitated, so that complete correction of hypothyroidism may be unwise.

d **True.** Because of high percentage (reversible) binding to thyronine binding proteins, neither free T_4 or TSH serum levels are affected by such short-term omissions.

e **False.** Except in the first 6 months of therapy, requirements alter only slowly: 6–12 month checks are adequate. Individual thyroxine dose changes should be rechecked by thyroid function tests only after 5–6 weeks to allow for equilibration. It is uncommon to require more than 150 μg thyroxine daily.

C.13 a **True.** A similar prevalence has been found among most ethnic/geographic groups: some variation may be due to choice of screening method (serum T_4 vs serum TSH).

b **False.** Screening programmes, whether using serum TSH or thyroid hormone assay are cost-efficient with a benefit ratio of around 10 (based on the prevalence and cost of institutional care for brain-damaged patients resulting from late diagnosis, compared with the cost of community screening programmes).

c **True.** This is the main consequence of delayed treatment, most marked with treatment delay beyond 2 months of age. However, severe cases have intrauterine hypothyroidism, so that even prompt neonatal thyroid replacement may not prevent brain damage.

d **False.** Neonatal hypothyroidism is a sporadic disorder. Multiplex families have not bee reported.

e **False.** The commonest causes are thyroid agenesis or ectopia possibly due to anomalies in thyroid transcription factors (TTF-1 and TTF-2) or mutations of the thyroid peroxidase (TPO) gene. Congenital dyshormonogenesis and transient hypothyroidism due to transplacental blocking antibodies are less frequent. Autoimmunity is a rare cause.

C.14 a **True.** Some cases of juvenile hypothyroidism are due to thyroid biosynthetic defects (mainly organification block), when thyroid antibodies will be negative. However, the majority of cases are due to autoimmune disease.

b **True.** Bone age is often markedly delayed, and to a greater extent than height age.

c **False.** Euthyroid replacement doses of thyroxine (sufficient to normalize serum TSH) will permit maximum catch-up growth. High (TSH-suppressive) doses risk the induction of premature epiphyseal fusion and ultimate short stature. Premature fusion of cranial sutures (cranial synostosis) may impair CNS development.

d **True.** Whether autoimmune disease or biosynthetic defect is the primary pathology, there is a high risk of multiplex families.

e **False.** Although some cases of adult hypothyroidism may remit spontaneously, perhaps because of a waning iodide inhibitory effect, this is very rare in childhood: thyroxine must be given lifelong, with annual biochemical monitoring of thyroid function.

C.15 a **False.** Parenteral or oral (naso-gastric tube) thyroxine or tri-iodothyronine should be given even on suspicion: thyroid function tests should always be available within 48 hours, and allow suspension of therapy if the diagnosis is excluded.

b **True.** Hyponatraemia is due to defective excretion of a water load and an inappropriate ADH (SIADH) syndrome due to the hypothyroidism. Hypercapnia (and hypoxia) are due to the hypoventilation associated with hypothermia, but are not specific to hypothroidism.

c **False.** Prevention of further heat loss by (unheated) blankets or foil are safer (external heating risks vasodilatation and cardiovascular collapse). Gradual rewarming using heated IV fluids (35–37°C) is much safer.

d **True.** The patient may have secondary hypopituitarism due to pituitary disease (and hence be ACTH-deficient). Furthermore adrenal responsiveness to stress is impaired in gross hypothyroidism. In either instance, giving cortisol is a safeguard.

e **False.** Survival rate is little more than 20%, even in experienced hands. Mortality is due to infection and occasionally adrenal failure: severe hypothyroidism impairs the pituitary adrenal response to stress.

C.16 a **True.** Dysphonia, dysphagia, as well as increasing nodule size over weeks or months justifies further investigation by fine needle aspiration biopsy (FNAB) irrespective of any other investigation findings.

b **True.** Hyperparathyroidism and medullary thyroid carcinoma are two components of the familial multiple endocrine neoplasia type 2 (MEN-2) syndromes. Calcitonin measurement is indicated!

c **True.** Regional lymphadenopathy should always be considered suggestive of malignancy until proven otherwise: FNAB of nodule and node(s) is needed.

d **False.** Decreased uptake ('cold nodule') represents a higher malignancy risk than increased uptake ('hot nodule'). However, in both cases FNAB is desirable to exclude malignancy.

e **False.** Multi-nodularity (found to be present with 50% of clinically apparent solitary nodules) does not exclude malignancy, but significantly reduces its likelihood.

C.17** a **False.** In Graves' hyperthyroidism, serum TSH is invariably suppressed by increased circulating levels of (free) T_3 and T_4.

b **True.** The results are entirely in keeping with this rare condition.

c **True.** A variety of genetic defects result in defective thyroid hormone receptor activity activity, commonly an anomaly of the thyroid hormone receptor beta gene. Defects may also be expressed in peripheral tissues, but the biochemical findings in this patient indicate an anomaly with associated resistance at the pituitary level.

d **False.** Increased thyronine binding proteins would explain neither the raised *free* T_3, nor the raised serum TSH.

e **True.** The iodine component of amiodarone can induce hyperthyroidism, particularly in antibody-positive individuals. Amiodarone itself inhibits peripheral tissue conversion of T_3 to reverse-T_3, and also inhibits pituitary thyroid hormone receptor activity: its chemical structure has certain homologies with thyroid hormones. Together, these actions may be responsible for a paradoxical rise in serum TSH.

C.18 a **True.** Iodide triggers an immune reaction in patients with underlying autoimmune thyroid disease. It can also trigger relapse in previously hyperthyroid patients who were in remission following a course of antithyroid drugs. These phenomena are together referred to as the Jod–Basedow effect.

b **True.** Hypothyroidism can be induced by the same immune-enhancing process as in a. Iodide in larger amounts also inhibits organification (Wolff–Chaikoff effect) and thyroidal hormone release.

c **True.** This is another example of the Jod–Basedow phenomenon, seen particularly where iodized oil (derived from standard radiological contrast medium) is used in large scale prophylaxis in endemic goitrous areas.

d **True.** Iodide competes with the effects of thiocarbamide drugs on thyroid peroxidase.

e **False.** No current thyroid hormone assay methodologies are affected by iodide.

SAQ Answers

C.19

CVS: (SY) palpitations (increased adrenergic tone), oedema (LVF and increased capillary permeability): (SI) elevated JVP (high output state and/or biventricular failure due to cardiomyopathy), systolic hypertension (peripheral vasodilatation and positive inotropic effect of adrenergic tone).

RS: (SY) breathlessness (cardiomyopathy): (SI) tachypnoea (hypermetabolism).

CNS: (SY) irritability, anxiety, tremor (all adrenergic effects), irritable or prominent eyes (conjunctival injection due to infiltrative ophthalmopathy): (SI) hyperkinetic behaviour (possible direct effect of thyroid hormones on brain function), lid lag/retraction (adrenergic tone or infiltration of levator palpebrae superiorus as part of infiltrative ophthalmopathy).

MSS: (SY) fatigue, difficult stair climbing (thyrotoxic myopathy): (SI) proximal muscle wasting (thyrotoxic myopathy).

GIS: (SY) diarrhoea (increased motility – adrenergic tone): (SI) splenomegaly (Graves' disease related lymphocyte proliferation).

SKIN: (SY) increased sweating (adrenergic), alopecia (abnormal telophase due to thyroid hormone excess): (SI) warm, moist extremities (adrenergic), infiltrative dermopathy (Graves' disease only).

REPRO: (SY) increased libido, amenorrhoea (cause unknown).

C.20

CVS:(SY) chest pain (increased CHD): (SI) bradycardia (low adrenergic tone and hypometabolism), pericardial effusion (increased permeability in serous cavities).

RS: (SY) breathlessness (cardiomyopathy): (SI) pleural effusion (as for pericardium).

CNS: (SY) slow mentation and bradykinesis (direct effect of low thyroid hormone), tremor and ataxia (reversible cerebellar syndromes of obscure pathogenesis): (SI) delayed relaxation reflexes (hypothyroid myopathy and abnormal neuromuscular endplate function due to low thyroid hormone).

MSS: (SY) pseudo-claudication (cause unknown).

GIS: (SY) constipation (low adrenergic tone, hypometabolism).

SKIN: (SY)dry skin hypohidrosis due to low adrenergic tone, direct effect of low thyroid hormone): (SI) cold extremities (hypothermia), dry sallow skin (carotenaemia).

REPRO: (SY) infertility (possible effect of high TRH and/or prolactin), polymenorrhoea/menorrhagia (cause unknown).

C.21

Blurring of vision due to lacrimation, in turn due to corneal/conjunctival exposure secondary to lid lag and retraction; diplopia due to infiltration/tethering of extra-ocular muscles; exposure keratitis due to incomplete lid closure (lid retraction and proptosis); traction on optic nerve (optic neuritis) and retinal artery ischaemia; increased incidence of glaucoma (intraocular pressure increase on upgaze).

C.22**

No treatment required for minor proptosis, lid lag, and retraction (beta-adrenergic blocking drugs can reduce the degree of lid lag/retraction in some cases); in symptomatic cases (soreness, sticky eyes on wakening, general ocular discomfort) artificial tears, head of bed on blocks and low-dose diuretic; micropore tape for incomplete lid closure at night (causing early morning eye dryness/stickiness); if ophthalmoplegia progressive consider systemic steroids (40–60 mg prednisolone daily, reducing over 3–5 months); cyclosporine or methotrexate possibly additionally useful; for more severe proptosis/exophthalmos consider external (cobalt source) irradiation as a steroid-sparing exercise and long-term control for ocular relapse; need to monitor visual acuity—decreasing acuity due to optic nerve ischaemia justifies high dose steroid or orbital decompression (usually trans-antral); for chronic disabling proptosis, consider orbital decompression, probably additionally requiring muscle surgery to correct diplopia.

C.23

No treatment required if pain minimal, since condition self-limiting, aspirin if mild pain is present; corticosteroid (prednisolone 20–40 mg/day or equivalent dosage of alternative oral steroid) if moderate or severe pain; beta-adrenergic blockers for symptomatic relief (antithyroid drugs ineffective); steroid drugs tailed off slowly (otherwise risk of rebound recurrence); follow-up for transient (20–40% risk) or permanent (5–10% risk) hypothyroidism (more common in the presence of thyroid antibodies); recurrent episodes (other than poststeroid rebound) very rare.

C.24**

Average relapse/persistence rate of 10–20%; need to check biochemically at follow-up; need to avoid excessively large thyroid gland remnant at surgery; re-operation generally unwise because of high risk of parathyroid and recurrent laryngeal nerve damage (these disabilities usually lifelong); if antithyroid drugs used, will probably need to be given lifelong; radioiodine is usual treatment option.

C.25**

Overall long-term relapse rate 50–80%; rate probably higher after courses of treatment less than 6 months; higher also in older patients, with ophthalmopathy and with larger goitres; impalpable goitre a good prognostic sign; role of iodine/iodide in precipitating relapse (sources of iodide in vitamins, cough medicine, etc.); need for close observation and biochemical testing in first 6 months following discontinuation of drugs (time of maximum relapse rate); controversy about relevance of antithyroid drug dosage in influencing relapse rate (higher dosages are immunosuppressant and therefore possibly result in higher remission rate); unsatisfactory predictive capacity of (current) thyroid-stimulating antibody assays (TSAB).

C.26

Iodine deficiency is the common factor due to leaching of iodide from soil and plants (hilly or mountainous locations); indigenous plants additionally responsible in some locations (brassica/cassava) producing defect in iodide trapping and/or organification; cretinism largely due to effect of iodide deficiency on brain development rather than deficient thyroid hormone levels; iodine repletion programmes valuable, but difficult and expensive to implement and maintain; comparatively ineffective for correcting pre-existing goitres; more effective as preventive when introduced in young populations; use of iodized salt, bread, and particularly depot injections of iodized oil; intellectual deficit of cretinism irreversible by iodide repletion; adverse effects of iodide repletion in the form of Jod–Basedow phenomenon (iodide-induced hyperthyroidism).

References

Physiology
Topic: Regulation of gene expression by thyroid hormones and their heterodimeric receptors.
Glass, C.K. (1996). *Journal of Endocrinology*, 150, 349–57.
Topic: Iodothyronines and male gonadal function.
Jannini, E.A. *et al.* (1995). *Endocrine Reviews*, 16, 443–59.
Topic: The ageing thyroid.
Mariotti, S. *et al.* (1995). *Endocrine Reviews*, 16, 686–715.

Clinical
Topic: Pathophysiology of auto-immune thyroid disease.
Dayan, C. *et al.* (1996). *New England Journal of Medicine*, 335, 99–107.
Topic: The sick euthyroid syndrome.
Docter, J. *et al.* (1993). *Clinical Endocrinology*, 39, 499–518.
Topic: Congenital hypothyroidism.
Dubuis, J.M. (1996). *Journal of Clinical Endocrinology and Metabolism*, 81, 222–7.

Topic: Subclinical thyroid disease.

Elte, J.W.F. *et al.* (1996). *Postgraduate Medical Journal*, 72, 141–6.

Topic: Management of hyperthyroidism.

Franklyn, J.A. (1994). *New England Journal of Medicine*, 330, 1731–8.

Topic: Controversies in the management of cold, hot and occult thyroid nodules.

Guiffrida, D. (1995). *American Journal of Medicine*, 99, 642–50.

Topic: The thyroid and pregnancy.

Hall, R. *et al.* (1993). *British Journal of Obstetrics and Gynaecology*, 100, 512–15.

Topic: Thyroid cancer management.

Hardy, K.J. (1995). *Clinical Endocrinology (Oxford)*, 42, 651–5.

Topic: Investigation and treatment of hypothyroidism.

Lazarus, J.H. (1996). *Clinical Endocrinology*, 44, 129–32.

Topic: Thyroid-associated ophthalmopathy.

Perros, P.E. *et al.* (1995). *Clinical Endocrinology*, 42, 45–50.

Topic: Thyroid disease and the TSH receptor.

Tonacchera, M. *et al.* (1996). *Clinical Endocrinology*, 44, 621–34.

9 Calcium regulation, bone, and its metabolic disorders (Physiology)

Multiple Choice Questions

P.1 In the body, calcium

    a is mostly stored in the bones

    b circulates in the blood partly bound to plasma proteins

    c is present in muscle cells as the crystalline complex hydrated calcium phosphate apatite salt

    d is generally present in cell cytoplasm at a concentration greater than in the blood

    e is an essential component of cell membranes

P.2 Calcium ions in the blood

    a are in dynamic equilibrium with the circulating bound calcium component

    b are transported mainly within the red blood cells in association with a globulin protein

    c are normally present at a concentration of approximately 1.2–1.3 mmol/litre

    d represent factor IV in the intrinsic pathway of the haemostasis cascade

    e are freely filtered by the renal glomeruli

P.3 Calcium ions

    a are essential for maintaining neuromuscular excitability

    b are absorbed from the colon

    c enter cells through calcium channels

    d are actively pumped into cells in exchange for sodium ions

    e act as second messengers within cells

P.4 The calcium ion concentration in the blood

    a is increased by the actions of parathormone

    b decreases when renal phosphate excretion increases

    c is increased by vitamin C metabolites

    d is the principal physiological regulator of calcitonin release

    e if raised is a cause of hypertension

P.5 *The parathyroid glands*

a are usually four in number

b are routinely removed following bilateral thyroidectomy

c produce hormones under the control of the hypothalamo–adenohypophysial axis

d if overstimulated produce a goitre

e if absent or not functioning can be life-threatening

P.6 *Parathormone*

a is a steroid hormone

b is synthesized by the thyroid follicular cells

c binds to its receptors on osteoblasts in bone

d stimulates an increase in the plasma calcium ion concentration

e stimulates phosphate excretion by the kidneys

P.7 *Parathormone*

a stimulates renal 1α-hydroxylase activity

b is produced in response to an increased plasma calcium ion concentration

c synthesis is inhibited by 1,25-dihydroxycholecalciferol

d increases osteoclast activity in bone

e is synthesized in response to an increased circulating catecholamine concentration

P.8 *Vitamin D*

a in animals is present in the form of vitamin D_3, called cholecalciferol

b is a water-soluble vitamin

c is mainly synthesized in the skin

d is a precursor of bioactive metabolites

e is stored in the liver as a 25-hydroxylated molecule

P.9 *The metabolite 1,25-dihydroxycholecalciferol*

a is an energy substrate in the blood

b stimulates phosphate absorption in the small intestine

c is synthesized in the kidneys

d maintains the calcium stores in the bone matrix

e if deficient is associated with the bone disorder, osteomalacia

P.10 *Calcitonin*

a is a polypeptide hormone

b release is stimulated by thyrotrophin from the pituitary

c decreases the blood calcium ion concentration

d stimulates osteblast activity

e is present in raised concentrations in the blood during lactation

Short Answer Questions

P.11

List three hormones whose main physiological role is to regulate the plasma calcium ion concentration, and identify where they are synthesized. *Briefly* explain which tissues/organs are of particular relevance to calcium ion control.

P.12

Briefly explain how parathormone influences calcium ion regulation.

P.13

Briefly describe how parathormone and 1,25-dihydroxycholecalciferol act together in order to regulate calcium and phosphate in the blood.

MCQ Answers

P.1   a   **True.** All cells contain some calcium (normal intracellular total concentration of the order of 0.3 μmol/litre, free calcium ion concentration of the order of 0.1 μmol/l), and the blood contains it at a concentration of approximately 2.5 mmol/litre. However, the rest of the calcium (99% of the total in the body) is indeed found in the bones (and teeth), representing about 1 kg in an average person.

      b   **True.** Of the calcium in the blood approximately 50% is present as free ions, 45% is bound to the plasma proteins (albumin and globulin fractions), and the remainder is in association with anions such as phosphate, lactate, and citrate.

      c   **False.** In muscle cells calcium is present in the sarcoplasm (muscle cell cytoplasm) as free ions or bound to proteins (e.g. calmodulin, a regulatory protein), or is stored in various intracellular organelles such as microsomes and mitochondria in the form of simple salts. Hydroxyapatite crystals are a stable, long-term form of calcium salt complex only found deposited in the bone matrix.

      d   **False.** As indicated above, the concentration in the blood is some 10,000fold higher than the total calcium concentration found in cells, measured (in muscle cells at least) in μmol/litre.

      e   **False.** Calcium, as free ions specifically, plays various important roles inside cells, from acting as a coenzyme to being a second messenger. It is not present to any major extent (and is certainly not an essential component) in cell membranes although it can enter or leave the cell through specific channels in the membrane—or be actively pumped across the membrane by certain calcium exchange mechanisms (e.g. in association with sodium ions for instance).

P.2 a **True.** As mentioned above, calcium in the free, ionic form, represents approximately 50% of the total calcium in the blood, being in dynamic equilibrium with the bound forms of calcium (in association with proteins or diffusible salts).

b **False.** Calcium is transported mainly in the plasma (see above). The main protein in the red blood cells (the erythrocytes) is called haemoglobin because it actually contains iron atoms (one within each of the four haem groups associated with the protein).

c **True.** Approximately half of the calcium in the blood is present as free ions at any instant, and the total calcium concentration is approximately 2.5 mmol/litre. In fact the blood calcium concentration normally is extremely well regulated, within a narrow range of between 2.2 to 2.6 mmol/litre.

d **True.** One physiological role for calcium ions in the blood is to participate in haemostasis (blood coagulation) acting as an important cofactor (factor IV) in the intrinsic and extrinsic pathways leading to the formation of a blood clot.

e **True.** Calcium ions are freely filtered by the renal glomeruli and are subsequently reabsorbed further along the nephron. The reabsorption of calcium is under hormonal regulation; parathormone, for example, stimulates this process in the distal convoluted tubule of the nephron.

P.3 a **True.** Calcium ions 'sit' over the sodium channels thereby decreasing the movement of sodium down their electrochemical gradient, into neurones and muscle cells (i.e. influencing the membrane permeability to sodium). In hypocalcaemia there is an increased movement of sodium ions into the cells resulting in increased neuromuscular excitability. This manifests itself clinically as an increased tendency for tetany to develop.

b **False.** Calcium is not absorbed in the colon but in the small intestine, at the greatest rate in the duodenum but with an important contribution occurring in the jejenum. It is chiefly under the control of the bioactive vitamin D_3 metabolite 1,25-dihydroxycholecalciferol which is, itself, regulated by parathormone and calcitonin (see *P.7a*, *P.10c*).

c **True.** Calcium ions enter cells through channels which may be voltage- or ligand-gated (i.e. opened by depolarizing stimuli or by molecule–receptor binding). The electrochemical gradient favours the movement of calcium into cells.

d **True.** In addition to the calcium channels mentioned above, calcium can enter cells by an active pump mechanism which exchanges the ion for sodium. This pump is activated by an ATPase situated in the membranes.

e **True.** One important function of calcium ions within cells is to act as a second messenger system. Either calcium moving into the cell through a channel (e.g. ligand-gated) can act directly, perhaps as a coenzyme, on a metabolic pathway within the cell, or it can be liberated from an intracellular storage site by another second messenger such as inositol triphosphate—in which case the calcium ions could be considered to be a third messenger system.

P.4   a **True.** Parathormone is a hormone primarily concerned with the regulation of the blood calcium ion concentration. This hormone acts directly on the kidneys and bone, and indirectly on the small intestine, to increase circulating concentrations of this cation.

b **True.** Calcium and phosphate ions are in dynamic equilibrium with calcium phosphate salts in the blood so that if there is a decrease in the concentration of one of the two free ions then the salts will dissociate more in order to restore the equilibrium state. As a consequence, more calcium ions become free and their concentration rises. If there is an increased renal excretion of phosphate then this initiates the dissociation process. An early action ascribed to parathormone was the decreased reabsorption of phosphate in the proximal tubule resulting in its increased excretion in the urine. The consequent increase in plasma calcium ion concentration was at the time believed to be due to an indirect effect of parathormone, and only subsequently was it found that the hormone also increased calcium directly.

c **False.** Vitamin C has various important effects in the body but an increase in blood calcium ion concentration is not one of them. Rather, it is vitamin D_3 metabolites, particularly 1,25-dihydroxycholecalciferol, which increase it.

d **True.** Calcitonin decreases the blood calcium ion concentration and so, not surprisingly, changes in the concentration of this divalent cation regulate the production of this hormone. The main physiological stimulus for calcitonin release is an increase in blood calcium ion concentration.

e **False.** Hypercalcaemia is not commonly associated with raised arterial blood pressure even though calcium plays an important role in muscle (e.g. arteriolar smooth muscle) contraction.

P.5   a **True.** There are usually four parathyroid glands, one located in each of the four poles of the thyroid lobes (i.e. one in each of the superior and inferior poles). However, the number of parathyroids can vary and be as few as two or as many as five (or even six). Therefore care is required to check the position of all parathyroids before performing a thyroidectomy.

b **False.** This could have serious consequences for physiological calcium regulation if the parathyroid glands were routinely removed along with the thyroid during a thyroidectomy.

c **False.** The parathyroid glands are not influenced by hormones from the anterior pituitary and consequently are not controlled by the hypothalamo–adenohypophysial axis. Parathormone secretion is mainly under the control of the circulating calcium ion concentration, a decrease in the latter stimulating production of the hormone.

d **False.** A goitre is an enlarged thyroid gland consequent upon over-stimulation of the follicular cells by the adenohypophysial hormone, thyrotrophin. The parathyroid glands are not influenced by thyro-trophin and do not contribute to the goitre.

e **True.** Without the parathyroid glands calcium ion regulation is disturbed, the calcium ion concentration will decrease and hypo-calcaemia if severe enough will result in increased neuromuscular excitability. Death may be caused by asphyxiation due to tetanic contraction of the bronchi and bronchioles.

P.6 a **False.** Parathormone is a polypeptide hormone 84 amino acids long, synthesized from a prohormone of 90 amino acids which itself is derived from an initial molecule of 110 amino acids containing the signal sequence.

b **False.** Parathormone is synthesized in cells (chief cells) in the parathyroid glands which are located on the lobes of the thyroid. The follicular cells of the thyroid gland synthesize the iodothyronines thyroxine and tri-iodothyronine (see Chapter 8).

c **True.** This is perhaps surprising, but true. Osteoblasts lay down new bone (i.e. they are involved in bone formation which is associated with decreased blood calcium levels), whereas osteoclasts are the bone cells which increase bone breakdown (resorption) liberating calcium into the blood in the process. However, the parathormone receptors are on the osteoblasts, and it now appears that these cells, when stimulated by parathormone, synthesize an osteoclast-stimulating factor which activates the osteoclasts.

d **True.** Parathormone has various effects which result in increasing the calcium concentration in the blood. For example, it increases calcium reabsorption in the distal convoluted tubules of the renal nephrons, and stimulates osteoclast activity.

e **True.** One renal effect of parathormone is to stimulate the excretion of phosphate by an action in the proximal tubules to inhibit its reabsorption.

P.7 a **True.** Parathromone stimulates 1α-hydroxylase activity in the proximal tubules of the renal nephrons resulting in increased synthesis of bioactive 1,25-dihydroxycholecalciferol (which stimulates intestinal calcium absorption).

b **False.** Parathormone, which acts to *increase* blood calcium levels, is stimulated by a *decrease* in calcium concentration. Thus, calcium exerts a direct negative feedback effect on the parathyroid glands, this being the principal controlling influence on parathormone production.

c **True.** Parathormone stimulates 1,25-dihydroxycholecalciferol production and therefore, not surprisingly, the latter exerts a negative feedback effect on the parathyroids.

d **True.** Parathormone stimulates the production of an osteoclast-stimulating factor by osteoblast cells in bone. This factor then stimulates the osteoclasts which produce and secrete various molecules which break down the surrounding bone matrix. These molecules include various proteases (e.g. collagease and acid phosphatase) and acids (.e.g citric and lactic acids) which together stimulate the degradation of the bone matrix liberating calcium in the process.

e **True.** Catecholamines, including dopamine, stimulate parathormone release through β receptors on the parathyroid chief cell membranes. The intracellular mechanism involves cyclic AMP and protein kinase A, and appears to cause the release of preformed parathormone from membrane-bound granules.

P.8 a **True.** There are two principal forms of vitamin D which are called vitamin D_2 and vitamin D_3. Vitamin D_2 is found in plants and is called ergocalciferol while vitamin D_3 is the form found in animals and is called cholecalciferol. Cholecalciferol is mostly synthesized in the skin from 7-dehydrocholesterol (see c below). Animals can also utilize ergocalciferol and so the diet is also a source of the vitamin.

b **False.** The various vitamin B molecules are water-soluble. Vitamin D is a steroid derived from the cyclopentanoperhydrophenanthrene nucleus common to all cholesterol-derived molecules.

c **True.** Cholecalciferol is synthesized in the skin in the presence of ultraviolet light (range 230–315 nm wavelength). Pigmentation influences the penetration of light through the outer layer of the skin.

d **True.** Vitamin D_3 is not bioactive itself. It has to be hydroxylated to bioactive forms. The first hydroxylation (in the presence of 25-hydroxylase) occurs in the liver forming 25-hydroxycholecalciferol. This molecule has limited bioactivity, but is itself the precursor of various metabolites formed in the kidneys, examples being 24,25-dihydroxy, 25,26-dihydroxy, and 1,24,25-trihydroxy cholecalciferols. The principal known bioactive metabolite, however, is the 1,25-dihydroxycholecalciferol molecule.

e **True.** The first hydroxylation of cholecalciferol to 25-hydroxycholecalciferol occurs in the liver. This 25-hydroxy metabolite is stored in this organ which is why liver is an important dietary source of the vitamin.

P.9 a **False.** This molecule is an important steroid hormone involved in calcium regulation. It is not an energy substrate.

b **True.** This vitamin D_3 metabolite is active in the small intestine where it stimulates both calcium and phosphate absorption. The absorptive process for phosphate is different from that for calcium since they can occur independently.

c **True.** This molecule is synthesized in the proximal tubules following the stimulation of 1α-hydroxylase enzyme by parathormone. Consequently, 25-hydroxycholecalciferol from the liver is hydroxylated in the carbon 1-position of the steroid molecule. Calcitonin may inhibit the 1α-hydroxylase enzyme activity.

d **True.** This is an important effect of the bioactive vitamin D_3 metabolite. In vitamin D deficiency, the bone matrix becomes decalcified, and the strength of the bone is lost. In children, the typical bowing of the legs due to the bone decalcification process in the absence of sufficient 1,25-dihydroxy vitamin D_3 is a characteristic feature of the disease called rickets.

e **True.** The softening of bone due to deficiency of vitamin D_3 (and more importantly its bioactive metabolites) in adults is called osteomalacia (see clinical section). This is the adult form of rickets seen in children. In early industrial cities of the 19th century in Britain, many children and adults received very little exposure to sunlight and ate a poor vitamin D-deficient diet. Consequently, rickets and osteomalacia were relatively common conditions of the time. Nowadays, Asian and Muslim communities in Britain and other western countries are potential victims of these clinical conditions either because the increased pigmentation of their skin, or the complete covering of the face and body in northern climates decreases the effect of ultraviolet light on the synthesis pathway.

P.10 a **True.** Calcitonin is a polypeptide hormone 32 amino acids long, synthesized in the parafollicular cells within the lobes of the thyroid. The parafollicular cells, or C (clear) cells, lie either singly or in small clusters in between the follicles. The precursor molecule, called procalcitonin, is 136 amino acids long.

b **False.** Thyrotrophin acts on the follicular cells of the thyroid to stimulate the synthesis and release of the iodothyronines. It has no effect on the parafollicular cells which are controlled mainly by the blood calcium ion concentration such that the stimulus for calcitonin synthesis and release is an increase in circulating calcium levels.

c **True.** Calcitonin acts mainly on bone and the kidneys to decrease the blood calcium concentration. In bone, calcitonin stimulates calcium deposition in the matrix while in the kidneys it inhibits 1α-hydroxylase activity (decreasing synthesis of 1,25-dihydroxycholecalciferol) and increasing calcium excretion (as well as having a natriuretic effect and also increasing the urinary excretion of phosphate, bicarbonate, and potassium).

d **True.** Calcitonin stimulates the osteoblasts in bone which secrete the enzymes necessary for bone formation, increasing collagen synthesis and the formation and deposition of calcium salts.

e **True.** Calcitonin levels in the blood rise during pregnancy (as do many other hormones during this event) and lactation. One physiological effect of the rising calcitonin levels is to protect bone from being excessively demineralized as a consequence of the raised circulating levels of parathormone released in response to an increased demand for calcium by the growing fetus.

SAQ Answers

P.11

While various hormones influence calcium regulation (e.g. oestrogens, iodothyronines, glucocorticoids) the three hormones whose *main physiological role* is to regulate the plasma calcium ion concentration must be: (a) parathormone, (b) 1,25-dihydroxycholecalciferol, and (c) calcitonin.

Parathormone (PTH) is a polypeptide synthesized in the chief cells of the parathyroid glands which are situated on the upper and lower poles of each of the two thyroid lobes. The main bioactive vitamin D_3 metabolite, 1,25-dihydroxy-cholecalciferol, is a steroid synthesized in the proximal tubular cells of the kidneys. Calcitonin is a polypeptide hormone synthesized in the parafollicular cells of the thyroid gland. These cells lie between the follicles which are associated with iodothyronine hormones.

While all cells and tissues contain calcium—because this ion has diverse actions—the tissues/organs which are particularly relevant to its control are: (i) the small intestine, particularly the duodenum and jejunum, which is the site of calcium absorption from the diet, (ii) the kidneys which are important because they are the site where calcium excretion is controlled, and (iii) the bones (and teeth) because these are the principal storage sites of calcium.

P.12

Parathormone (PTH) acts to increase the blood calcium concentration if it falls below a concentration normally regulated between 2.2 and 2.6 mmol/litre. It acts on the three main tissues involved in calcium metabolism in the body: (i) the bone where 99% of the calcium is stored, (ii) the small intestine where calcium is absorbed into the body, and (iii) the kidneys, first by stimulating calcium reabsorption (thereby decreasing its urinary loss), then by stimulating 1α-hydroxylase activity (which stimulates the synthesis of 1,25-dihydroxycholecalciferol, see below), and also by increasing the urinary phosphate excretion which alters calcium levels in the blood indirectly.

The direct effects of parathormone on calcium in the kidneys are more complex than indicated above. For instance, it is likely that the reabsorption of calcium is actually inhibited in the proximal tubules resulting in an increased presentation of the ion to more distal segments of the nephron. In the distal tubule, PTH stimulates calcium reabsorption; perhaps because there is a greater amount of calcium arriving at the distal nephron there is an overall reabsorption by the kidneys. By stimulating the synthesis of 1,25-dihydroxycholecalciferol in the proximal tubules, PTH also contributes (indirectly) to calcium absorption in the intestinal tract.

In bone, PTH stimulates osteoblasts to produce osteoclast-stimulating factor which then stimulates osteoclast activity. Consequently, there is an increased breakdown of bone matrix resulting in the liberation of calcium into the extracellular fluid. Osteoblast activity is otherwise depressed by PTH.

P.13

Parathormone (PTH) and 1,25-dihydroxycholecalciferol $(1,25(OH)_2D_3)$ act together to raise the blood calcium ion concentration. In vitamin D deficiency, however, PTH is unable to exert its normal effects on bone. Since $1,25(OH)_2D_3$ increases calcium absorption from the small intestine it provides the calcium which is necessary for the normal mineralization of bone. Consequently, part of the interaction is probably the necessity for sufficient calcium deposition in bone which is more a function of the steroid hormone. However, other direct interactive effects actually on bone cells are probably operational also.

Regarding phosphate, however, the two hormones counteract each other; thus PTH stimulates the loss of phosphate by decreasing its reabsorption in the proximal tubules, while $1,24(OH)_2D_3$ independently stimulates phosphate absorption in the small intestine. In the kidneys the vitamin D_3 metabolite also increases calcium reabsorption. Therefore, the two hormones work together to increase calcium ion concentration in the blood but oppose each other with respect to phosphate, preventing the excessive loss of this anion when calcium is required.

Calcium regulation, bone, and its metabolic disorders (Clinical)

Multiple Choice Questions

C.1

A 65-year-old Asian woman has long-standing currently well-controlled diabetes, but complicated by nephropathy and retinopathy. She presents with one-year's increasing hip girdle pains, weakness, and tiredness, and is found to have a serum calcium of 2.03 mmol/litre (NR 2.2–2.55) and serum phosphate of 0.7 mmol/litre (NR 0.8–1.4). Which of the following would represent an explanation?

a The hypocalcaemia is due to hypoalbuminaemia secondary to diabetic nephropathy
b She has vitamin D-deficient osteomalacia
c The changes would be consistent with chronic renal failure
d The abnormalities could be explained by a low calcium diet
e She has primary hypoparathyroidism

C.2

In the same patient, the serum 25-hydroxycholecalciferol (25 $(OH)D)_3$ level is found to be 6 nmol/litre (NR 15–50). Serum albumin was in fact normal (38 g/l), repeat serum calcium 1.96 and serum phosphate 0.6 mmol/litre. Serum creatinine was 90 μmol/litre (NR 70–120) and alkaline phosphatase 680 units (N < 300). With a provisional diagnosis of vitamin D-deficient osteomalacia, which of the following statements is/are true?

a Bone radiology is necessary to confirm the diagnosis
b Measurement of serum PTH should be performed
c A bone biopsy should be carried out for confirmation that her pains are indeed due to osteomalacia
d Treatment with vitamin D should be lifelong
e Her family members should be checked for vitamin D deficiency

C.3

Which of the following conditions may be responsible for causing osteomalacia?

a Chronic renal failure
b Ulcerative colitis
c Chronic alcoholic liver disease
d Anticonvulsant therapy
e Vitamin D-resistance syndromes

C.4

A 25-year-old woman complains of increasing paresthesiae and cramps. She is quite short (60 inches: 152 cm), but otherwise has no abnormality clinically. Serum calcium is 1.93 mmol/litre (NR 202–2.55), serum phosphate 2.0 mmol/litre (NR 0.8–1.4) with similar results on repeat assessment. Serum alkaline phosphatase is 270 iu/litre (N < 300). Which of the following diagnoses is/are consistent with these findings?

a Chronic renal (glomerular) failure
b Idiopathic hypoparathyroidism
c Malabsorption syndrome secondary to gluten-sensitive enteropathy
d Pseudo-hypoparathyroidism
e Pseudo-pseudo-hypoparathyroidism

C.5

A 55-year-old lifelong heavy smoker presents with a 5-month history of increasing malaise, nocturia, and a past history of right renal calculus surgically removed 15 years previously. Clinical finding are otherwise negative. Her serum calcium is 3.3 mml/litre (NR 2.2–2.55), serum phosphate 0.6 mmol/litre (NR 0.8–1.4), and serum creatinine 105 μmol/litre (NR 50–110). What diagnosis would you consider to be consistent with this presentation?

a Hypervitaminosis D due to 'abuse' of self-prescribed multivitamin pills
b Primary hyperparathyroidism
c Tumour-associated hypercalcaemia (ectopic PTH syndrome)
d Sarcoidosis
e Familial hypocalciuric hypercalcaemia

C.6

In this same patient, serum immunocreative PTH (iPTH) is subsequently found to be 185 ng/ml (NR 10–50), thereby confirming the diagnosis of primary hyper-parathyroidism and excluding other causes (at lower values of iPTH, familial hypocalciuric hypercalcaemia would still need some consideration). Which of the following approaches is/are now appropriate?

a Await spontaneous resolution of his hypercalcaemia
b Parathyroidectomy after attempted localization of the presumptive parathyroid adenoma
c Drug treatment to lower serum calcium as a definitive long-term strategy
d Investigate for possible causes of tertiary hyperparathyroidism
e Initiate family studies

C.7**

In the course of a routine 'executive screen' carried out as part of a pre-employment medical check, a 49-year-old woman is found to have a raised serum calcium of 2.8

mmol/litre (NR 2.2–2.55). She is asymptomatic, except for occasional hot flushes associated with her recent menopause. Biochemical screen is otherwise normal. Repeat serum calcium is 2.7 mmol/litre, serum phosphate 0.8 mmol/litre (NR 0.8–1.4) and serum iPTH 95 ng/ml (NR 10–50). Which of the following approaches is/are appropriate?

a No action. Simply observe and recheck clinical state and serum calcium 6-monthly
b Parathyroidectomy after attempted localization of the presumptive parathyroid adenoma
c Bone densitometry to assess extent of parathyroid-related demineralization
d Treat with oestrogenic hormone replacement therapy (HRT)
e Treat with a bisphosphonate or phosphate in order to normalize serum calcium

C.8
In relation to the behaviour of bone mass (density), which of he following statements is/are true?

a Density equates to the strength of bone
b Bone density increases in both sexes until the fifth decade, from whence it progressively declines
c The rate of decline from the end of the fifth decade is broadly similar in males and females
d The rate of decline in bone mass is similar in wrist, hip, and spine
e Conventional lateral thoracolumbar spine radiology identifies a visually appreciable reduction in density when 10–15% of mineral loss has been lost

C.9
Which of the following factors may impair the achievement of peak bone mass?

a Dietary calcium deficiency
b Reduced physical activity
c late menarche
d Corticosteroids
e Adverse genetic determinants

C.10
Which of the following factors accelerate the decline of bone density following achievement of peak mass?

a Hypothyroidism
b Therapeutic corticosteroids
c Vitamin D overdosage
d Early menopause
e Decreased physical activity

C.11

In relation to the risk of fractures, which of the following statements is/are true?

a The lifetime risk of symptomatic fracture in women is 30%
b The risk of hip fracture in women by age 85 is approximately 15%
c The fracture rate in the elderly has been progressively decreasing since 1970
d The fracture threshold is a realistic concept in the screening process of bone densitometry
e The existence of a vertebral fracture does not affect the lifetime risk of femoral fracture

C.12

In clinically profiling the biochemical and structural aspects of bone disease, which of the following statements is/are true?

a The only currently available marker of osteoblast-mediated bone formation is serum osteocalcin
b Osteoclastic bone resorption is accurately reflected by serum alkaline phosphatase
c Fasting urine calcium/creatinine ratio is a useful index of abnormal bone resorption
d Dual energy X-ray absorptiometry (DEXA) is more precise than quantified computerized tomography (QCT) in the detection of altered bone density
e Repeat bone densitometry within 3 months is capable of identifying significant response to introduction of treatment

C.13

A 75-year-old nun from a local Catholic convent presents with increasing low- and mid-spinal pain. Her only past history is hypothyroidism which was diagnosed and treated 1 year previously. Her periods ceased at age 46. Lateral spine radiology shows compression fractures of D10, D12. The remaining spine appears osteopenic. She has a body mass index (BMI) of 18, and clinical examination is normal except for some kyphosis and angulation of the spine at D12. Which of the following represent major diagnostic possibilities?

a Metastatic carcinoma of the spine
b Osteoporosis secondary to overtreated hypothyroidism
c Osteomalacia
d Primary hyperparathyroidism
e 'Simple' osteoporosis of ageing

C.14

In the above patient, treatment decisions need to be taken. Which of the following would be logical, given the components responsible for her vertebral collapse?

a Oestrogen replacement
b A spinal support brace
c Calcium and vitamin D therapy
d An exercise enhancement programme
e An oral bisphosphonate

C.15

A fit and asymptomatic 50-year-old woman without significant past history is persuaded to have bone density assessment, based on her perimenopausal status and a family history of spinal osteoporosis in her mother (onset age 65), and a fatal femoral neck fracture in one aunt (age 82). Bone densitometry on DEXA scan reveals both her spinal (L2–4) and hip densities to be reduced by 1.8 and 2.1 SD respectively. Which of the following statements do you consider to be valid?

a Checking her bone density was not indicated
b She should be screened for underlying, potentially correctable disorder of bone chemistry
c Administration of postmenopausal oestrogen should be advised
d An exercise programme should be instituted
e A DEXA scan should be performed in 12 months

C.16

A 60-year-old woman complains of pain in the left thigh area extending down to the knee. On examination the femur is bowed, and there is swelling and crepitus on moving the left knee joint. Paget's disease of bone (osteitis deformans) is suspected, and radiologically confirmed. Which of the following statements apply in this case?

a Whole body isotope scan is a useful investigation in this patient
b There is a high risk of malignant change in the dominantly affected bone
c The pagetic involvement of her left femur reduces its fracture risk
d Treatment is possible with bisphosphonates
e The knee pain is likely to respond to non-steroidal anti-inflammatory drugs

Short Answer Question

C.17

A 74-year-old heavy smoker had a pituitary adenoma removed trans-frontally 10 years previously and is on phenytoin for recurrent fits following this procedure. He is on replacement therapy with thyroxine and hydrocortisone (cortisol). He stumbles down two steps on the way out of his favourite pub and is admitted to hospital with a fractured neck of femur. Itemize the elements which may have rendered his bones susceptible to trauma. *Briefly* identify the mechanism(s) which underlie each element.

MCQ Answers

C.1 a **True.** In the presence of diabetic nephropathy, proteinuria often leads to hypoalbuminaemia. Since serum calcium is almost always measured in its protein-bound form, anomalously low levels of serum calcium may be due to this phenomenon: the metabolically significant ionized calcium fraction is normal in this situation. To correct for this anomaly, add 0.02 mmol to the measured serum calcium level for every gram/litre of serum albumen below 40. A similar 'false hypocalcaemia' is seen in hypoalbuminaemia of any cause.

b **True.** Vitamin D deficiency occurs in up to 10% of Asians, particularly if vegetarian (prevalence up to 20%). This is due to the combined effects of low vitamin D intake (mainly present in meat, fish, and eggs), and reduced solar vitamin D skin synthesis due to skin pigment and traditional clothing coverage. It is more common in immigrant Asians because of lower solar exposure, particularly in more northern latitudes. Hypophosphataemia often coexists. The resulting osteomalacia is responsible for the generalized pains and weakness.

c **False.** In chronic renal (glomerular failure), hypocalcaemia does occur, partly because of failed conversion of $25(OH)D_3$ to $1,25(OH)_2D_3$ by defective renal dihydroxylation and consequently reduced calcium absorption. However, this patient does not have the hyperphosphataemia which is characteristic of chronic renal failure, and is due to impaired glomerular phosphate clearance.

d **False.** A low calcium diet does not produce hypocalcaemia. Any tendency to a low calcium recruits a parathyroid response (secondary hyperparathyroidism). Consequent bone resorption subsequently restores/maintains normocalcaemia.

e **False.** In primary hypoparathyroidism, serum phosphate is almost invariably raised, consistent with the absent phosphaturic effect of parathormone.

C.2 a **False.** One might see microfractures (Looser's zones) in the femoral necks, but this would not alter management.

b **True.** Vitamin D deficiency can only be deemed to be clinically significant (in terms of explaining her symptoms) if there is secondary hyperparathyroidism. It is important to note that in many patients this secondary hyperparathyroidism is sufficient to normalize the serum calcium. Accordingly, *normocalcaemia does not exclude vitamin D deficiency.*

c **False.** Although biopsy (usually taken from the iliac crest) would most certainly show thickened osteoid seams, this procedure is unnecessary in the presence of diagnostic serum bone chemistry as in this patient. The procedure is uncomfortable and the processing of undecalcified sections and their interpretation is not a universally available facility. Low serum $25(OH)D_3$ and raised serum PTH are together sufficient to make the diagnosis.

d **True.** Oral medication with 800 IU daily of cholecalciferol or ergo-calciferol (usually with calcium) is sometimes adequate. However, compliance is poor. Intramuscular depot calciferol 3.75 mg, repeated every Autumn, provides adequate lifelong treatment without risk of hypervitaminosis. Serum calcium, $25(OH)D_3$, PTH, and alkaline phosphatase levels normalize within 4 months. It has been suggested that 'at-risk' populations should receive such repletion on a preventive basis, since clinical onset is subtle and often overlooked.

e **True.** In principle, this is a good idea, since population studies show as many as 50% of first degree relatives have low $25(OH)D_3$ levels (although not necessarily with raised serum PTH). Treatment of this subclinical state is justified.

C.3 a **True.** Bone disease in chronic renal failure is complex: defective hydroxylation of $25(OH)D_3$ to $1,25(OH)D_2D_3$ interferes with calcium absorption and bone mineralization, producing osteomalacia. The hyperparathyroid response is often extreme: the bones show evidence of further resorption due to this. In addition, prolonged stimulation of the parathyroids leads to autonomy and hyperplasia/adenoma formation, with the development of hypercalcaemia. The collective term, 'renal osteodystrophy' is applied to this constellation of findings.

b **False.** The large bowel has no function in terms of either vitamin D or calcium processing. The small bowel, however, is critical to calcium homeostasis. Any diffuse small bowel defect interferes with vitamin D absorption, which usually cannot be compensated by solar-skin synthesis. Similarly, chronic pancreatic disease and any other cause of steatorrhoea can lead to osteomalacia because of defective absorption of (fat-soluble) vitamin D.

c **True.** The liver is responsible for 25-hydroxylation. Any diffuse hepatic disease is associated with osteomalacia (hepatic osteodystrophy), most marked in the case of chronic biliary obstruction/cholestasis or biliary cirrhosis where steatorrhoea is additionally present,

d **True.** Defective 25-hydroxylation of vitamin D can be caused by long-term therapy with drugs (particularly barbiturates and phenytoin) which induce P-450 microsomal enzymes and enhances the production of (metabolically inactive) polar metabolites such as $24,25(OH)_2D_3$. Alcohol also induces P-450 microsomal enzymes, contributing to the hepatic osteodystrophy referred to in c above. The process affects all steroids, but feedback pathways ensure that cortisol and sex hormone levels are maintained. No such feedback applies to cholecalciferol metabolism so that osteomalacia (or rickets in children) develops in up to 50% of treated patients. In addition, phenytoin also directly inhibits intestinal calcium absorption.

e **True.** Vitamin D resistance presents either as childhood rickets or as osteomalacia, and is due to vitamin D receptor abnormalities which are either familial (X-linked) or due to sporadic receptor mutations. Patients are strikingly hypophosphataemic: phosphate therapy is required as well as high-dose vitamin D.

C.4 a **True.** As mentioned in C.3, this combination of findings would be consistent with chronic renal failure, although as a result of secondary hyperparathyroidism, a raised serum alkaline phosphatase level is more likely to be present. Short stature may accompany chronic renal disease of long standing, due both to reduced somatomedian (IGF-I) levels and defective bone response (abnormal hGH and IFG-I bone receptor affinity). Serum creatinine would clinch the diagnosis.

b **True.** This uncommon condition often manifests itself first is this age group, and is due to autoimmune destruction of the parathyroids, often associated with other organ-specific immune disorders, especially hypothyroidism, Addison's disease, and pernicious anaemia (see Chapter 14). Apart from the clinical effects of neuromuscular excitability, basal ganglia occasionally calcify and some (rare) patients develop extra-pyramidal symptoms. Cataract also occurs. The identical clinical syndrome occurs following accidental damage to parathyroids following thyroidectomy. Treatment is by the (unphysiological) use of vitamin D analogues (alfacalcidol or calcitriol), since PTH cannot be administered by mouth because of enzymic degradation.

c **False.** Although presentation with short stature and hypocalcaemic symptoms is not unusual in gluten-sensitive enteropathy (even sometimes without symptomatic diarrhoea), serum phosphate would be expected to be low, not only due to defective vitamin D-mediated absorption but also due to secondary hyperparathyroidism, which enhances renal tubular phosphate excretion.

d **True.** This familial syndrome (PHP) is due to defective parathormone receptor function with subsequent reduced intracellular cyclic AMP synthesis, a mediator of PTH function. A number of developmental features are associated, although inconsistently. These include a round face, short stature, subnormal intelligence, and a short 4th or 5th metacarpal bone. Serum PTH levels are accordingly raised. Rare variants have isolated renal tubular PTH resistance: accordingly the raised serum PTH may then induce hyperparathyroid-type bone lesions.

Surprisingly, quite modest doses of calcitriol restore biochemical normality in many cases.

e **False.** This familial syndrome (PPHP) has the clinical characteristics of PHP, but without the biochemical changes. Since the clinical anomalies are clearly not due to the biochemical disturbance, the disorder is undoubtedly a genetic variant of PHP with intact bone an renal tubular PTH receptor function. Some cases have an XO karyotype (see Chapter 12), and indeed the somatic characteristics are similar in many respects to gonadal dysgenesis (Turner's syndrome).

C.5 a **False.** This is likely to produce hyper phosphataemia: vitamin D enhances phosphate as well as calcium absorption. However, renal calculi sometimes figure in the past history of such patients, due to resulting hypercalciuria. Nephrocalcinosis may also be found.

b **True.** This is a typical presentation. The distant past history of renal calculi may be significant, since the condition has often been present for many years in asymptomatic form before it becomes clinically apparent. The hypopphosphataemia is due to PTH-induced renal tubular phosphate loss, and the nocturia due to (often reversible) hypercalcaemia-dependent renal tubular ADH resistance. The weakness is due to hypercalcaemic myopathy, occasionally with a component of hypomagnesaemia (also due to renal tubular loss).

c **True.** As a heavy smoker, the common bronchogenic carcinoma must be considered. As with many other tumours, a PTH-related peptide (PTH-RP) is produced by the tumour (see Chapter 12) which has identical biochemical actions. Serum PTH levels are consistently suppressed by the hypercalcaemia. The renal calculus may be incidental: less than 5% of patients with renal calculi have a readily identifiable metabolic abnormality as a cause.

d **False.** The biochemical picture is similar to that of vitamin D excess. The sarcoid granulomas are capable of synthesizing $1,25(OH)_2D_3$ so that hypercalcaemia (and hyperphosphataemia) are usual. Renal calculi can occur in sarcoid, because of the hypercalciuria resulting from calcium hyperabsorption.

e **True.** This uncommon condition is readily confused with primary hyperparathyroidism. It represents a mutation of the gene encoding calcium 'recognition' by the parathyroid. The threshold reset phenomenon results in the need for higher PTH levels to maintain higher calcium levels. Either medical means or total parathyroidectomy are needed for correction of hypercalcaemia. Surprisingly, the converse 'low reset' phenomenon has not yet been reported.

C.6 a **False.** Spontaneous resolution is rare. At this serum calcium level, increasing and often irreversible glomerular damage occurs. The additional risk is dehydration, either by co-incidental disease or by vomiting due directly to hypercalcaemia. Dehydration potentiates hypercalcamia by reducing renal calcium clearance. This calcium rise may lead to coma and death.

b **True.** Parathyroidectomy is essential. Some surgeons do not require preoperative localization studies: the tumour associated with this degree of hypercalcaemia is likely to be readily identified inrtraoperatively. Ultrasound, isotope, or MRI scanning and neck vein catheterization (for iPTH concentration gradient) are sometimes performed with an overall 80% chance of localization. The usually multiple gland parathyroid hyperplasia (responsible for less than 10% of cases) cannot usually be identified by these means, but is identified by the surgeon who systematically examines the 4 main parathyroid 'beds'.

c **False.** With higher serum calcium levels than in this patient, preoperative reduction of serum calcium is wise in order to avoid cardiovascular (arrythmia) and anaesthetic (dehydration) complications of surgery. Definitive medical treatment would only be indicated if the patient refused surgery; a medical contra-indication to surgery would be rare. Hydration with saline, bisphosphonates, or calcitonin (which impair PTH-mediated bone resorption) and oral phosphate can be used, but never produce long-term satisfactory or safe control of hyper-calcaemia, however caused.

d **True.** Renal failure-associated secondary hyperparathyroidism quite often becomes autonomous with either hyperplasia or adenoma formation. In turn, this causes hypercalcaemia (tertiary hyperpara-thyroidism). Similarly, chronic hypocalcaemia due to vitamin D deficiency (nutritional or due to malabsorption syndrome) sometimes results in transition of secondary to tertiary hyperparathyroidism. In some cases such an underlying cause is worth pursuing.

e **False.** Hyperparathyroidism may be familial (see Chapter 14), but is not usually worth pursuing unless there is a more suggestive family history of parathyroid-related symptoms or other endocrinopathy.

C.7** a **True.** This is an acceptable approach: studies of the natural history of so-called asymptomatic hyperparathyroidism (serum calcium usually < 2.8 mmol/l) indicate minimal increases over many years. However, there is a small increased risk of pancreatitis and progressive renal dysfunction and an increased bone turnover with net loss of bone mass (and strength). Surgery is in most circumstances a preferred option.

b **True.** This is the optimal approach, but depends on available surgical skills, in view of the small size of the likely causative tumour. Post-operative hypoparathyroidism resulting from inadequate surgical skill is a very poor exchange for aymptomatic hyperparathyroidism! Attempted preoperative localization is probably worthwhile (see C.6b).

c **True.** This may be a pivotal evaluation. If bone mass is reduced in this woman already at menopause, the likely further reduction due to the combined effects of menopausal hypooestrogenaemia, and increased bone loss due to (untreated) hyperparathyroidism could put her bones at serious risk of fracture in later life. If bone mass were normal, a more conservative approach, as in (a) above, might be acceptable.

d **True.** HRT would probably help this woman's flushes. In addition, oestrogen reduces bone receptor affinity for PTH, so that parathyroid-dependent bone loss would be reduced and serum calcium is likely to fall to some extent. If her bone density were normal, use of HRT might again justify a non-operative approach.

e **False.** Bisphosphonates may reduce the rate of bone loss in the long term in this condition. It would not be justified to use either of these drugs simply to reduce serum calcium.

C.8 a **False.** Bone density depends on calcium content, while its fracture resistance depends to some extent on the geometry of trabecular structure (loss of horizontal trabeculae affect 'cross-bracing'). For example, fluoride excess (fluorosis) results in markedly increased density, with much less impressive increase in fracture resistance because of the abnormal bone quality. The broad correlation between these two variables nevertheless underlies the role of bone densitometry in screening for potential 'bones at risk'.

b **False.** Bone density increases until the third decade (peak mass) and declines thereafter, according to a variety of factors. Within a population, this decline is probably more variable than the peak mass achieved.

c **False.** In males the rate of loss from the fifth decade onwards averages 0.5% per annum: in females (untreated postmenopausal), the rate is approximately 2% per annum.

d **True.** Density in all 3 sites tends to decline with age. However, density at the wrist (which measures cortical bone) correlates only poorly or not at all with vertebral fracture risk (which reflects density of cancellous bone).

e **False.** It is necessary to lose 30–40% of bone calcium before even skilled assessment of plain radiographs (e.g. spine) confidently identify abnormality. Such reduction is close to the fracture threshold. However, precise measurements of anterior compared with mid and posterior vertebral height can be carried out on high quality lateral radiographs of the spine. Such measurements help to identify the earliest stages of vertebral collapse.

C.9 a **True.** Dietary calcium intakes below 1000 mg daily statistically reduce peak bone mass, with a greater effect in the 25% of women from most European countries who consume below 500 mg daily. Correlations are made more difficult by the confounding effects of calorie-containing nutrients and the effect of body weight: slimness is associated with lower peak bone mass, while obesity is protective. Smoking and alcohol are further variables adversely affecting peak bone mass by inhibiting osteoblast activity.

b **True.** Exercise is a critical determinant of peak bone mass, thought to reflect biophysical factors. A lack of 'muscle pull' on tendon insertions critically impairs structural integrity and calcium content of bone. At high exercise (competitive athletic) levels, hypothalamic gonadotrophin 'turn-off' in women paradoxically impairs peak mass due to oestrogen deficiency.

c **True.** Anabolic effects of oestrogen critically affect formation. A late menarche results in a lower exposure to this anabolic effect leading up to bone maturity/peak mass. Delayed puberty has a similar effect in males.

d **True.** The reduced bone formation/increased bone resorption profile of (therapeutic) corticosteroids significantly impairs peak bone mass.

e **True.** The dominant effect is ethnic, with blacks having age-specific densities consistently higher than whites (and a correspondingly lower fracture incidence). In addition, there are almost certainly other genetic variables, suggested by a higher concordance of bone density in identical compared with non-identical twins. Genetic variation in vitamin D receptor affinity may prove to be one such variable.

C.10 a **False.** Hyperthyroidism increases bone turnover, but dominantly resorption leading to reduced bone density. Significant overreplacement of hypothyroid patients with thyroxine has a similar but less dramatic effect.

b **True.** There is a substantial variability in the bone resorptive effects of corticosteroids. Pathological fractures can occur in quite young people after a course as short as 6 months. Orally, daily doses of 5 mg prednisolone or above put the patient at risk. This risk extends to topical and inhaled corticosteroids although at a much lower level.

c **False.** Experimentally, vitamin D toxicity does marginally increase bone resorption. However, of greater significance is the contribution of vitamin D *deficiency*, causing osteomalacia. In the elderly (especially institutionalized), between 10% and 20% have a significant component of osteomalacia contributing to reduced bone density, and hence fracture proneness.

d **True.** Loss of menopausal oestrogen is the largest determinant of the increased fracture proneness of elderly women. Premature menopause further exacerbates this phenomenon. After age 60, 66% of women with documented premature menopause have bone density below 'fracture threshold' compared with 18% of women with normal age at menopause. Oestrogen loss from other causes is also relevant, as in anorexia nervosa (which also affects peak bone mass) and the hypooestrogenaemia associated with athletic 'excess'.

e **True.** Moderate physical activity is as important in reducing decline of bone density as in the achievement of peak mass. There is a great variability in the ability to regain bone mass after prolonged immobilization due to illness. This is also germane to the zero-gravity effects of space travel.

C.11 a **True.** This high prevalence contributes in a major way to mortality as well as morbidity. It is important to stress that falls constitute an important component of the 'fracture syndrome'.

b **True.** The prevalence rate is about 3 times higher than in men, a difference which can be almost entirely attributed to loss of bone mineral density secondary to hypo-oestrogenaemia.

c **False.** The age-specific hip fracture rate is increasing progressively for reasons which are not clear.

d **True.** As long as the arbitrariness of this concept is accepted, it forms a useful point of reference. An approximate 40% reduction from the median population sex-specific peak bone mass is often quoted as the 'fracture threshold'. Clearly, behavioural and mechanical factors, and specifically falls are of equal importance.

e **False.** The presence of a vertebral fracture on plain lateral spine radiography doubles the risk of subsequent hip fracture.

C.12 a **False.** Osteocalcin is an osteoblast-specific protein which can be used for monitoring purposes. Alkaline phosphatase is also produced by osteoblasts but is less sensitive. Serum C-terminal pro-peptide of type-I collagen (P1CP) is a more precise indicator of bone formation, but will be superseded in accuracy by 24-hour urine assay which will smooth out within-day fluctuations.

b **False.** Although serum alkaline phosphatase appears to increase with osteoclastic activity, this is due to the phasic linkage of osteoblastic to osteoclastic activity. Urinary hydroxyproline (a collagen metabolite) and deoxypyridinoline cross-links together with serum C-terminal teleopeptide of type-I collagen (1CTP) represent the current best markers for bone resorption.

c **True.** Although not frequently used, this simple index of calcium excretion after an overnight fast is a useful marker for both individual and epidemiological studies.

d **False.** DEXA scans are actually less *precise* than QCT scans, since only the latter measures purely trabecular bone: DEXA quantifies a mixture of trabecular and compact (cortical) bone. However, DEXA scans are more reproducible, and are therefore valuable for longitudinal studies. The radiation dosage is also only 1% of that produced from QCT. Ultrasonic densitometry may eventually replace both methods.

e **False.** Most current DEXA scanning equipment allows accurate identification of a 2% change in density (recently bordering on 1%).

The rates of density change which occur spontaneously or in response to therapy are around 2% per annum, so that a 6–12 month period represents the shortest interval likely to reveal a significant change.

C.13 a **True.** This diagnosis must *always* be considered. However, a normal ESR, serum calcium, and lack of obvious destructive lesions of the pedicles of affected vertebrae confirmed from MRI scanning made this unlikely, as did densitometry of the spine which showed that bone density was 3 SD below the mean for (normal) young females [T-value of −3.1 at apparently uninvolved L2 and L3 vertebrae].

b **False.** Such a short course of treatment of thyroxine could not adversely affect spinal density, even if overtreatment was gross. However, auto-immune hypothyroidism is often associated with premature menopause: although not unduly early, oestrogen lack may be a significant factor, contributing to the demineralization.

c **True.** Osteomalacia must be considered as a possible component in every patient with 'thin bones', and most especially in the elderly and institutionalized: radiologically no confident distinction can be made between osteomalacia and osteoporosis. Nuns are prone to vitamin D deficiency based on skin cover from traditional clothing and frequent dominance of indoor activity. Her serum $25(OH)D_3$ level was indeed 8 nmol/litre (NR 15–100).

d **False.** It would be unusual for this condition to present with vertebral collapse and no other symptoms. However, serum iPTH was 150 ng/m litre (NR 10–50) and serum calcium was 2.25 mmol/litre. This is not *primary* hyperparathyroidism but secondary hypoparathyroidism consequent on her vitamin D deficiency.

e **True.** As in so many cases of 'thin bones', multiple factors are operative, in this case including age, slimness, marginally early menopause, relative inactivity, osteomalacia, and possibly genetic factors. Some studies involving bone biopsy suggest an osteomalacic component in up to 20% of cases of apparently 'simple' osteoporosis.

C.14 a **True.** Oestrogen at any age inhibits bone resorption (but with some secondary reduction in bone formation). At this age, however, the slight benefits may not justify the possible risk of oestrogens, even if given continuously with a progestogen to avoid withdrawal bleeding. Tibolone (which has both oestrogenic and androgenic effects) may be preferable, and will also avoid withdrawal bleeding.

b **False.** These are not often helpful, reducing spinal mobility, compressing the abdomen and providing little pain relief except in the severest cases.

c **True.** This can be provided as in C.2d and probably continued lifelong. Serum $25(OH)D_3$ and iPTH levels need to be monitored until normality is restored within a 4–6 month period. Some thought should be given to any other causative factor such as clinically inapparent adult coeliac disease.

d **True.** Evidence is conflicting about the benefits of exercise with the exception of high-impact weight-bearing or impact training such as jumping and jogging, which would be clearly inappropriate in this patient. However, the potential preventive role of walking and swimming is still unclear, and could prove of longer-term value. There are certainly no side-effects from such low-impact exercise! Furthermore, studies show reduced fracture rates in exercising women without improvement in bone density. This suggests that activity improves co-ordination, muscle tone, and body control, thereby minimizing the risk of falls.

e **True.** Continuous or cyclical bisphosphonate (depending on type) should be introduced. Many studies show either reduced rate of bone mineral loss or even increase of density, together with a reduced spinal fracture rate. The drugs are well tolerated and in a number of studies provide significant pain relief compared with placebo. Increasing data support low-dose parathormone as beneficial in rebuilding destroyed trabecular architecture, but at present, this therapy is not practicable.

C.15 a **False.** Family history of osteoporosis or early menopause (or a period of at least 6 months of otherwise unexplained amenorrhoea) are prime indications for bone densitometry. Given the accelerated bone loss which predictably follows the menopause, the correct investigation is being done at the correct time. By definition, density between 1.0 and 2.5 SD below the peak female mean, the T-value, classifies her as 'osteopenic' (below 2.5 SD identifies 'osteoporosis').

b **True.** As indicated in C.13, exclusion of possible underlying causes is comparatively inexpensive and reassuring, irrespective of the presence of a family history.

c **True.** Irrespective of any other contributory factor, this woman cannot afford to lose further bone mass in view of her osteopenia. Depending on her personal preference, either cyclical or continuous oestrogen (with progestogen) is indicated, ideally lifelong: the precise duration of treatment needed to offer optimal protection is currently unknown.

d **True.** The fact that she is 'fit' allows one to propose a high-impact exercise programme, best supervised from a health and fitness club oriented towards such programmes.

e **True.** It is always useful to know that a particular treatment plan is effective. Furthermore, it enhances compliance.

C.16 a **True.** Isotope concentration is typical with high uptake into affected areas. It also gives a more precise indication than radiology of the extent of an individual lesion. In the context of this patient, her knee pain may be due either to Pagetic joint involvement, or to simple degenerative changes secondary to altered weight-bearing characteristics of genu varum deformity. Furthermore, a whole body scan will reveal all sites of currently asymptomatic bone involvement (polyostotic disease).

b **False.** Although Paget's disease does increase the risk of malignant change in the affected bone, the actual risk of fibrosarcoma has been previously exaggerated: bias was introduced in earlier studies by the pattern of presentation to orthopaedic clinics. Paget's disease can be identified in more than 5% of the population over age 60. Malignant change is thought to occur in approximately 1% of *symptomatic* cases.

c **False.** The bone is often denser and associated with cortical thickening in the more advanced (sclerotic) stage of the disease. In the early stages, there is increased vascularity and abnormal bone architecture (porotic stage) which increases fracture risk.

d **True.** Bisphosphonates given either by mouth or (alternatively) by infusion suppress both the increased bone resorption and secondarily bone formation. Pain is reduced and indices of bone turnover (serum alkaline phosphatase and other bone formation and resorption markers) are reduced.

e **True.** In this patient NSAID-type drugs are likely to benefit the pain, whether it is due to Pagetic or osteoarthritic changes.

SAQ Answer

C.17

Age: progressive resorption without compensatory bone formation.

Smoking: for every 10-pack years of smoking, bone density is 2% lower than controls: osteocalcin levels (bone formation) lower. Smoking increases SHBG, and thus reduces free sex hormone concentration.

Alcohol: acute reduction in osteocalcin after alcoholic binge, possible cumulative. Also effect on normal pulsatility of LH, reducing androgen levels (loss of anabolic function).

Possible overreplacement with thyroxine: increased bone resorption.

Possible cortisol overdosage: increased bone resorption.

Phenytoin: P-450 microsomal enzyme induction; generation of polar calciferol metabolities with reduced activity: osteomalacia component to osteopenia.

Hypogonadism: effect of alcohol excess, interfering with oestrogen degradation plus no replacement being given following induction of surgical hypopituitarism.

Growth hormone deficiency: almost certainly present following pituitary surgery.

References

Physiology

Topic: Hormonal regulation of renal calcium transport.
Friedman, P.A. *et al.* (1995) *Physiological Reviews*, 75, 429–64.
Topic: Seasonal variation in vitamin D stores.
Haddad, J.G. (1996). *Trends in Endocrinology and Metabolism*, 7, 209–12.
Topic: Vitamin D receptor defects and rickets.
Hochberg, Z. *et al.* (1995). *Trends in Endocrinology and Metabolism*, 6, 216–20.
Topic: Osteoclasts and factors influencing their function.
Roodman, G.D. (1996). *Endocrine Reviews*, 17, 308–32.

Clinical

Topic: Management of hypercalcaemia.
Bilzekian, J.P. (1993). *Journal of Clinical Endocrinology and Metabolism*, 77, 1445–9.
Topic: Asymptomatic hyperparathyroidism.
Birkenhaeger, J. *et al.* (1996). *Postgraduate Medical Journal*, 72, 323–6.
Topic: Corticosteroid-induced bone disease.
Canalis, E. (1996). *Journal of Clinical Endocrinology and Metabolism*, 81, 3441–7.
Topic: Localization of parathyroid tumours.
Heath, D.A. (1995). *Clinical Endocrinology*, 43, 523–4.
Topic: Aetiology of osteoporosis.
Marcus, R. (1996). *Journal of Clinical Endocrinology and Metabolism*, 81, 1–5.
Topic: Prevention and therapy of osteoporosis.
Riggs, B. *et al.* (1993). *New England Journal of Medicine*, 327, 620–7.
Topic: Hyperparathyroidism.
Silverberg, S. *et al.* (1996). *Journal of Clinical Endocrinology and Metabolism*, 81, 2036–40.
Topic: Paget's disease.
Siris, E. *et al.* (1996). *Journal of Clinical Endocrinology and Metabolism*, 81, 961–7.
Topic: Investigation of osteoporosis.
Smith, R. (1996). *Clinical Endocrinology*, 44, 371–4.
Topic: Tumour-induced osteomalacia.
Wilkens, G.E. *et al.* (1995). *Journal of Clinical Endocrinology and Metabolism*, 80, 1628–34.

10 The Pancreas (Physiology)

Multiple Choice Questions

P.1 Glucose

a is transported in the blood mainly bound to proteins
b can be synthesized from certain amino acids
c is stored in cells as the polymer, glycogen
d enters hepatocytes by an active transport mechanism
e is the principal source of metabolic energy in the central nervous system

P.2 The arterial blood glucose concentration

a in fasting conditions is normally over 12 mmol/litre
b is increased by catecholamines
c tends to decrease in stressful situations
d if it falls, and stays below 2 mmol/litre can result in coma
e increases with hypertension

P.3 The pancreas

a is mainly composed of endocrine tissue
b secretes a bicarbonate-rich fluid into the blood
c contains distinctive clusters of cells distributed within the main tissue
d has a venous outflow into the hepatic portal vein
e is innervated by autonomic nerve fibres

P.4 The islets of Langerhans

a consist of at least four different cell types
b contain cells which are connected to each other by gap junctions
c secrete hormones which influence metabolic processes
d control blood flow to the gastrointestinal tract
e are chiefly controlled by the hormones of the hypothalamo–adenohypophysial axis

P.5 Insulin

a is synthesized in α cells of the pancreatic islets
b is formed from a precursor by the removal of a connecting peptide

c shares some of its effects with insulin-like growth factors (IGF-I and IGF-II)

d is stored in granules inside the cells where it is synthesized

e coexists with another molecule called amylin

P.6 *Insulin release*

a is calcium-dependent

b occurs within 15 minutes after ingestion of food

c following appropriate prolonged stimulation occurs in early and late phases

d is mainly by diffusion through insulin channels

e is induced by metabolism of glucose within the cell of production

P.7 *Insulin's physiological actions*

a occur following binding of the hormone to its membrane receptor

b on carbohydrate metabolism result in an increased blood glucose concentration

c include the stimulation of protein synthesis

d result in increased urine excretion (diuresis)

e are mediated by stimulation of adenyl cyclase and cyclic AMP synthesis

P.8 *The release of insulin*

a is stimulated by increased sympathetic activity via adrenergic α receptors

b is controlled primarily by an adenohypophysial insulin-stimulating factor

c is stimulated by the paracrine effect of somatostatin

d is inhibited by amino acids such as arginine

e is greater for a given glucose load when administered intravenously than when taken orally

P.9 *Glucagon*

a is a glycoprotein hormone

b is released throughout the day at a steady basal rate

c is transported in the blood mainly bound to albumin

d enters its target cells by an active transport mechanism

e activates the phospholipase C–inositol phosphate pathway

P.10 *The physiological effects of glucagon*

a overall are to increase the blood glucose concentration

b include the stimulation of hepatic glycogenolysis

c are associated with increased distal tubular sodium reabsorption

d include the inhibition of the facilitated diffusion of glucose into muscle cells e are produced by a direct inhibition of insulin's actions on glucose metabolism

P.11 *Glucagon synthesis*

    a is inhibited by increased vagal nerve activity
    b is increased by the gastrointestinal hormone, cholecystokinin
    c is suppressed by raised circulating blood glucose concentrations
    d is partly under paracrine inhibitory control by somatostatin
    e is stimulated by certain amino acids such as arginine

P.12 *Somatostatin*

    a is produced by δ cells of the islets of Langerhans
    b is a polypeptide
    c is synthesized in certain hypothalamic neurones
    d decreases the rate of gastric emptying
    e inhibits the inflammatory response

P.13 *Somatostatin*

    a mediates the actions of somatotrophin (growth hormone)
    b is synthesized in response to an increase in the blood glucose concentration
    c coexists with pancreatic polypeptide in the same cells
    d has a half-life estimated to be less than 3 minutes
    e is present in considerably higher concentrations in men than in women

Short Answer Questions

P.14

Briefly explain why the blood glucose concentration requires regulation, and why hypoglycaemia and hyperglycaemia can both be associated with coma.

P.15

Identify three principal hormones of the pancreas indicating *briefly* how they influence glucose metabolism, and each other.

P.16

List four physiological effects of insulin and briefly explain why lack of the hormone, as in diabetes mellitus, is associated with polyuria and polydipsia.

P.17

Briefly describe how insulin production is regulated, using a labelled diagram if desired.

MCQ Answers

P.1 a **False.** Glucose is mostly transported in the plasma unbound. However, some proteins (e.g. plasma albumins and globulins) can contain small amounts of carbohydrate such as glucose in which case they are called glycoproteins. Some glycoprotein formation is enzymatically induced, and this process is called glycosylation. However, most glycoproteins are formed by the non-enzymatic covalent linkage of hexoses such as glucose to the protein in a reaction called glycation. This process occurs in proportion to the plasma glucose concentration so that when it is chronically raised (e.g. in diabetes mellitus), the amount of glycosylated haemoglobin becomes a good indicator of glucose metabolism and its control.

b **True.** Certain amino acids are called 'glucogenic' because they can be converted ultimately to glucose in the liver by a gluconeogenic pathway. Alanine is one particularly good example of a glucogenic amino acids.

c **True.** Most, if not all, mammalian cells can store small amounts of glucose in the form of glycogen. Muscle and liver cells probably account for most of the stored glycogen. The liver is particularly important because the breakdown of glucose in this organ results in the formation of glucose which can be released into the blood for general use by other cells. The breakdown of glycogen in muscle cells produces glucose for intracellular use only, playing an important role as the source of energy for the contractile process.

d **False.** Glucose enters cells by a diffusion process involving glucose transporter (GLUT) molecules which carry the glucose across the cell membranes and into the cell cytoplasm. Once inside the cell the glucose is rapidly converted to glucose-6-phosphate, and this consequently maintains the concentration gradient favouring glucose movement into the cell. Because the glucose moves down its concentration gradient by a diffusion process which does not involve the use of metabolic energy but simply relies on the presence of GLUT molecules in the membrane, the process is called *facilitated diffusion*. There are at least 4 different GLUT molecules which have been identified in different cell membranes, only one of which (GLUT 4) is sensitive to the pancreatic hormone insulin.

e **True.** The importance of glucose as an energy substrate is mainly due to its vital role in the central nervous system. In conditions of hypoglycaemia, ketones can be utilized instead of glucose to a limited extent.

P.2 **False.** The normal fasting arterial blood glucose concentration is usually around 4–5 mmol/litre, a value of 12 mmol/litre indicating hyperglycaemia and probably diabetes mellitus. The renal threshold for glucose (i.e. the blood glucose concentration at which the reabsorption mechanism becomes saturated) is normally approximately 10–12 mmol/

litre, so that any increase in blood glucose concentration above this level will result in increasing quantities of glucose being excreted in the urine (glycosuria), a good indicator of diabetes mellitus.

b **True.** The blood glucose concentration will be increased by catecholamines acting directly via β receptors on glycogenolysis, and indirectly by stimulating the release of other hormones (e.g. glucagon) which increase glycogenolysis and/or gluconeogenesis.

c **False.** Stressors generally are associated with an increase in blood glucose concentration following the release of various hormones which stimulate glucose anabolism by increasing hepatic glycogenolysis and gluconeogenesis.

d **True.** A persistent blood glucose concentration below 2 mmol/litre may be insufficient to provide the glucose required by the central nervous system in which case a coma can develop.

e **False.** There is no general association between the arterial blood glucose concentration and hypertension. The latter is usually defined as a diastolic blood pressure above 90 mmHg (or 12 kPa, where 1 mmHg = 133.3 Pascals). However, *insulin resistance* is associated with hypertension suggesting that metabolic abnormalities contribute to the development of a chronically raised arterial blood pressure.

P.3 a **False.** About 98% of pancreatic tissue is exocrine, composed of acinar cells which secrete into small intercalated ducts forming the main pancreatic duct which passes the secretions directly into the duodenum. The acinar cells synthesize digestive enzymes, including proteolytic enzymes produced as inactive proenzymes which normally only become activated in the duodenum. The remaining 2% of the pancreatic tissue is composed of small clusters of cells lying within the exocrine tissue. These cells are granular endocrine cells which secrete into the extracellular fluid, particularly the general blood circulation.

b **False.** The cells lining the intercalated ducts synthesize a large volume of bicarbonate-rich (i.e. alkaline) fluid into the pancreatic duct, *not* into the blood. The final pancreatic duct fluid contains the enzyme secretions of the acinar cells as well as the bicarbonate which neutralizes the acidic chyme reaching the duodenum from the stomach.

c **True.** These clusters of cells are called islets of Langerhans and represent the endocrine part of the pancreas. There are approximately one million islets distributed throughout the pancreas with greatest density in the tail of the organ.

d **True.** The hormones secreted by the islet cells are particularly important regulators of metabolism, exerting many important effects in the liver. Secretion of these hormones into the hepatic portal vein directs them directly to this crucial metabolic organ along with the absorbed digestive products.

e **True.** The vagus nerve is a mixed nerve containing many para-sympathetic fibres some of which innervate endocrine islet cells (particularly the α and β cells, see below) as well as the exocrine acinar cells. There is also a sympathetic innervation of the islet cells.

P.4 a **True.** The four main cell types present in islets of Langerhans are called alpha, beta, delta, and F cells (α, β, δ, and F). The core of each islet is made up predominantly of β cells (approximately 60%) with α cells mainly around the periphery (25%) and δ cells scattered more randomly throughout (10%) with F cells making up approximately 3% of the remainder. The composition of the islets regarding the different cell types varies, so that it appears that the islets in the tail have a greater proportion of α cells than those in the head of the pancreas, for example.

b **True.** The gap junctions can be detected in electron micrographs, and are approximately 25 nm wide. These junctions are gaps in adjacent cell membranes which provide a direct (though restricted) link between the cytoplasm of the two cells. Ions and small molecules have been shown to pass from one cell to the other through these gap junctions.

c **True.** As mentioned above, the endocrine role of the pancreas is related to the secretion of hormones by the cells of the islets of Langerhans. The α cells synthesize glucagon, the β cells insulin (and a recently identified molecule called amylin), the δ cells somatostatin, while the F cells synthesize a molecule called pancreatic polypeptide. Glucagon and insulin are particularly important metabolic regulators; somatostatin has many effects and is found in various other parts of the body (see later) while the function of pancreatic polypeptide is still unclear.

d **False.** None of the islet cell hormones has clearly defined effects on the cardiovascular system, so at present there is no evidence for any influence on blood flow to the gastrointestinal tract.

e **False.** The pancreatic hormones are controlled by a variety of stimulatory and inhibitory factors, certainly, but there is no major influence exerted by hormones from the hypothalamo–adenohypophysial axis.

P.5 a **False.** As mentioned above, insulin is synthesized by the β cells along with amylin, while the α cells synthesize glucagon. Amylin is a polypeptide which is released with insulin.

b **True.** Insulin is synthesized first as a larger precursor molecule called pre-proinsulin which loses its signal (or leader) peptide sequence to leave a polypeptide proinsulin molecule of 86 amino acids. This molecule folds spontaneously such that two disulphide bonds are formed. Once inside the granules a peptide sequence (called cleavage, or C, peptide) is removed leaving the final product, the two-chain polypeptide insulin. The α and β chains consist of 21 and 30 amino acids linked together by the disulphide bridges.

c **True.** The membrane receptors for insulin and the two insulin-like growth factors (also known as somatomedins, see Chapter 4) belong to a related family of proteins which have some homology with each other. Both IGF-I and IGF-II have a limited binding affinity for insulin receptors, and this probably accounts for their insulin-like effects.

d **True.** Insulin is mostly stored in granules within the cytoplasm of the β cells partly complexed with zinc. Release is by exocytosis of granule contents into the surrounding extracellular fluid. The process of exocytosis is associated with a depolarization of the cell membrane and an influx of calcium ions (reminiscent of neuronal transmitter release) although calcium ions are equally likely to come from intracellular stores within the cell.

e **True.** As mentioned above, amylin is released together with insulin by exocytosis from the granules. It may counteract the effects of insulin (e.g. by stimulating glycogenolysis), although such effects only occur when non-physiological concentrations are present. Other effects such as an inhibition of gastric emptying may be more physiological.

P.6 a **True.** The essential intracellular mediator of the insulin release process is an increase in calcium ion concentration, and this may be involved in the transport of the granules along microtubules towards the membrane where exocytosis occurs.

b **True.** The release of insulin usually occurs within 10–12 minutes of food ingestion. This ensures that insulin is already increasing in the hepatic portal blood when the various digested by-products are being absorbed along the small intestine.

c **True.** If glucose is infused at a prolonged and maintained rate, there is an initial acute rise in insulin concentration in the blood (the early phase) after which the insulin concentration decreases towards basal before a second, more gradual increase (late phase) which is then maintained for as long as the glucose infusion. It is believed that the early phase represents the exocytotic release of insulin from granules close to the cell membrane while the later phase is associated with the movement of granules from within the cell and the subsequent release of newly synthesized hormone.

d **False.** As discussed earlier, insulin is contained in granules from which it is released by the process of exocytotis. However, it should be noted that it is possible that a small component of the intracellular insulin may be present free, or complexed with zinc, in the cytoplasm. How these molecules would be released—if they exist at all—is unknown.

e **True.** Glucose is the major stimulus for insulin release. It is quite possible that a true glucose receptor is present in the β cell membrane but none has been identified so far. This would probably be linked to an intracellular mechanism of action involving an increase in intracellular calcium ion concentration. An alternative mechanism actually involves the entry of glucose into the β cells (involving glucose transport molecule GLUT 2) followed by its metabolism which is linked in some way with the increase in calcium ion concentration.

P.7 a **True.** The insulin receptor consists of a dimeric molecule spanning the target cell membrane, with extracellular domains to which insulin and other ligands (e.g. IGF-I and IGF-II) bind, and intracellular domains which have intrinsic tyrosine kinase activity.

b **False.** Insulin's overall effects on carbohydrate metabolism are to remove glucose from the blood, for instance by increasing glucose uptake by muscle cells and increasing glycogenesis (i.e. storing glucose). The blood glucose concentration consequently *decreases* with insulin.

c **True.** This is another important physiological action of insulin. It is indeed a growth hormone, and it influences protein synthesis directly (mRNA activity increases after insulin administration) as well as by increasing substrate (i.e. amino acid) availability inside cells through an action on amino acids transport across cell membranes by facilitated diffusion.

d **False.** Indeed a diuresis (or polyuria) is a presenting symptom of diabetes mellitus which is the disease associated with absence, or lack of, insulin or its physiological actions. In this instance, the diuresis is due at least partly to the increased loss of glucose in the urine causing an accompanying loss of water (osmotic diuresis).

e **False.** As indicated above, the insulin receptor has intrinsic tyrosine kinase activity which, when stimulated, results in phosphorylation of intracellular proteins (e.g. other kinase enzymes and transporter molecules).

P.8 a **False.** The β cells are innervated by splanchnic sympathetic fibres, and there are α and β receptors on the cell membranes. However, the overall effect of sympathetic stimulation of the β cells is an *inhibition* of insulin release, mediated via the α receptors. In contrast, stimulation of β receptors is associated with an increased release of insulin in response to another subsequent stimulus, suggesting that this pathway is involved in insulin synthesis rather than release of preformed insulin.

b **False.** The pancreatic islet β cells are not influenced by any specific insulin-stimulating factor from the adenohypophysis (nor are the α and δ cells influenced by specific glucagon- or somatostatin-stimulating factors).

c **False.** Somatostatin is an ubiquitous molecule which generally seems to have inhibitory effects. In the pancreas it inhibits both insulin and glucagon release, and it is believed that these effects are likely to be paracrine.

d **False.** Certain amino acids, particularly arginine in humans, stimulate insulin release. Insulin in turn 'removes' the amino acid stimulus from the blood by increasing protein synthesis.

e **False.** The same glucose load when taken orally produces a greater insulin release than the same load given intravenously. This is because various gastrointestinal hormones (e.g. gastrin, cholecystokinin-pancreozymin, secretin) released by the oral load stimulate insulin release. The initial signal is thus greatly amplified by the release of many stimulating molecules.

P.9 a **False.** Glucagon is a 29 amino acid polypeptide initially synthesized as a much larger prohormone molecule of 160 amino acids in the α cells of the islets of Langerhans. It is stored in granules together with other by-products formed from the proglucagon molecule such as the glucagon-like polypeptides, and is released by exocytosis of the granule contents. Another molecule with glucagon immunoreactivity is synthesized by the gastrointestinal tract.

b **False.** Most hormones have a basal release and larger pulses released by specific stimuli or at certain times of day. Glucagon is released basally (normal basal concentrations estimated to be around 50 ng/litre) but in greater amounts during fasting (e.g. when blood concentrations need to be maintained).

c **False.** Glucagon is not believed to be bound to plasma proteins, certainly not to any large extent. It is, in fact, quite rapidly removed from the blood partly by a plasma enzyme system and partly by the liver. It has a half-life of less than 5 minutes.

d **False.** Glucagon binds to specific membrane receptors on its target cells (e.g. hepatocytes).

e **False.** Glucagon exerts its physiological effects by stimulating the catalytic unit adenyl cyclase with the subsequent generation of cyclic AMP. There is some evidence that an increased intracellular calcium ion concentration is also necessary, but activation of the inositol phosphate pathway has not been associated with glucagon.

P.10 a **True.** Glucagon's principal physiological effect is to increase the blood glucose concentration.

b **True.** The stimulation of glycogenolysis in the liver is undoubtedly the main physiological effect of glucagon. However, glucagon also stimulates hepatic gluconeogenesis. Indeed, it is generally believed that the liver is the only target organ for this hormone.

c **False.** Glucagon has no clear effect on renal function.

d **False.** Glucagon has no effect on the various glucose-transporting (GLUT) proteins in cell membranes, particularly those in muscle cells which only respond to insulin stimulation.

e **False.** Certainly, overall the effect of glucagon on glucose metabolism is to increase the blood glucose concentration which is counter to the overall effect of insulin, and it can be said that the two hormones function in direct opposition to each other regarding glucose metabolism. However, the effects of glucagon and insulin on the hepatic glycogenolysis pathway are not necessarily via opposing actions on the same enzymes (i.e. either to stimulate or inhibit). For example, insulin stimulates those enzymes involved in the synthesis of glycogen (glycogenesis) as well as inhibiting the enzymes involved in glycogen catabolism (glycogenolysis), while glucagon only stimulates the glycogenolytic process.

P.11 a **False.** Both vagal and sympathetic stimulation of the islet α cells results in an increased production of glucagon. This is not surprising for sympathetic stimulation since all other aspects of increased sympathetic activity (in response to a stressor, for example) will be to increase the blood glucose concentration, including release of catecholamines from the adrenal medulla and inhibition of insulin release. However, increased vagal activity also increases insulin release, so a simultaneous release of glucagon appears paradoxical. It must be appreciated that many stimuli are common to both the release of insulin and the release of glucagon, examples being certain amino acids and gastrointestinal hormones. A possible teleological explanation might be that there are situations when the blood glucose concentration requires stabilizing (as a result of insulin and glucagon actions on glucose) but protein synthesis can proceed under the influence of insulin.

b **True.** Certain gastrointestinal hormones such as cholecystokinin (also known as pancreozymin, or cholecystokinin-pancreozymin) stimulate the release of both insulin and glucagon.

c **True.** The principal stimulus for glucagon release is a decrease in the blood glucose concentration. An increase, not surprisingly, suppresses glucagon release.

d **True.** Somatostatin inhibits both insulin and glucagon at concentrations which are very high in the peripheral blood but are probably readily reached locally (i.e. it probably has a paracrine effect).

e **True.** Certain amino acids such as arginine and leucine stimulate the α and β cells to produce glucagon and insulin, respectively.

P.12 a **True.** Somatostatin is synthesized in various parts of the body, one being the δ cells of the islets of Langerhans.

b **True.** It is a tetradecapeptide.

c **True.** Somatostatin was first identified in the hypothalamus. It was found to act as an inhibitory factor for somatotrophin (growth hormone) release, being released from certain nerve endings terminating in the median eminence. The hypothalamo–adenohypophysial portal system transports this molecule down to the somatotrophs in the adenohypophysis.

d **True.** Somatostatin is found in endocrine cells of the gastric mucosa. It appears to inhibit the release of a variety of other gastrointestinal hormones including gastrin and secretin. It inhibits acid secretion into the stomach and decreases the rate of gastric emptying. It also decreases the rate at which various digested carbohydrate and protein end-products are absorbed along the small intestine.

e **False.** Somatostatin has not yet been shown to have any effect on the inflammatory response.

P.13 a **False.** Somatostatin inhibits somatotrophin release from the adeno-hypophysis; the somatomedins IGF-I and IGF-II mediate at least some of the effects of somatotrophin.

b **True.** Somatostatin is released by the same stimuli for insulin release, and this includes an increase in the blood glucose concentration.

c **False.** Somatostatin is produced by the δ cells while pancreatic poly-peptide is synthesized by the F cells which represent about 3% of the islet cells.

d **True.** Somatostatin is rapidly removed from the blood, its metabolic half-life in humans being less than 2 minutes.

e **False.** There is no evidence for any sexual dimorphism with respect to circulating somatostatin concentrations in the blood.

SAQ Answers

P.14

Glucose is a generally available, widely used energy substrate; it is a particularly important molecule because it happens to be the principal energy substrate for the neurones of the central nervous system. The mechanism for getting glucose across membranes (or the blood–brain barrier) is generally by facilitated diffusion, which involves a suitable concentration gradient favouring the movement of glucose into cells (or into the brain extracellular fluid) and the presence of glucose transporter (GLUT) proteins in the membranes.

Hypoglycaemia (i.e. a lower than normal blood glucose concentration, (e.g. < 2 mmol/l) can result in a coma and ultimately in death simply because the central nervous system becomes deprived of sufficient nutrient for its normal functioning. This is an occasional dangerous complication associated with certain insulin preparations currently used for the treatment of patients with diabetes mellitus.

Hyperglycaemia (i.e. a higher than normal blood glucose concentration, (e.g. > 12 mmol/l) can also result in coma, but for a very different reason. This is generally associated with diabetes mellitus which is due to a lack or absence of insulin (or its physiological effects). The renal threshold for glucose reabsorption is surpassed, so it is excreted in the urine. Because it exerts an osmotic effect, increased volumes of water are excreted with it (polyuria) and dehydration develops resulting in hypovalaemia. A second consequence of insulin lack is the increased formation of ketone bodies (acetoacetic acid, β-hydroxybutyric acid, and acetone) from the increased lipolysis. This acidosis combined with the hypovolaemia together result in cellular changes which, in the central nervous system, again can manifest in the development of a coma.

P.15

The endocrine part of the pancreas is represented by the islets of Langerhans. Each islet consists of at least four types of cell, three of them being associated with hormones which are important in metabolic regulation.

1. The α cells, which tend to lie more in the periphery of the islet, synthesize glucagon which is a 29 amino acid polypeptide acting mainly on the liver where it stimulates glycogenolysis and gluconeogenesis. These two effects result in an increase in the blood glucose concentration. Glucagon stimulates the release of insulin and somatostatin, and it is generally believed that these are paracrine effects within the islets.

2. The more centrally situated β cells synthesize the two-chain (21 and 30 amino acids) polypeptide hormone, insulin. Insulin is the only hormone which decreases the blood concentration of glucose, other metabolically active hormones increasing it, for instance as part of the normal adaptive response to stressors. Insulin decreases the blood glucose concentration in various ways, including the inhibition of glycogenolysis and gluconeogenesis, the stimulation of glycogenesis and glycolysis, and the increased uptake of glucose by peripheral cells in muscle and adipose tissue. Insulin inhibits glucagon production by a paracrine effect, and this may explain why, in diabetes mellitus, there is an inappropriately high glucagon concentration for the rise in blood glucose.

3. The third type of cell, representing approximately 10% of the total, are scattered more randomly throughout the islets and are called δ cells. These cells synthesize the tetradecapeptide, somatostatin, which has various effects in the body (generally inhibitory) and these include the inhibitory paracrine control of both insulin and glucagon from the islets. Another, peripheral, effect of somatostatin is the delayed glucose absorption from the small intestine that it induces.

P.16

Insulin has numerous effects, particularly on the metabolic processes involving protein, carbohydrate and lipids. Below, under general headings, are listed a few of these effects, any four of which would suffice.

Protein metabolism: increased amino acid transport into cells (e.g. muscle); increased genomic effect on protein synthesis (via activated intracellular transcription factors).

Carbohydrate metabolism: increased glucose transport into cells (e.g. muscle) involving the GLUT 4 protein molecules; increased glycogenesis; increased glycolysis; decreased glycogenolysis.

Lipid metabolism: increased lipogenesis; decreased lipolysis.

Other effects: maintenance of intracellular potassium ion concentration.

The reason why a lack of insulin, as in untreated diabetes mellitus, is associated with polyuria and polydipsia is essentially because of the raised blood glucose concentration since it is no longer adequately moved into muscle and adipose tissue, nor is it stored as glycogen. A high blood glucose concentration (over 12 mmol/l) is associated with so much glucose in the glomerular filtrate that the proximal tubular transport system for glucose, a secondary active transport mechanism involving sodium ions and a carrier molecule, becomes saturated. Consequently, glucose remains in the tubular fluid and is excreted in the urine, which is large in volume because of the induced osmotic diuresis. The extracellular fluid volume is reduced and the hypovolaemia normally stimulates the thirst centre in the hypothalamus resulting in an increased drinking (polydipsia).

P.17

Figure 10.1 illustrates the principal stimulatory and inhibitory influences acting on the β cells altering insulin production. Stimulatory and inhibitory effects are indicated by + and − respectively; (+) for the β receptor-mediated response to sympathetic stimulation indicates that this effect is not the primary response (the inhibitory effect via the α receptors is the primary response).

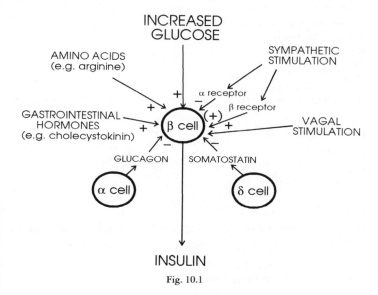

Fig. 10.1

The pancreas (Clinical)

Multiple Choice Questions

C.1

Which of the following biochemical phenomena is/are a direct consequence of insulin deficiency?

a Increased hepatic gluconeogenesis
b Decreased serum free (non-esterified) fatty acid levels
c Increased levels of circulating glucagon
d Increased non-enzymic glycosylation of proteins
e Increased activity of the aldose reductase pathway

C.2

Which of the following conditions may cause hyperglycaemia and precipitate or unstabilize diabetes mellitus?

a Phaeochromocytoma
b Growth hormone deficiency
c Pharmacological use of corticosteroids
d Haemochromatosis
e Chronic pancreatitis

C.3

Which of the following represent direct consequences of hyperglycaemia?

a Polyuria
b Visual blurring
c Weight loss
d Drowsiness and confusion
e Nausea and vomiting

C.4

Which of the following factors are relevant to the aetiology of insulin-dependent (type 1) diabetes mellitus?

a The presence of islet cell antibodies
b Presence of class 1 and class 2 antigens
c Antibody-mediated destruction of β cells
d Infection of pancreatic islets
e Increased insulin resistance

C.5

Which of the following factors are relevant to the aetiology of non-insulin-dependent (type 2) diabetes mellitus?

a Defective intracellular glucose signalling in the β cell
b Abnormal intracellular enzyme activity
c Defective cleavage of proinsulin to insulin
d Increased insulin resistance
e Reduced β-cell responsiveness to normal insulin secretagogues

C.6**

In relation to the genetics and epidemiology of insulin-dependent (type 1) diabetes, which of the following statements is/are true?

a There is a single peak age of onset at around age 24 years in males and females
b There is no seasonal variation in onset
c The overall population prevalence of around 0.5% is remarkably uniform across ethnic and national groups
d The concordance rate in identical twins is about 30%
e The risk of diabetes developing in a sibling is approximately 10%

C.7**

In relation to the genetics and epidemiology of non-insulin-dependent (type 2) diabetes, which of the following statements is/are true?

a There is a progressive age-related increase in prevalence
b There is no seasonal variation in onset
c The overall population prevalence of around 2% is remarkably uniform across ethnic and national groups
d The concordance rate in identical twins is about 80%
e The risk of diabetes developing in a sibling is at least 10%

C.8

In the diagnosis and monitoring of diabetes which of the following statements is/are true?

a A random blood glucose of 8 mmol/litre (140 mg/100 ml) excludes diabetes
b A random blood glucose of 12 mmol/litre (215 mg/100 ml) confirms diabetes
c The main criterion of diabetes during (75 gram dextrose) oral glucose tolerance testing is a (venous or capillary) blood glucose exceeding 11.1 mmol/litre (200 mg/100 ml) at 2 hours
d The main criterion of 'impaired glucose tolerance' (IGT) is a (venous or capillary) blood glucose between 7.8 and 11.1 mmol/litre (138–200 mg/100 ml) at 2 hours
e Haemoglobin A1c (HBA1c) is a useful method of screening populations for the presence of diabetes

C.9

A 55-year-old woman weighing 73 kg (161 lb: BMI = 28) presents with polyuria and polydipsia and is found to have glycosuria. There is no significant past history. Which of the following approaches to diagnosis would you endorse?

a   No further tests are required: a diagnosis of diabetes has been established
b   A random laboratory blood glucose should be checked, before treatment is commenced
c   An oral glucose tolerance test should be performed for confirmation
d   The presence of ketonuria provides a guide as to whether she has type 1 or type 2 diabetes
e   Measurement of serum insulin provides a guide as to whether she has type 1 or type 2 diabetes

C.10

For the above patient, diabetes has now been confirmed: a random blood glucose is 18 mmol/litre (325 mg/100 ml), and urinary ketones are absent. On your assessment, her current 'diet' seems reasonable. What is your chosen strategy for treatment?

a   Introduction of strict dietary controls
b   Commencement of an oral sulphonylurea (e.g. glibenclamide)
c   A combination of diet and a sulphonylurea
d   A combination of diet and a biguanide (e.g. metformin)
e   Temporary treatment with insulin for symptomatic control

C.11

What form of monitoring of glycarmic control would it be reasonable to introduce into this patient's management profile, in order to assess her response to the treatment you have initiated?

a   Assessment only of her symptomatic response to your treatment schedule
b   A single laboratory-based fasting blood glucose measurement prior to her next visit to you
c   Self-monitoring of urinary glucose by the patient once or more daily
d   Self-monitoring of blood glucose by patient (SMBG) once or more daily
e   Measurement of glycated haemoglobin (HbA1c) or fructosamine now, and again prior to her next visit to you

C.12

In this same patient treated with diet alone, weight has decreased by 4 kg (9 lb) 3 months later to 69 kg. There is persisting intermittent glycosuria and HbA1c is 8.5% (NR 4.2–6.1%). What would represent acceptable next options?

a   Continuing the previous strategy for a further 6 months
b   Implementing a further dietary review
c   Adding an oral sulphonylurea or biguanide drug

d Adding an α glucosidase inhibitor drug
e Adding insulin therapy

C.13

In regard to the above index patient, HbA1c remains between 8% and 8.5% after a further 6 months despite combining maximum dose sulphonylurea drug with maximum dose metformin (3 g daily). Supplemental acarbose (α-glucosidase inhibitor) is only tolerated in low dose because of excessive flatus. Weight remains static between 67 kg and 70 kg (BMI = 27) despite apparent dietary compliance. Which of the following strategies would be appropriate to consider?

a Accepting this level of control on a long-term basis
b Re-referring for dietary and exercise advice
c Supplementing current oral drugs with once-daily insulin
d Transferring to definitive mono-therapy with insulin alone twice or more daily
e Considering addition of drugs (e.g. thiazolidine-diones) with specific action on reducing insulin resistance

C.14

In regard to the use of the oral sulphonyurea drugs, which of the following statements is/are true?

a They act mainly by enhancing insulin response to glucose
b The therapeutic range of all sulphonylurea drugs is similar when used in maximum doses
c Hypoglycaemia is a rare side-effect
d The addition of a biguanide represents a logical step if treatment objectives are not achieved with suphonylurea alone
e Once or twice daily dosage suffices in all cases

C.15

In regard to the use of the biguanide, metformin, which of the following statements is/are true?

a It acts primarily by decreasing small intestinal absorption of monosaccharides
b It should not be used in patients with known ischaemic heart disease
c It is a safe drug to use in the presence of impaired renal function
d The commonest side-effect is epigastric discomfort and diarrhoea
e Hypoglycaemia risk is greater than with sulphonylurea drugs

C.16

A 25-year-old man presents with general debility, polyuria, polydipsia, and 7 kg weight loss over the last 3 weeks, to his current weight of 60 kg (132 lb: BMI = 18). He has heavy glycosuria, no ketonuria, and a random laboratory blood glucose of 18 mmol/litre. Which of the following treatment strategies would be appropriate?

a Defer decision on treatment or referral for 1–2 weeks pending a glucose tolerance test, full biochemical assessment, and assay for islet cell antibodies
b Commence 'strict' diet and prescribe an oral sulphonylurea drug in maximum dose
c Employ strategy b above, but in addition prescribe metformin 850 mg daily
d Refer to a diabetes centre with a view to commencing insulin in a b.d. (twice-daily) regimen
e Refer to a diabetes centre with a view to commencing insulin in a q.d.s. (4 times daily) regimen (short-acting before meals and intermediate-acting) insulin at bedtime

C.17

What form of monitoring of glycaemic control would it be reasonable to introduce into this patient's management profile, in order to assess his response to the treatment you have initiated?

a Assessment only of his symptomatic response to your treatment schedule
b A single laboratory-based fasting blood glucose measurement prior to his next visit to you
c Self monitoring of urinary glucose by the patient once or more daily
d Self-monitoring of blood glucose by patient (SMBG) once or more daily
e Measurement of glycated haemoglobin (HbA1c) or fructosamine now, and prior to his next visit to you

C.18

In this patient, which of the following nutritional schedules can be accommodated, without sacrificing the quality of his glycaemic control?

a Freedom to eat and drink as and when desired
b Three regular meals of similar carbohydrate distribution, plus mid morning, mid afternoon, and bedtime snacks
c Three meals at varying times, and of continuously varying carbohydrate content, plus a bedtime snack
d As in c above, but with occasional meals missed altogether
e 'Crash' dieting for a day or two at a time to make up for indulgences during the rest of the week

C.19

The same patient is an active and occasionally competitive sportsman. What adaptations to his schedule would you advice?

a Giving up the competitive, more intensive aspect of his sport
b Omitting or reducing his insulin doses before commencing physical exercise
c Continuing the same doses of insulin but supplementing his diet with extra food before and/or after the sport
d Combining both b and c above

e Continuing his usual standard insulin regimen, but carrying lump sugar or Dextrosol during the sport, to be taken if necessary

C.20

Hypoglycaemia is an occasional or even recurrent problem in many diabetics. In regard to this problem, which of the following is/are true?

a Most early warning symptoms of hypoglycaemia are a direct result of reduced glucose supply to the brain
b Unless an episode of hypoglycaemia is treated promptly, brain damage is a significant risk
c The early warning symptoms of hypoglycaemia may be lost as a result of excessively tight control (low blood sugar levels)
d Hypoglycaemia is often followed by a spontaneous rise of blood glucose to hyperglycaemic levels
e Recurrent episodes of hypoglycaemia may result in permanent brain damage

C.21

For the avoidance and management of hypoglycaemia, which of the following is/are true?

a Calcium channel blockers should be avoided as hypotensive agents, since they can potentiate hypoglycaemia
b Because of their caloric content, alcoholic drinks are an adequate substitute for food in the insulin-requiring diabetic
c In the mildly exercising insulin-requiring diabetic, it is safer to wait for hypoglycaemic symptoms to occur rather than anticipating by reducing dosage in advance
d Glucagon is a useful standby for more severe hypoglycaemia occurring remote from access to medical care
e Dextrosol or lump sugar should be carried by patients on sulphonylurea drugs as well as those having insulin

C.22

In relation to the cause of so-called microvascular complications (retinopathy and nephropathy), which of the following statements is/are true?

a The risk of these complications is related directly to duration of diabetes and the quality of glycaemic control
b There are independent genetic factors controlling susceptibility to these complications
c Both the aldose reductase and non-enzymic glycosylation pathways are likely to be major contributors to microvascular pathology
d Improving glycaemic control after long-duration poor control does not influence progression of these complications

e Hypertension and its treatment influence the development, but not the progression of the complications once they are present

C.23

In background diabetic retinopathy, which of the following statements is/are true?

a It consists only of miroaneurysms, and dot and blot haemorrhages
b Visual acuity is not affected
c About 20% of patients progress to proliferative retinopathy
d It is not possible to identify a 'pre-proliferative' phase
e Skilled examination of the retina is only required once visual acuity has been shown to be affected

C.24

In proliferative diabetic retinopathy, which of the following statements is/are true?

a It consists of mainly of new vessel formation, subsequently leading to preretinal (vitreous) haemorrhages
b Once proliferative retinopathy occurs, laser therapy does not reduce the risk of subsequent vitreous haemorrhages and visual loss
c The 5-year risk of blindness in untreated cases is 50%
d The blindness is untreatable
e The presence of glaucoma reduces the severity of retinopathy

C.25

In diabetic nephropathy, which of the following statements is/are true?

a Its pathological basis is abnormal structure and function of the glomerular basement membrane
b The earliest biochemical abnormality is an increase in urinary albumin excretion (microalbuminuria)
c End-stage renal disease due to diabetic nephropathy is now an uncommon indication for dialysis and renal transplantation
d Lowering of blood pressure in normotensive patients with microalbuminuria will not reduce the risk of progression to overt nephropathy
e Macrovascular disease (especially stroke and myocardial infarction) occurs with increased frequency in patients with diabetic nephropathy

C.26

In the practical management of diabetic nephropathy, which of the following statements is/are true?

a An early morning semi-quantitative test for microalbuminuria (Micral test or similar) or urine albumin/creatinine ratio should be performed annually in every diabetic
b Once either test is positive, this is sufficient to classify the patient as having 'microalbuminuria'

c Once 'microalbuminuria' is confirmed, an ACE inhibitor should be prescribed only if the blood pressure is 160/90 or higher

d Serum creatinine measurements should be performed annually in all diabetics

e A serum creatinine of 150 μmol/litre is an indication for referral for specialist renal opinion

C.27

In the management of hypertension in people with diabetes, which of the following statements is/are true?

a There is an approximate 5% prevalence of hypertension after diabetes duration of 10 years

b Treatment of coexistent hypertension reduces the rate of decline of renal function, but not of stroke or heart attack

c Blood pressure should be checked annually in all diabetics, and at least 4-monthly once hypertension has been identified and treated

d The indication for treatment is a blood pressure at or above 160/90 which is also the maximum for all patients on treatment

e As long as the treatment target is achieved, the type of hypotensive drug used is irrelevant

C.28

In relation to the pathogenesis of diabetic neuropathy, which of the following statements is/are true?

a The aldose reductase pathway plays a significant part in the aetiology of this complication

b Occlusive disease of the vasa nervorum is responsible for some components of diabetic neuropathy

c Changes in nerve conduction velocity in both sensory and motor nerves can be reversed in recently diagnosed diabetics by restoring euglycaemia

d Even long-standing distal sensory neuropathy is reversible by restoration of good glycaemic control

e Presence of sensory neuropathy is related to the duration of diabetes but not to preceding levels of glycaemic control

C.29

In relation to clinical aspects of diabetic neuropathy, which of the following statements is/are true?

a Sensory neuropathy is usually recognized by the patient before it is identified by the doctor

b Symmetrical sensory neuropathy is most readily identified by absence of vibration sense and/or ankle reflexes

c Sensory neuropathy represents an important factor identifying feet 'at risk' of developing ulceration and gangrene

d Painful paresthesiae are reversible by improved glycaemic control
e Motor neuropathy rarely involves the cranial nerves

C.30

Which of the following statements is/are true in relation to the pathogenesis of arteriosclerotic macrovascular disease in diabetes?

a It is about twice as common in diabetics as in an age-matched population
b Glycaemic control is the most important determinant of its extent and severity
c Hyperlipidaemia is less relevant to its development in diabetes than in the general population
d Microalbuminuria is related to the risk of macrovascular occlusive events
e Given the high vascular risk resulting from diabetes itself, cigarette smoking does not materially add to this risk

C.31

Which of the following statements is/are true in relation to the clinical effects of arteriosclerotic macrovascular disease in diabetes?

a Myocardial infarction is not only more common than in non-diabetics but is also more frequently unrecognized
b Mortality of myocardial infarction is greater than in non-diabetics
c Proximal arteries are more seriously affected than distal arteries in lower limb vascular disease of diabetics, when compared with non-diabetics
d Involvement of renal arteries may be responsible for (potentially) surgically remediable hypertension
e Aspirin has been shown to reduce incidence of macrovascular occlusive events

C.32

Which of the following factors has been shown to contribute to the risk of infection/ulceration and gangrene in the diabetic?

a The use of enclosed shoes with leather soles and soft uppers
b Daily washing of the feet
c Reliance on chiropody/podiatry care in the elderly
d Barefoot walking indoors
e The use of over-the-counter callus and corn cures

C.33

A 70-year-old man with non-insulin-dependent diabetes presents with a one centimetre weeping abrasion on the medical aspect of his big toe. Excessive wearing of new shoes is identified as the primary cause. Which of the following would you advise?

a The shoes should be taken to a shoemaker/repairer for stretching

b The feet should be examined there and then for evidence of neuropathy and vascular disease
c The patient should be advised to leave the lesion uncovered to allow it to dry
d A topical antibiotic cream should be applied
e If the lesion has not healed in one week, the patient should be asked to re-attend

C.34

On return of the above patient 5 days later, the surface of the abrasion is purulent and the toe is now swollen, red and uncomfortable, but not painful (presumably because he was found by you to have neuropathy at his last visit). The swab culture showed a mixed growth, including a staphylococcus which is sensitive only to flucloxacillin. Which of the following steps would be appropriate?

a Commence the patient on oral flucloxacillin in high dose
b Arrange an X-ray of the foot
c Check current glycaemic control by getting the result of HbA1c/fructosamine
d Suggest warm water soaks of the foot to make the toe more comfortable
e Refer the patient for expert diabetic or vascular opinion

C.35**

Which of the following is/are true in relation to hyperlipidaemia in diabetes?
a 10% of patients with non-insulin- dependent diabetes (NIDDM: type 2 diabetes) have an abnormal serum lipid profile
b Insulin resistance plays a major part in the genesis of the lipid abnormalities in NIDDM
c Uncontrolled insulin-dependent diabetes (IDDM: type 1 diabetes) causes a rise of total and LDL cholesterol
d Diabetic nephropathy is associated with a worsening atherogenic lipid profile
e Alpha-adrenergic blocking drugs, calcium channel blockers, and ACE inhibitors may all further worsen the lipid profile in diabetes

C.36

A moderately obese 50-year-old woman with non-insulin diabetes treated with diet alone smokes 15 cigarettes a day. Her blood pressure is 180/100 on the calcium channel blocker, amlodipine. Biochemical assessment at the time of her 'annual review' examination reveals an HbA1c of 8.5% (NR 4.4–6.1), serum triglyceride level is 5.3 mmol/litre (N < 1.8), cholesterol 7.4 mmol/litre (N < 5.6), and HDL cholesterol is 0.6 mmol/litre (NR 1.1–2.5), with a normal serum creatinine of 89 μmol/l. She has a strong family history of myocardial infarction in the 5th decade. With a main target of reducing her own cardiovascular risk, which of the following strategies would be appropriate?

a Arrange for a dietary review and commence a sulphonylurea oral hypoglycaemic drug
b Advise her to cease smoking

c Commence a statin drug
d Change her hypotensive drug to atenolol
e Advise commencement of aspirin

C.37

In relation to the effects of diabetes on pregnancy, which of the following is/are true?

a Fertility is impaired in insulin-requiring diabetics
b Glycaemic control of diabetes at the time of conception affects the incidence of congenital abnormalities
c There is a greater risk of miscarriage
d Large babies are more likely if diabetic control is too 'tight'
e Once delivered, the baby of a diabetic is at no greater risk than that of a non-diabetic

C.38

In relation to the effects of pregnancy on diabetes, which of the following is/are true?

a Diabetes tends to become more stable in pregnancy
b Women previously receiving oral hypohlycarmic drugs may continue these throughout pregnancy, providing glycaemic control is maintained
c Diabetic retinopathy and nephropathy usually remain stable, unless glycaemic control is lost during pregnancy
d Women receiving insulin usually require larger doses during pregnancy to maintain control
e Ketosis in pregnancy diabetics is of lesser significance than in non-diabetics

C.39

Which of the following facts concerning gestational diabetes is/are true?

a It occurs in about 5% of pregnancies
b It can usually be predicted by appropriate antenatal tests
c It carries the same pregnancy risks as diabetes which antedated the pregnancy
d Insulin is required for treatment in all cases
e Not all cases return to normal glucose tolerance postpartum

C.40

An insulin-dependent diabetic woman age 71 develops polyuria and polydipsia in the course of an episode of severe acute bronchitis. Her urine tests have become positive for ketones, and blood glucose is 20 mmol/litre (360 mg/100 ml). Which of the following approaches are appropriate?

a Await improvement in her diabetes control over the next 1–2 days, following introduction of antibiotics
b Increase her insulin doses the next day by 30%

c Ask her to recheck her urine ketones again 4–6 hours later

d Advise her to drink clear non-caloric fluids only and stop all solid food

e Admit her to hospital for stabilization

C.41

The same patient rings you 8 hours later. She feels nauseated, and has vomited once. When you get to her home, she seems a bit drowsy, her urinary ketones are still positive, but her blood glucose has fallen to 13 mmol/litre (235 mg/100 ml). She makes it clear to you that she does not even wish to consider the possibility of hospital admission, since it is 12 miles distant and she is afraid to leave her cats alone! Which of the following would represent important steps in her immediate management?

a Give her a further 4–12 units of soluble (clear, regular) insulin subcutaneously

b Call the ambulance for urgent admission

c Give her an intramuscular anti-emetic (e.g. metoclopramide)

d Give her intravenous antibiotics

e Insert an intravenous line to commence rehydration

C.42

The same patient is finally admitted to hospital, rather more drowsy than when seen at home. Which of the following statements is/are true in relation to the treatment of diabetic ketoacidosis which was indeed confirmed, superimposed on extensive bilateral bronchopneumonia?

a Slow infusion of insulin (4–6 units/h) is less effective than a large (50–100 unit) bolus

b Hyperkalaemia is a significant complication of treatment

c Acidosis should not be treated with alkali (sodium bicarbonate) unless blood pH is less than 7.0

d Intravenous colloid (e.g. 5% human serum albumin) should be used if she is hypovolaemic and persistently hypotensive

e A naso-gastric tube should be inserted if she vomits

C.43**

In the syndrome of hyperosmolar non-ketotic coma (HONK), which of the following statements is/are true?

a The condition is mainly found in type 2 (NIDDM) patients

b There is a high risk of occlusive vascular episodes

c Patients tend to have higher blood glucose levels than in diabetic ketoacidosis (DKA), and be less sensitive to insulin

d Hypotonic solutions (e.g. half-normal saline) are preferred for prompt correction of hyperosmolarity

e Following recovery, almost all patients can be controlled on diet and oral hypoglycaemic agents

Short Answer Questions

C.44

'The centrepiece of diabetes care is the adherence to dietary principles.' In *note* form, outline the basis of this statement in relation to the management of the non-insulin-dependent (type 2) diabetes.

C.45**

Provide a synopsis of 3 manifestations of diabetic autonomic neuropathy. For each, provide a *brief* outline of possible therapeutic measures which are available.

C.46**

'The education of the patient with diabetes is central to reducing the cost of diabetes, both in terms of human suffering as well as financial burden on the community.' Illustrate this principle, by writing *short* notes on 6 important aspects of such education.

C.47**

Write *brief* notes on 3 skin disorders encountered in association with diabetes mellitus.

MCQ Answers

C.1 a **True.** Fasting hyperglycaemia is an early manifestation of diabetes, due to increased hepatic gluconeogenesis resulting from a lack of the inhibitory action of adequate insulin concentrations.

    b **False.** Fatty acid levels are increased. Insulin directly inhibits lipolysis and increases lipogenesis: insulin deficiency results in hypertriglyceridaemia, and increased free fatty acid and ketone formation.

    c **True.** Hyperglucagonaemia occurs (paradoxically) in IDDM and to a lesser extent in NIDDM. Insulin has a paracrine inhibitory effect on α-cell glucagon release. In insulin deficiency, hyperglucagonaemia is responsible for a significant part of resulting ketogenesis, and can be (experimentally) reversed by somatostatin infusion.

    d **False.** Non-enzymic glycosylation, leading to glycoprotein formation and deposition in basement membranes is entirely independent of insulin action. It is dependent directly on blood glucose levels.

    e **False.** The activity of aldose reductase, the consequent synthesis of sorbitol, and its subsequent reduction to fructose (via alcohol dehydrogenase) are all dependent on glucose and unaffected by insulin or its lack.

C.2 a **True.** Although unlikely to cause clinical diabetes, hyperglycaemia is often found during investigation. Catecholamines stimulate glycogenolysis and gluconeogenesis, and also lipolysis. Complete remission of long-standing diabetes has been described following removal of a phaeochromocytoma.

b **False.** Growth hormone deficiency causes (fasting) *hypoglycaemia*, especially in adults. Hyperglycaemia is seen in chronic growth hormone excess, as exemplified by acromegaly, and often reversible by successful treatment of acromegaly. Growth hormone increases lipolysis and indirectly (via enhanced glycerol synthesis) gluconeogenesis. More acutely growth hormone increases glycogenolysis.

c **True.** Hyperglycaemia and induction of more permanent diabetes are frequent and serious complications of both acute and long-term corticosteroid therapy. Corticosteroids increase insulin resistance in muscle and liver cells by decreasing insulin receptor affinity. They also directly enhance gluconeogenesis. Stimulation of appetite with resultant increased food intake is an additional factor. All these factors are also operative in (non-iatrogenic) Cushing's syndrome of any cause.

d **True.** The increased iron absorption in this condition leads to deposition in many organs, including the pancreas. The islets are rarely affected histologically, so that the pathogenesis of the frequently encountered hyperglycaemia is not clear.

e **True.** Diabetes is a consequence of both acute and chronic pancreatisis. Inflammation and fibrosis affects dominantly exocrine pancreatic tissue, and it is assumed that islet function is compromised either by direct involvement of islets in the acute form, or by effects on the microcirculation of islets in the chronic form.

C.3 a **True.** The increased glucose concentration in the glomerular filtrate leads to an osmotic diuresis: water content of glomerular filtrate exceeds the tubular reabsorption capacity.

b **True.** Glucose accumulates in the lens and cornea causing a refractive change based on osmotically based water accumulation. Some of the osmotic effect is contributed by (insulin-independent) formation of sorbitol by the aldose reductase pathway.

c **True.** Daily urinary glucose excretion often exceeds 5 grams per 100 ml in untreated or uncontrolled diabetes. Together with an increased daily urine output of 3 litres or more, upwards of 150 grams of glucose (equivalent to 600 kcal) accordingly can be lost daily. In addition, dehydration from the glycosuria-related osmotic diuresis contributes to weight loss. A major additional factor (but related to insulin deficiency rather than hyperglycaemia itself) is increased tissue catabolism, including lipolysis, secondary to insulin deficiency.

d **True.** Glucose transporters in neural tissue are independent of insulin action, and cell glucose entry is maintained only by the concentration gradient across the cell membrane. Osmotic accumulation of water in the brain (cerebral oedema) therefore occurs. Some of the osmotic (and neurotoxic) effects are due to sorbitol accumulation as in b above.

e **False.** Nausea and vomiting are features secondary to severe or protracted insulin deficiency causing ketogenesis and subsequent ketoacidosis. It may develop in parallel with hyperglycaemia, but is not due to it. Ketoacidosis may occur with a normal blood glucose level.

C.4 a **True.** Islet cell (ICA) and insulin (IAA) antibodies are found in more than 50% of newly diagnosed type 1 diabetics. Antibodies to a 64 kDa β-cell antigen (glutamic acid dehydrogenase: GAD) are also frequently present.

b **True.** DR-3, DR-4 (also B-8 and BW-15) among class I and a variety of DQ haplotypes (class II) are seen with increased frequency in type 1 diabetes.

c **False.** β-cell destruction is a cell-mediated rather than antibody-mediated phenomenon. The presence of antibodies as in (a) above, represents an epiphenomenon of antigen presentation/expression and abnormal immune response without representing a pathogenetic action.

d **True.** Maternal rubella classically transfects fetal islets and leads to β-cell destruction and later development of type 1 diabetes. An immune component may be present. Coxsackie, mumps, and CMV infection in childhood have been similarly implicated, but the overall contribution of infective agents to aetiology of type 1 diabetes is still not known.

e **False.** Insulin resistance is not an aetiological factor for type 1 diabetes, although it may supervene in the later course of the disease, due to exogenous insulin-mediated down-regulation of its own receptor affinity and number. It may also develop as a consequence of subsequent obesity.

C.5 a **True.** This phenomenon is almost certainly due to abnormal function of glucokinase and glucose transport, rendering the β cell unresponsive to ambient glucose concentration.

b **True.** Abnormal glucokinase activity has been reported in some families with type 2 diabetes. Other enzyme defects due to gene mutation are likely to be responsible for some familial cases.

c **False.** Although this is a theoretical possibility, there is no evidence for such a defect as a significant cause of diabetes.

d **True.** This is a major factor in most if not all cases. Abnormal glucose transporter function (specifically GLUT-4) may be mediated by a number of genetic or acquired factors. Insulin resistance is closely linked to hyperlipidaemia and to the increased incidence of macrovascular disease (Reaven's syndrome 'X'), although the key link between these components is still unknown.

e **True.** The defective β-cell response is not unique to glucose, involving also amino acids and peptides, including secretin and the most potent insulin secretagogue—glucagon-like peptide (GLP-1).

*C.6*** a **False.** There are peaks of onset at ages 5, 13, and 18 in both sexes which dominate the age-of-onset profile. These correspond with changes of educational environment, and may give a clue to a potential infective or other environmental (?chemical) agent.

b **False.** Peak months of onset in most populations studied have been during Autumn and early Winter in both northern and southern hemispheres, again adding support to possible infective agent(s).

c **False.** Although a prevalence of 0.5% applies to many national and ethnic groups, there are major departures. In Sicily and Finland, prevalence is six times higher, although no responsible factors have been identified. A high prevalence in Iceland has been attributed to a possible chemical diabetogenic agent in smoked fish which is consumed in large amounts in this ethnic group.

d **True.** This concordance rate of 30% in identical twins should be compared to the 10% concordance rate in non-identical twins, and highlights the significant, but not overwhelming genetic factor in type 1 diabetes. Environmental factors are almost certainly of greater importance in the aetiology of this type of diabetes.

e **True.** The sibling prevalence rate is (not surprisingly) identical to that between non-identical twins (see above). It should also be noted that diabetes risk is 50% higher if the father has type 1 diabetes rather than the mother. This observation remains unexplained.

*C.7*** a **True.** However, there is an uncommon variant, maturity onset diabetes of the young (MODY), probably representing a range of gene mutations affecting insulin action, glucose transport, and intracellular processing.

b **True.** However, there is an apparent peak in *diagnosis* due to the aggravation of diabetes symptoms by intercurrent respiratory infections which are more prevalent in Winter months. Because of its invariably insidious onset, true time of onset of non-insulin-dependent diabetes is impossible to identify.

c **False.** Variation between ethnic groups is even greater than in type 1 diabetes. Nauruans, Australian Aborigines, and certain North American Indian tribes have prevalence rates exceeding 20%. Whereas the figure of 2% holds true for most of Europe, USA, and other developed countries, immigrant Asians in the UK have a prevalence exceeding 10%. There is evidence that both genetic and environmental factors are responsible for this variation; particularly obesity (which is the major determinant of insulin resistance). In developing countries, prevalence is well below 1%, probably due to low levels of nutrition and comparative absence of obesity. In most studies world-wide, population screening identifies approximately one new case for every known case of type 2 diabetes.

d **True.** Some studies show even higher concordance rates, identifying the dominant genetic determinant of type 2 diabetes. This is notwithstanding the clear role of diet and obesity as environmental factors.

e **True.** In fact, when glucose tolerance tests are performed in siblings, 'impaired glucose tolerance' (see later) is found in a further 30% of siblings: only 60% of siblings have normal glucose tolerance by World Health Organization criteria.

C.8 a **False.** A 'random' venous plasma glucose may be equivalent to a fasting level if taken 3 hours or more after food: a value of 8 mmol/litre (145 mg/100 ml) may rise to well above 11.1 mmol/litre (200 mg/100 ml) in response to food or glucose and therefore cannot exclude diabetes. Random (and fasting) levels below 6.4 mmol/litre (115 mg/100 ml) *do* exclude diabetes.

b **True.** Ideally a 'random' blood glucose should be done about 1 hour after a main meal. Most diabetics will have a blood glucose above 12 mmol/litre (215 mg/100 ml). Only levels of 7.8–11.1 mmol/litre (140–200 mg/100 ml) justify proceeding to glucose tolerance testing.

c **True.** The fasting and 1 hour (peak) blood glucose levels are of lesser significance, and do not materially affect the diagnostic classification, although a fasting blood glucose below 6.5 mmol/litre (115 mg/100 ml) excludes diabetes. A number of factors, including smoking, stress, drugs (phenytoin, diuretics, oestrogens, steroids), and previous low carbohydrate intake impair glucose tolerance. The GTT is an imprecise test with reasonable sensitivity but low specificity, and 'border values' should therefore be interpreted with caution.

d **True.** This diagnosis is of increasing importance since: (i) around 50% of such patients will undergo transition to overt diabetes within their lifetime; and (ii) patients with IGT have almost identical prevalence of macrovascular events to that seen in overt diabetes. Finally, IGT can be found in approximately 30% of the first degree relatives of patients with non-insulin-dependent (type 2) diabetes, raising important questions concerning population screening. It has been suggested that the lower limit of the IGT blood glucose range should be reduced to 6.7 mmol/litre (120 mg/100 ml).

e **False.** HbA1c may be normal with significant glucose intolerance at either IGT or diabetic levels. This low sensitivity (but high specificity) does not put it into a useful category for screening purposes.

C.9 a **False.** Although it is likely that she has diabetes on this evidence, commencement of a lifelong management programme justifies greater certainty. Her dry mouth could result from a blocked nose and the urine test container may have been contaminated!

b **True.** In symptomatic diabetes, a random blood glucose, especially sampled within 2 hours of eating is almost always above 12 mmol/litre (215 mg/100 ml). In non-diabetics, this value would never exceed 9 mmol/litre (160 mg/100 ml).

c **False.** Only in the unlikely event of a random blood glucose level between 9 and 12 mmol/litre (160–215 mg/100 ml) would this be necessary. A glucose tolerance test (GTT) is otherwise unnecessary, since it provides no additional information and is time-consuming and uncomfortable for the patient. Even in an asymptomatic patient with chance finding of glycosuria, a random blood glucose usually provides the answer. A GTT is useful for diagnosis of diabetes in pregnancy where renal threshold for glucose is low.

d **True.** Mild to moderate ketonuria on a fasting specimen may be a normal finding. In a non-fasting specimen, ketonuria indicates inappropriate lipolysis. In the context of this patient, this indicates insulin deficiency. Although not an absolute indicator of type 1 diabetes, most of such patients will require insulin.

e **False.** On theoretical grounds, type 1 diabetics may be expected to have absolute insulin deficiency. In practice, significant insulin production may continue for up to 3 years or so. However, islet cell antibodies are present in 70% of type 1 diabetics at diagnosis, and by definition are not found in type 2 diabetes. Although the use of insulin is usually decided on more pragmatic grounds (such as presence of ketonuria), measurement of islet cell antibodies is helpful in some cases.

C.10 a **True.** Despite your own assessment, she is in fact overweight. A trained dietitian can usually identify 'hidden' calorie sources. Dietary restriction immediately lowers blood glucose with resulting symptom control, even before weight reduction occurs. Despite the initially high random blood glucose level, 20–30% of such patients may achieve optimal control on diet alone.

b **False.** This is only a supportable strategy if the patient was of normal weight and had convincingly instituted a 'diabetic diet' prior to her being seen.

c **False.** This strategy is only justified at the time of diagnosis if osmotic symptoms are disabling, or if there is associated infection or other illness which makes prompt control essential. Immediate commencement of an oral hypoglycaemic agent (OHA) may diminish the patient's perception of the pivotal role of diet: dietary compliance tends to be less good. Despite the apparent safety of OHA, side-effects are still common, and problems resulting from long-term use not entirely dismissed.

d **False.** A similar line of reasoning to (c) above applies. However, immediate blood glucose lowering is less likely to be achieved with biguanides.

e **False.** This is not a reasonable first step unless the presenting symptoms are very disabling, or the patient is being prepared for surgery or has just been admitted with a recent myocardial infarct: in both these latter situations, uncontrolled diabetes carries additional risks.

C.11 a **False.** Although it is reassuring to know that a patient may feel better, this is too imprecise. Furthermore, some more immediate and objective day-to-day monitoring is required to ensure that glycaemic control is improving, to achieve motivation and reassurance for your patient.

b **False.** Although more objective than symptom assessment, a single fasting blood glucose level is non-indicative of overall trends in glycaemic control and is often very misleading. Patients also try to impress by complying only in the days leading up to their next assessment!

c **True.** Since the renal glucose threshold for most patients is around 9 mmol/litre (160 mg/100 ml), urinary glucose measurement is a reasonable and economical approach. Progressive reduction and eventual abolition of glycosuria in (especially post-prandial) specimens is likely to signify reasonable control.

d **True.** This is a perfectly satisfactory alternative to (b) above (but much more expensive by a factor of 10). For less skilled and motivated patients there is also more opportunity for measurement error, whether using a visual strip or meter reading technique. There is little proof from randomized studies that patients using SMBG are eventually better controlled than those using urine monitoring.

e **True.** This should be seen as supplementary to patients' own self-monitoring assessments. Serum fructosamine reflects the integrated blood glucose over a 10–14 day interval, and glycated haemoglobin reflects the last 8–10 weeks. Choice of these tests therefore depends on the period over which evaluation is intended. Many assays for HbA1c give artificially low values in the presence of haemoglobinopathies (present in 10–15% of African-Caribbeans).

C.12 a **False.** It is very unlikely that your present strategy will bear fruit! The next assessment is likely to be similar and 6 months will have been lost.

b **True.** A single session of dietary instruction rarely suffices: many additional minor points often emerge at a 3-month dietetic review: if not, then an alternative strategy (below) needs implementing. A build up of physical activity (energy expenditure) complements diet in a weight loss strategy. Exercise also has independent effects on increasing muscle–cell glucose uptake and reducing insulin resistance.

c **True.** This is a logical next step, adding a drug from either group in increasing doses until the patient is free of glycosuria or maximum doses are reached. Glycosylated protein measurements should be within 15% of the upper limit of the normal range (and ideally actually within the normal range). Biguanides are preferred in the presence of more substantial obesity, on which it has some additional benefit. Combined sulphonlyurea and biguanide therapy is needed to achieve optimal control in about 20% of patients.

d **True.** This group of drugs has the advantage of safety (excessive flatus is the only major side effect!). When used alone, average reductions of HbA1c of around 1% are achieved. It is more useful as supplemental to other oral drugs rather than as monotherapy.

e **False.** This decision is premature. Indeed, weight (re)gain is often a consequence. It is nevertheless an ultimate treatment decision in 10–20% of patients with type 2 (apparently non-insulin-dependent) diabetes, either supplementing a sulphonylurea or biguanide drug as a nocturnal bolus to normalize fasting blood glucose, or as definitive mono-therapy. Drugs which reduce insulin resistance (thiazolidine-diones: glitazones) are being introduced. They may reduce the need for insulin in this situation, and indeed may prove useful as first-line therapy.

C.13 a **False.** This should only be a total default option. The patient is often not feeling 100% well because of poor metabolic control. The risks of complications and infection and of acute (and dangerous) loss of glycaemic control due to superimposed stress of any type are substantial. This option should only then be accepted after full discussion with the patient herself.

b **True.** Although it is unlikely that there is room for manoeuvre, the discussion of (a) above may lead to higher motivation and compliance with both a tighter dietary and more ambitious exercise programme.

c **True.** This strategy sometimes works, with administration of a medium-acting insulin with a bedtime snack, with increasing doses aimed at normalizing fasting blood glucose (the patient will need to acquire SMBG testing technique).

d **True.** This is a realistic option, and may follow (c) above. Patient acceptance is assisted by presenting the insulin regimen as a 'trial run' rather than as an irreversible step: in practice, improved well-being (often at the expense of weight gain) ensures ongoing insulin therapy as definitive.

e **True.** This group of drugs is not generally available, but may provide a useful additional approach, since insulin resistance is such an integral component of type 2 diabetes itself, as well as being a consequence of superimposed obesity.

C.14 a **True.** This is the major effect, although they also increase insulin-dependent cell glucose uptake, and may reduce degradation of insulin by hepatic insulinase.

b **True.** There is little to choose between these drugs in terms of hypoglycaemic action. Some oral sulphonylurea drugs were thought to have specific effects on inhibiting platelet aggregation and other prothrombotic blood components, but this has been largely disproven.

c **False.** This is a major problem, particularly in the elderly (who may omit to eat and are also more prone to neuroglycopenic brain damage). It is also more common with more potent and longer-acting sulphonylureas such as glibenclamide (as compared with tolbutamide). The risk of hypoglycaemia rises with the development of renal failure as a result of the combined effects of reduced insulin and sulphonylurea clearance.

d **True.** Biguanide and sulphonylurea drugs have synergistic actions. Such combined therapy sometimes obviates the need for a transfer to insulin.

e **True.** Single (morning) doses suffice in many patients, and reduce the risk of nocturnal hypoglycaemia.

C.15 a **False.** One major action is to increase non-insulin-dependent glucose uptake into muscle cells by enhancing anaerobic glycolysis. Insulin resistance (one of the major components of type 2 diabetes) is thereby reduced. it also reduces hepatic gluconeogenesis, and impairs monosaccharide absorption to a minor extent. By an incidental anorexigenic action, it prompts a reduction in food intake to the benefit of any weight reduction programme.

b **True.** As a consequence of enhanced anaerobic glycolysis, lactate levels are higher in patients on metformin, which also inhibits lactate uptake in the liver. Supplemental lactic acidaemia resulting from an ischaemic myocardial episode can induce (occasionally fatal) lactic acidosis.

c **False.** Renal failure impairs lactate excretion and metformin clearance, and so predisposes to lactic acidosis in the presence of superimposed lactic acidaemia (usually as a consequence of a myocardial, peripheral vascular or mesenteric occlusive vascular event).

d **True.** Nausea and anorexia, epigastric discomfort and diarrhoea are common when metformin is initiated in too large a dose. Low starting doses (500 to 850 mg daily) and time-related tolerance to the drug often, but not invariably avoids these adverse effects.

e **False.** Metformin is virtually free of hypoglycaemia risk, probably because of the absence of any stimulating effect on pancreatic insulin release (thereby allowing reduction of insulin secretion to occur in the presence of any trend to hypoglycaemia). However, it will potentiate the risk of hypoglycaemia if used in conjunction with a sulphonylurea drug (or insulin).

C.16 a **False.** There is no doubt about the diagnosis with a random blood glucose as high as 18 mmol/litre. Indeed, you could acutely worsen his metabolic state by giving him the standard 75 g dextrose load used for a glucose tolerance test. Again, although a positive islet cell antibody result may give you a more confident diagnosis (of type 1 diabetes), it is not worth the risk of leaving such a patient untreated.

b **False.** This may well lower his blood glucose levels temporarily, but almost certainly not into the normal range. Although patients with maturity onset of the young (MODY) present at this age (and are controllable by sulphonylurea drugs) they do not have the weight loss and debility of this patient. Deferring the commencement of insulin may soften the blow of the diagnosis, but is probably not worth the risk of sudden metabolic decompensation (even ketoacidosis), which may occur spontaneously or with an intercurrent infection. He will also not feel 'back to normal' until he is appropriately treated.

c **False.** As in (a) above. Your chances of temporarily controlling him are marginally better. The lack of ketonuria should not deter you: in the early stages of insulin-dependent diabetes (IDDM: type 1 diabetes) there is often just enough residual endogenous insulin secretion to suppress ketogenesis: but this is temporary.

d **True.** This is an acceptable approach, and for some patients more easy to accept than the immediate introduction of a q.d.s. regimen.

e **True.** This is marginally preferable. Control can usually be achieved more quickly and effectively. Some studies suggest that such 'tight' control immediately following diagnosis helps to maintain endogenous insulin secretion for a longer period (with the implication of overall better control in the crucial early years of diabetes).

C.17 a **False.** Some form of self-monitoring is essential.

b **False.** Single blood glucose levels are of no value at all in assessing the progress of treatment in a patient such as this, in whom blood glucose levels probably fluctuate very widely.

c **False.** An unsatisfactory second-best approach. Urinalysis is far too indirect and imprecise a method of identifying glycaemic control, considering inter- and intra-individual variation in renal glucose threshold. However, some patients find finger-pricking more painful than insulin injections!

d **True.** This is the only useful form of monitoring, providing feedback to your patient of his individual responses to food, exercise, and stress. Only in this way can he learn to modify doses in anticipation of changes to his routine. Use of meters rather than visual strip testing does not appear to significantly benefit control. Maintenance of (near) normo-glycaemia must be the goal, in view of studies showing medium- and long-term microvascular, neuropathic, and even macrovascular risk reduction by this means (particularly bearing in mind his age).

e **True.** Some patients check (and record) their blood glucose levels 'selectively' (i.e. when they are thought to be running high, or in other patients running low). Only Hba1c provides a properly integrated picture (2–3 months retrospective control). It should ideally be performed every 4 months, again with 'feedback' to your patient.

C.18 a **False.** Although it is theoretically possible to match the carbohydrate content or the 'glycaemic index' of any meal with an appropriate short-acting insulin dose, in practice, the doses are difficult to calculate and anticipate. The level of control will be poor, with increased risk of hypoglycaemia.

b **True.** This regular pattern of eating can be followed by many people. Twice-daily insulin (usually mixed short-acting/medium-acting combinations) doses can be adjusted to achieve excellent control. The between-meal and bedtime snacks are *essential* to avoid the risk of hypoglycaemia in the majority of patients.

c **True.** This pattern of eating is favoured by many people, due to demands of both work and leisure. It can normally be matched by a regimen involving short-acting insulin pre-prandially, and medium-acting insulin given at bedtime *with a snack to avoid nocturnal hypoglycaemia*. Between-meal snacks are usually not required. Patients have to acquire the skill of anticipating the insulin requirement for the meal which is to follow. Intelligent use of this approach by doctor and patient allows maintenance of excellent control, sometimes with normal HbA1c levels.

d **True.** This is one of the advantages of the q.d.s. regimen, although repeated exercises of this type are discouraged. The dose of short-acting insulin is omitted before the meal to be missed. Some patients however require a smaller dose of insulin at the usual time to avoid hyperglycaemia before the next meal.

e **False.** This eating pattern is sometimes favoured by 'figure-conscious' patients. There is no insulin regimen which can be safely adapted to it.

C.19 a **False.** This advice would be unwarranted. There are few, if any activities which cannot be handled safely by a correctly informed diabetic.

b **True.** Many sports people find this approach perfectly satisfactory. Even mowing a lawn, or a walk which is longer or brisker than usual often calls for a reduction in the *preceding* insulin dose. In some people, the hypoglycaemic effect of exercise carries on for 12–18 hours. By trial and error a reduction in one or two of the following insulin doses is then also necessary.

c **True.** This approach works well for some patients, although there is a tendency to overdo the caloric replacement, with consequent weight gain.

d **False.** Only in very exceptional cases is this necessary. High intensity, short duration competitive sport is perhaps the only situation where it may be needed.

e **False.** Except for the most low intensity sport (e.g. rambling or leisurely golf), this approach is not likely to work safely. Anticipating blood sugar changes is a safer strategy. Taking along fruit or a sandwich may be useful.

C.20 a **False.** The common and early symptoms of hypoglycaemia (tremor and sweating) are due to the release of catecholamines from adrenergic nerve endings and adrenal medulla. Only stimulation of appetite can be attributed to cerebral (strictly hypothalamic) glucopenia at these early stages. Confusion and coma are later and (fortunately) much less common features of hypoglycaemia, and are then due to the direct cerebral effects of low blood glucose.

b **False.** Brain damage is very rare after an individual hypoglycaemic episode, unless resulting from intentional and massive overdose of insulin (or occasionally oral hypoglycaemic drugs). Its rarity is due to the release of catecholamines, growth hormone, glucagon, and cortisol in response to the hypoglycaemia, all of which tend to rapidly restore blood glucose to normal by enhancing gluconeogenesis.

c **True.** The ability to maintain blood glucose at near-normal and often subnormal levels, using multiple daily insulin doses and conscientious self-monitoring often results in blunting of the adrenergic warning symptoms. This is possibly due to down-regulation of adrenergic receptors by chronically elevated plasma catecholamine levels. Similar loss of warning symptoms is also seen in long-standing diabetes, and is due to autonomic neuropathy, which inhibits catecholamine release.

d **True.** Post-hypoglycaemic hyperglycaemia (Somogyi effect) occurs frequently, and is due to the excessive release of the homeostatic hormones mentioned in (b) above. In its nocturnal form, it is referred to as the 'dawn effect'. It is often not recognized because the hypoglycaemic 'trigger' is inapparent. The phenomenon is important since the hyperglycaemia is treated (paradoxically) by reducing rather than increasing insulin dosage.

e **True.** Even subclinical episodes can cause brain dysfunction in a cumulative manner. Psychological studies reveal loss of cognitive function in such patients. Dementia is an occasional additional consequence in (particularly) older patients where the process of brain damage is accelerated by the coexistence of cerebrovascular disease.

C.21 a **False.** Only beta-adrenergic blockers (particularly non-selective ones like propranolol and nadolol) potentiate hypoglycaemia, by blocking the restorative action of catecholamines. No other hypotensives have this effect. For this reason it is safer to avoid beta-adrenergic blockers in diabetics on insulin.

b **False.** All alcoholic drinks, whether 'neat' (as in brandy or whisky) or diluted (mixers or beers) block the breakdown of glycogen to glucose (glycogenolysis) which is so essential to the body's response to hypoglycaemia, should it occur. For safety, food should always accompany alcohol on every occasion.

c **False.** It is always safer to anticipate the effect of exercise rather than treating the resulting hypoglycaemia.

d **True.** Glucagon is available in travel packs for this purpose. An accompanying person need to be shown the procedure in advance.

e **True.** Unless being treated on diet alone or with metformin, *every* diabetic should carry Dextrosol or lump sugar *at all times*. With the progressively greater emphasis on achieving normoglycaemia, even in non-insulin-dependent diabetes, the chance of inducing hypoglycaemia is greater.

C.22 a **True.** The development of both retinopathy and nephropathy is time-related, approaching a plateau of maximum prevalence of 80% and 60% respectively, after approximately 25 years duration. Both cross-sectional and longitudinal studies confirm that glycaemic control is the principal determinant of expression of both retinopathy and nephropathy in both IDDM and NIDDM. It has been estimated that for each 1% reduction in HbA1c, microvascular risk may be reduced by as much as 50%.

b **True.** Studies show familial clustering of proneness to microvascular complications. The existence of a maximum prevalence of these complications at the 25-year 'plateau' (often despite lifelong poor glycaemic control) represents additional circumstantial evidence for genetic modification of complication proneness. The determinants probably represent protective genes whose phenotypic pathways have not yet been identified.

c **True.** Both pathways are well recognized as being relevant. However, there are no clear data about activity of specific pathways, which might determine the component of the variance in complication development not determined by the level of glycaemic control.

d **False.** The Diabetes Control and Complication Trial (DCCT) study (USA) and a smaller study in Sweden have both shown that irrespective of the duration of previous poor glycaemic control, improved control statistically improves outcome in both retinopathy and nephropathy. Occasionally, there is a temporary worsening of retinopathy when good control replaces a long period of very poor control.

e **False.** The primary role of hypertension in the *development* of these complications is still somewhat unclear, although achievement of normal blood pressure in patients with microalbuminuria delays progression to overt renal disease. Once complications are established, however, treatment of hypertension has been clearly shown to retard progression of retinopathy and reduce the rate of progression to renal failure and the need for dialysis and transplantation.

C.23 a **False.** Exudates also occur. Some represent true diffusion of protein through effective capillary walls. Others are in fact areas of ischaemic retina due to capillary (and arteriolar) underperfusion or occlusion.

  b **False.** It is the exudates (and only to a much lesser extent larger haemorrhages) which affect vision, principally if located on the macula (diabetic maculopathy). In addition, the condition of macular oedema can supervene in retinopathy of all types.

  c **True.** The progression from background to proliferative retinopathy is influenced in part by the quality of glycaemic control and possibly by blood pressure. Furthermore, appropriately timed laser therapy also reduces the rate of progression to the proliferative phase. This underlies the importance of systematic and skilled annual retinal review, so that the earliest phases of preceding background changes can be tracked and treated at the appropriate time.

  d **False.** Pre-proliferative retinopathy is an important entity, represented mainly by intraretinal microvascular abnormalities (IRMA).

  e **False.** Altered visual acuity in diabetes always justifies specialist appraisal unless the changes are confidently due to refractive error (confirmed by restoration of visual acuity using a pinhole). However, serious pathology can occur in the retina without visual impairment, highlighting the essential nature of skilled annual retinal review.

C.24 a **True.** These are the key features. New vessel formation is promoted by incompletely characterized vascular growth factors which are released from ischaemic retina.

  b **False.** This stage of proliferative retinopathy is eminently treatable: laser therapy does indeed reduce the risk of preretinal haemorrhages (and subsequent risk of visual loss).

  c **True.** See (b) above. Laser therapy of new vessels and active bleeding sites, sometimes extending to panretinal grid laser application, has substantially improved the visual prognosis.

  d **False.** In a limited number of cases, vitreous surgery and treatment of retinal detachment may improve visual acuity, even when seriously impaired.

  e **True.** Raised intraocular pressure reduces the pressure gradient across capillary, venular, and arteriolar walls, thereby lessening the severity of haemorrhage in both background and proliferative retinopathy. However, glaucoma can also be the result of proliferative eye disease: new vessels in the iris (rubeosis iridis) may bleed and cause obstruction of the drainage angle.

C.25 a **True.** Abnormal and increased glycoprotein (advanced glycosylation end-products: AGE) and mucopolysaccharide deposition in the glomerular basement membrane are responsible for altered biophysical characteristics, allowing glomerular protein escape and later hypoalbuminaemia and subsequent nephrotic syndrome. The same process results in progressive glomerular sclerosis, potentially resulting in renal-failure.

b **True.** Albumin excretion of 30–300 mg per 24 hours characterizes microalbuminuria. Its presence relates strongly to later development of hypertension, overt nephropathy (dipstick-positive proteinuria and impaired creatinine clearance) as well as hyperlipidaemia and macrovascular disease (stroke, myocardial infarction, and peripheral vascular disease).

c **False.** End-stage diabetic renal disease is still a common indication both for dialysis and for transplantation. The effect of prompt recognition and earlier treatment at the microalbuminuric stage should reduce this rate.

d **False.** Even in originally normotensive diabetics with microalbuminuria, lowering of blood pressure (especially with ACE inhibitors) reduces the risk of developing renal dysfunction. Target blood pressures of 120–130 mm systolic have been advocated.

e **True.** These macrovascular events occur more frequently in the presence of microalbuminuria, and with even higher frequency in 'overt' nephropathy. The raised LDL– and reduced HDL–cholesterol together with increased serum triglyceride levels regularly identified in nephropaths may partly explain this relationship.

C.26 a **True.** This is the only current way of screening for early diabetic renal involvement.

b **False.** It needs two tests to be sure, since temporary increases of urine albumin occur with fever, exercise, and urinary tract infection. If a single screening test is positive, a repeat single specimen test should be performed within 6 months, or ideally a 24-hour laboratory-quantified urine albumin estimation. Key values for Micraltest are: >20 μg/litre, for urine albumin/creatinine ratio: >2.0 mg/μmol, and for 24-hour urine: 30–300 mg/24 hours.

c **False.** Irrespective of the presence of hypertension, treatment of patients with microalbuminuria significantly reduces the rate of development of overt nephropathy (dipstick-positive proteinuria and reduced creatinine clearance/glomerular filtration rate).

d **True.** This is necessary irrespective of whether microalbuminuria, proteinuria, or hypertension is present. Among other factors it influences the choice of oral hypoglycaemic agent and a variety of other drugs.

e **True.** Although this cut-off point is arbitrary, it is wise for such patients to have follow-up in a specialist unit. Patients may be alarmed by this, but it is important for them to recognize that they are at risk. There may also be other (readily remediable) causes for their glomerular dysfunction.

C.27 a **False.** As many as 20% of diabetics are hypertensive (= or >160/90) after 10 years duration. Only some cases of hypertension appear to be associated with nephropathy, suggesting 'clustering' of genes determining diabetes and essential hypertension.

   b **False.** Treatment of hypertension certainly reduces the rate of development of renal failure. In diabetics as in non-diabetics, it also reduces the risk of stroke, and to a lesser extent of myocardial infarction.

   c **True.** The annual check of blood pressure is essential. Apparent 'white coat hypertension' should not be dismissed as insignificant: data suggest that many cases become 'permanent': interim measurements by practice nurse or electronic self-monitoring equipment are advised. Once hypertension is identified and treated, minimum 4-monthly checks are essential to confirm compliance and continued control.

   d **False.** Whereas 160/90 is widely accepted as 'safe' in non-diabetics, data support a target pressure of 140/80 in diabetics, and ideally 120–130/80 in younger diabetics, particularly in the presence of microalbuminuria.

   e **False.** Although correction of hypertension by any of the major groups of hypotensives has been shown to be beneficial, current research shows better responses with ACE inhibitors. Part of this benefit may accrue from the lower adverse effect profile of ACE inhibitors, leading to better compliance. For the moment, this appears to be the drug group of choice, particularly the longer-acting analogues which can be administered once daily.

C.28 a **True.** The enzyme aldose reductase is widely distributed in neural tissue. Sorbitol, the sugar alcohol resulting from the action of aldose reductase on glucose, is neurotoxic. Experimentally, neuropathy can be prevented by aldose reductase inhibitors. Clinically, there is little or no benefit on established neuropathy, presumably because or irreversibility of pre-existing nerve damage.

   b **True.** Nerve biopsy shows frequent occlusive lesions, which probably contribute to the irreversible nature of most neuropathic findings.

   c **True.** Both motor and sensory nerve conduction velocities are slowed in acute hyperglycaemia, and are reversible by restoration of normoglycaemia.

   d **False.** Long-standing neuropathy of this type is associated with demyelination and axonal death. Little if any improvement can be expected even with restoration of normoglycaemia.

   e **False.** Prevalence of neuropathy is related both to the duration of diabetes as well as the integrated level of preceding glycaemic control.

C.29 a **False.** Paresthesiae may occur early in neuropathy. However, in most cases of symmetrical sensory neuropathy, objective changes are present before the patient volunteers any sensory symptoms. This highlights the importance of regular neurological review.

b **True.** Although loss of modalities of light touch, pain, and temperature all may occur in sensory neuropathy, they are inconstant and often late-appearing. Accordingly, identification of neuropathy by loss of vibration perception and ankle reflexes are more helpful as a 'hallmark' of neuropathic change.

c **True.** Peripheral vascular disease alone is rarely a cause of ulceration and gangrene. It is the associated sensory neuropathy which predisposes to unnoticed minor injury which in turn often triggers major foot problems.

d **True.** Improved glycaemic control does benefit some patients: more often, paresthesiae are persistent. Some benefit accrues from the use of topical capsaicin cream, or the use of carbamazepine, tricyclic antidepressants, and octreotide injections. Lignocaine infusions also help some patients.

e **False.** Cranial nerves, especially the 3rd, 4th, 6th, and 7th are typically affected, sometimes at the onset of diabetes, or during a period of poor glycaemic control. Cranial neuropathy is almost always (spontaneously) reversible. Whether vascular or metabolic factors predominate is unknown.

C.30 a **False.** Most studies place the relative risk as high as 8 times that of the general population. Macrovascular occlusive events are the major cause of morbidity and mortality, particularly in NIDDM, and contribute the highest cost factor to the diabetes care budget.

b **False.** It was thought that glycaemic control was irrelevant to the development risk of macrovascular disease. Recent studies show a significant, albeit minor contribution. The diet which predisposes to diabetes either directly or via hyperlipidaemia, may itself be atherogenic. Insulin resistance which is commonly present in type 2 diabetes links with hyperlipidaemia and hypertension to produce a particularly atherogenic profile (variously termed the insulin-resistance or metabolic syndrome, or (Reaven's) syndrome 'X'.

c **False.** Although intervention (prevention) studies are not yet available to assess the effect of lipid-lowering medication on the natural history of occlusive vascular disease, cross-sectional studies reveal a very strong association between hyperlipidaemia and macrovascular disease.

d **True.** The presence of microalbuminuria further increases the risk of occlusive events, especially myocardial infarction by about 20 times. A variety of factors, including fibrinogen, plasminogen activator inhibitor (PAI), and other haemorheological variables are known to be abnormal in microalbuminuric patients. The nature of this link is not yet known.

e **False.** Smoking contributes a significantly greater vascular risk to the diabetic than to the non-diabetic. Because other treatment strategies for diabetes have at best a minor benefit on *macrovascular* risk, it is even more important to avoid smoking as a contributory factor.

C.31 a **True.** Myocardial infarction is painless (and therefore often unrecognized) in approximately 20% of episodes in diabetics, compared with 10% of episodes in non-diabetics. This is due to the high incidence of subclinical autonomic neuropathy.

b **True.** The reason may relate to a relative lack of coronary anastomotic/collateral vessels in diabetic macrovascular disease, multi-vessel disease, or to pre-existing myocardial damage from previous subclinical ischaemic episodes. Metabolic factors may be significant, since prompt treatment of patients suffering from recent infarction with glucose and insulin infusions reduces the mortality rate, but not to that level seen in non-diabetics.

c **False.** Distal vessels are more seriously affected in diabetic vascular disease. This renders bypass surgery for gangrene and intermittent claudication somewhat less successful in diabetics.

d **True.** Hypertension is common in diabetes. In some cases this is due to a renovascular aetiology based on atherosclerotic segmental renal artery stenosis. Nevertheless, only occasionally is it possible to correct hypertension by surgical correction (or retrograde balloon angioplasty).

e **False.** Current data in diabetics are circumstantial rather than definitive. However, as in non-diabetics the likelihood of benefit in terms of reduced occlusive episodes is high. Accordingly, unless there are contra-indications (known gastroduodenal ulceration: aspirin-precipitated asthma) aspirin is now often recommended in NIDDM patients as primary prevention.

C.32 a **False.** This is exactly the type of footwear recommended for diabetics. Open-toed shoes, hard uppers, and thin soles liable to penetration represent an unnecessary hazard. This practice should start early, so that when feet are or become 'at risk' from neuropathy/vascular disease, this preventive strategy is already in place.

b **False.** Feet *should be* washed daily, and carefully inspected at the same time for minor injury or infection (e.g. fungal). Only if incompletely dried does this practice present a hazard. *Modest* use of talcum powder avoids this risk.

c **False.** Over age 60, decreasing visual acuity (presbyopia, cataract, and retinopathy) and less steady hands, coupled to the likelihood of 'feet at risk' (peripheral vascular disease/peripheral neuropathy) are a collective hazard. Although a capable friend or relative may suffice, professional (state-registered) chiropody/podiatry is preferred, *even for basic nail cutting.* Such visits also help to re-inforce healthy foot-care practice.

d **True.** Even indoors there are hidden hazards: splinters, pins, and even sharp-edged cardboard in carpet pile. Barefoot walking is universally unwise in diabetics.

e **True.** Although often advertised as being safe, even the mildest foot problem should be attended to by a chiropodist/podiatrist.

C.33 a **False.** The shoes may be totally unsuitable or far too tight. Either the doctor (if he/she feels confident) or preferably a chiropodist/podiatrist should examine the shoes in question. They may need to be discarded.

b **True.** Because of the inherent risks of these underlying complications, it is wise to check at this stage whether these, or any other factors are present which might delay healing. A check of HbA1c or fructosamine may be wise, since poor glycaemic affects tissue repair and proneness to infection.

c **False.** Unnecessary exposure may risk infection. A simple dry dressing is required.

d **False.** There is no evidence that application of antibiotic creams or ointments is helpful. However, a swab for culture and sensitivity would be wise, even if the lesion is not clinically considered to be infected.

e **False.** Relying on a patient of this age, possibly with suboptimal vision, to make a decision on healing represents an unnecessary risk. The potential for serious consequences is such that the lesion should be professionally reviewed within a week to confirm that healing is occurring. This provides the opportunity of ensuring that the culture report is seen and that the result of HbA1c or fructosamine is actually reviewed.

C.34 a **True.** The toe is clearly infected: immediate commencement of antibiotics is essential. Additional metronidazole might be wise, even in the absence of positive identification of anaerobic organisms on culture, since these often coexist, particularly with deeper infection. Anaerobic infection may have occurred in the last few days since the original swab was taken.

b **True.** Although it is probably too early to show change, a baseline X-ray of the foot should be done. Sometimes early osteomyelitis may be seen, probably because the lesion has been present for longer than the patient is aware (or admits to!).

c **False.** HbA1c and fructosamine, although useful do not reflect *current* control (i.e. that day!). Infection of this type can destabilize diabetes very rapidly. Blood glucose and urinary ketones should be checked: immediate changes in diabetes treatment may be needed.

d **False.** Because of his neuropathy, his heat perception may be seriously defective. Scalding could further compromise his toe. The toe should also be kept dry at this stage.

e **True.** He should be seen within 24 hours, and probably admitted to hospital forthwith. Close monitoring of progress with high-dose antibiotics (possibly given IV) is essential. The risk of septicaemia is high. In the presence of peripheral vascular disease, even amputation may prove necessary.

*C.35*** a **False.** In most studies, the figure is closer to 30%. Raised serum triglycerides and reduced HDL cholesterol are the common abnormalities, less so in well-controlled (normoglycaemic) cases, and contribute to enhanced atherogenesis in NIDDM patients. Hypercholesterolaemia may be present as an associated risk factor, but is no more frequent than in similar weight non-diabetics, unless in the presence of poor glycaemic control.

b **True.** In the presence of insulin resistance, lipolysis increases with associated increased free fatty acid delivery to the liver resulting in increased triglyceride synthesis. Reduced lipoprotein lipase activity (also a consequence of insulin resistance) further reduces VLDL clearance.

c **False.** Poor glycaemic control, whether in IDDM or NIDDM, increases triglyeride levels as a consequence of enhanced lipolysis. Although triglyceride represents a less important lipid than cholesterol in the process of atherogenesis, these changes are nevertheless likely to be the basis of the enhanced atherogenesis now known to occur in sub-optimally controlled diabetes.

d **True.** The nephrotic syndrome of diabetic nephropathy causes rises in total and LDL–cholesterol, possibly due to non-specific activation of hepatic protein synthesis by hypoalbuminaemia. Progression to chronic renal failure causes striking reductions in hepatic lipase and postheparin lipolytic activity. VLDL and triglyceride levels rise.

e **False.** It is precisely these drugs which have no adverse lipid effects, and are therefore preferred in the treatment of hypertension and cardiac problems which occur in people with diabetes. Loop and thiazide diuretics, as well as beta-adrenergic blocking drugs elevate LDL and reduce HDL levels, and may raise triglyceride levels as well. Low-dose thiazide diuretics (equivalent to 2.5 mg bendrofluazide daily) are probably immune from these consequences.

C.36 a **False.** Dietary review is clearly sensible, both to review the potential for calorie restriction as well as ensuring appropriate diet in relation to her hyperlipidaemia. However, metformin is preferred to a sulphonylurea, since it may help her to lose weight, and also reduces insulin resistance, the main factor in her lipid profile. There are no contra-indications in her case.

b **True.** Its worth a try! She has a 'full hand' of coronary risk factors and is otherwise destined to share the fate of her relatives. She should be motivated to make some changes to her lifestyle.

c **False.** Not yet. First, the hypercholesterolaemia may be partly due to poor glycaemic control (which you are correcting). Second, improved control, weight loss (one hopes), and the reduction in insulin resistance produced by metformin may help other aspects of her lipid profile. In fact, after achieving control, it is likely that her cholesterol will fall: with her low HDL, use of a fibrate may prove more successful than a statin.

d **False.** Changing to a beta blocker will make it harder for her to lose weight, and may worsen her hyperlipidaemia. Either increase the dose of amlodipine, or use alpha blockers or an ACE inhibitor, both of which are 'inert' as far as lipids are concerned.

e **True.** Certainly. There is no contra-indication. HRT should also be considered, unless there are any contra-indications. Current data suggest an important additional reduction in coronary risk of 20–30%.

C.37 a **False.** Fertility is quite normal in diabetics (male and female), and any infertility has to be ascribed to other causes.

b **True.** Prevalence of both mild and severe congenital abnormalities has decreased with the improved levels of glycaemic control achieved *before* conception. The correct strategy is for diabetics to be told of this risk, and advised to avoid becoming pregnant until informed that glycaemic control is optimal.

c **True.** Not only miscarriage, but also pre-eclampsia, hydramnios, intrauterine death, still-birth, and prematurity occur more frequently. Better glycaemic control during pregnancy has been shown to decrease the frequency of all these complications.

d **False.** Large babies are a consequence of poor glycaemic control. High maternal blood glucose levels transplacentally stimulate fetal hyperinsulinaemia. It is this which acts as the main growth-promoting stimulus to the fetus, affecting all organs (fetal macrosomia).

e **False.** Neonatal hypoglycaemia (due to the same mechanism as in (d) above), and hypocalcaemia (cause uncertain) are quite common. Of greater seriousness is the sometimes fatal neonatal respiratory distress syndrome due to abnormalities in pulmonary surfactant. Diabetes itself, together with Caesarean section and any prematurity separately or together contribute to this risk.

C.38 a **True.** In terms of glycaemic fluctuation and HbA1c, there are few pregnancies in which improvement is not seen. A significant proportion of this phenomenon is due to greater commitment of the woman and the higher professional input. The pregnancy itself appears to have some stabilizing effect, although the mechanism is not understood.

b **False.** Continuation of oral hypoglycaemic drugs is considered unwise. Trans-placental passage of the drug risks fetal β-cell stimulation, with hyperinsulinaemia and its consequences listed in 37d and e (above). There is also uncertainty about the potential teratogenicity of sulphonylurea drugs.

c **False.** Proliferative retinopathy often deteriorates during pregnancy with a proneness to retinal haemorrhage. This tendency has been less obvious since the provision of better antenatal ophthalmic assessment and laser therapy to affected retinae. Nephropathy substantially worsens fetal prognosis, particularly if serum creatinine is already raised. In turn, possibly because of altered renal haemodynamics, renal function may deteriorate in pregnancy.

d **True.** The mechanisms of 'insulin resistance' in pregnancy are multiple, including placental secretion of human placental lactogen/somatotrophin (hPL), increased free cortisol levels (partly stimulated by an apparent placental ACTH-like peptide). Pituitary somatotrophin (hGH) is also raised and the placenta expresses insulinase activity.

e **False.** Ketogenesis in pregnancy is increased, partly because of lipolysis secondary to hPL secretion. Ketonuria may also be sue to insufficient calorie intake. Ketoacidosis is particularly serious with a 20–50% risk of intrauterine death if late-recognized or suboptimally treated.

C.39 a **True.** At least 1 in 20 pregnancies (5%) are complicated by gestational diabetes, as identified by post-prandial blood glucose screening and glucose tolerance testing at the 28th week of pregnancy. This procedure has become routine in most obstetric units.

b **False.** Unfortunately, there is no genetic or immunological marker for what is essentially an early presentation of non-insulin-dependent diabetes in most cases (the immuno-tolerant state of pregnancy make the onset of insulin-independent (type 1) diabetes during pregnancy a rate phenomenon).

c **False.** The incidence of all complications (see 37c–e) is higher than in non-diabetic pregnancy, but not to the levels encountered in pre-existing diabetes.

d **False.** Many cases are controllable on diet alone initially: however, over 50% ultimately require insulin in due course based on unacceptable blood glucose and HbA1c levels.

e **True.** Between 5% and 10% of women with gestational diabetes remain glucose-intolerant postpartum, and are then treated as 'conventional' non-insulin-dependent diabetes. However, even after initial postpartum normalization, 50% of women undergo a spontaneous transition to non-insulin-dependent diabetes within their lifetime. This aspect justifies regular and lifelong review of all women with gestational diabetes, ideally with annual post-prandial blood glucose screening. Diabetes is thus identified at the earliest possible time, and should minimize the risks of diabetic complications.

C.40 a **False.** Relying on antibiotics alone is hazardous. The response is likely to be slow at this age, and the uncontrolled diabetes may impair the cell- and antibody-mediated response to her infection. It is very possible that her diabetes control may further worsen, with the development of ketoacidosis.

b **False.** This action is not sufficient. She has clearly become insulin resistant as a consequence of the infection. It is better to give her a 'stat' dose of 4–12 units of IM (not subcutaneous) soluble insulin, 4-hourly monitoring of blood glucose, and a further similar dose in 4 hours if the blood glucose is not falling. *In addition*, an increased dosing strategy as outlined (or one which the patient herself knows will work) should be implemented already at the time of the next regular dose.

c **True.** Transient ketonuria is not uncommon in infection, especially if samples after an overnight fast, or if food intake is reduced. A positive re-test 4–6 hours later might be negative, and therefore identify a less worrying scenario.

d **False.** This step is not necessary. Calories are required for sick patients! If she cannot take solids, orange juice or similar sources of liquid calories are needed.

e **True.** This would be a perfectly appropriate step, if in-house supervision and your ability or availability to monitor her are less than ideal.

C.41 a **False.** You are taking a big risk: the fall in blood glucose should not lull you into a false sense of security. She almost certainly has ketoacidosis. In this age group even successful treatment in hospital carries a mortality risk of at least 10%. You have to convince her somehow of the need for hospital admission. Ideally, give 20 units IV and 20 units IM (or 40 units IM alone): in ketoacidosis this is quite safe. Subcutaneous insulin may not be absorbed at all if she is dehydrated and hypotensive. Even if the dose given is too much, she should be in hospital by the time any hypoglycaemic reaction occurs.

b **True.** Yes! Most of the mortality of ketoacidosis is a consequence of undue delay in making the diagnosis and getting the patient into hospital.

c **True.** This is probably worthwhile. You must not risk her vomiting and aspirating (a major complication of ketoacidosis). Make sure that the ambulance keep her airway clear, and are prepared to apply oral suction.

d **False.** An hour or two delay will not worsen her prognosis. Further inpatient assessment may identify an infection for which an alternative antibiotic may be preferable.

e **True.** If you have this handy, it should be done straight away. The ambulance crew will certainly have the necessary items once it arrives. At this age, correction of dehydration is a crucial issue in survival, and at least another hour is likely to pass until she reaches a casualty department, and can be reassessed and treated.

C.42 a **False.** Single boluses are usually less effective than an insulin infusion, due to heptic degradation and renal clearance of large doses. Infusion rates above those stated can be used if blood glucose is not falling progressively (approximately 20% per hour).

b **False.** The administration of insulin causes massive intracellular shifts of glucose, accompanied by potassium (and magnesium). *Hypokalaemia* is the risk. In the elderly, this may induce fatal arrhythmias, particularly in the presence of digoxin. Potassium should be added to the infusate prophylactically, even if the patient is initially hyperkalaemic. Hyperkalaemia is due to extracellular movement of potassium induced by acidosis: whole body potassium is invariably low in DKA.

c **True.** Insulin alone will suppress lipolysis, and in turn ketogenesis, raising blood pH in all but the most severe cases. Excessively rapid normalization of blood pH produces CSF/blood pH disequilibrium which can further impair consciousness.

d **True.** This is a more sensible strategy than simply accelerating crystalloid (e.g. saline) infusion. Although many patients with diabetic ketoacidosis (DKA) are 6 or more litres in negative fluid balance, in this age group overhydration with its consequences of cerebral and pulmonary oedema is a real risk. Colloid helps to achieve intravascular volume expansion, maintaining all-important cerebral, coronary, and renal perfusion.

e **False.** Once she vomits and aspirates, it may be too late! A naso-gastric tube (correctly positioned) is essential as an immediate admission procedure. The airway must be protected during insertion.

C.43 a **True.** The very reason for the 'non-ketotic' state is the continued presence of insulin which inhibits ketogenesis. A common scenario is the precipitation of HONK by thiazide diuretics even in a previously undiagnosed diabetic. The thiazide both elevates the blood glucose as well as causing dehydration. The polyuria is taken for granted as an effect of the diuretic!

b **True.** The serum hyperosmolarity and dehydration increase blood viscosity and increase platelet aggregation, predisposing to thrombosis in key major vessels. It is these occlusive/ischaemic events which dictate the 50% mortality of HONK.

c **False.** The absence of acidosis renders patients with HONK relatively insulin-sensitive. Although blood glucose levels are sometimes well above 50 mmol/litre (900 mg/100 ml), there is no urgency about lowering these levels, providing that the patient is being rehydrated. Glucose reduction rates of 10–15% per hour suffice. Excessively rapid correction of hyperosmolarity can contribute to cerebral oedema (see d below).

d **False.** Although replacement with hypo-osmolar fluid seems rational in the presence of what is usually marked hypernatraemia, patients with HONK are in fact sodium-depleted. Progressive reduction of blood glucose and rehydration with saline (and later dextrose or dextrose–

saline) usually suffices to normalize serum osmolarity. Hypotonic fluids seriously risk cerebral oedema.

e **True.** The episode of HONK has in no way altered the fundamental biochemistry of type 2 diabetes (NIDDM).

SAQ Answers

C.44

Prevalence of diabetes is directly related to prevalence of obesity. Correction of obesity is fundamental to control of diabetes. Calorie restriction is essential component (coupled to increased physical activity). Avoidance of refined carbohydrate (sugar, sweet biscuit, soft drinks) with some allowance if sugar is taken simultaneously with other foodstuffs. Avoidance of excess fat intake (9 calories/gram! compared with 4 calories/gram for carbohydrate and protein). Fat limited to 40% of total calories consumed. Preference for vegetable (polyunsaturates) and low dietary cholesterol (eggs specifically). Maintenance of high fibre intake (ideally more than 15 g daily). Supplemental high fibre products (and drugs) to supplement fibre intake.

C.45

The five commonest manifestations of autonomic neuropathy:

Postural hypotension: relevant when patients have symptoms suggesting hypoglycaemia (but actually due to BP fall). Important to recognize when hypertensive diabetics are on treatment (risk of overtreatment). Possibly relevant to development of stroke in older patients. Symptoms treatable by head-up bed-tilt (to 'train' baroreceptors); fludrocortisone, ephedrine, and occasionally elastic stockings. Some cases apparently reversible by immaculate glycaemic control.

Impotence: only about 50% of cases in diabetics due to this aetiology: others due to arterial insufficiency and psychological causes. Both erectile and ejaculatory forms recognized (the latter with retrograde ejaculation as well, causing infertility). Treatment by topical glyceryl trinitrate, vacuum methods, intracavernosal papaverine, and prostaglandin, and occasional insertion of semi-rigid prosthesis.

Bladder dysfunction: causing outflow obstruction and incomplete bladder emptying (consider with recurrent urinary tract infection). Some cases respond to triple voiding plus suprapubic pressure, avoiding residual urine and its consequences. Alpha-adrenergic blockers sometimes helpful, but bladder neck resection sometimes required.

Diabetic diarrhoea: increased bowel frequency, often with characteristics of steatorrhoea. Due to reduced bowel motility and secondary bacterial overgrowth. Most cases respond to either metronidazole or teteracyclines, in short repeated or continuous courses.

Gastroparesis: more common than clinically recognized (gastric motility and isotope clearance) studies confirm. Responsible for irregular food (and drug) absorption, diabetic instability, as well as more obvious symptoms of epigastric discomfort/ distension and occasionally vomiting. Cisapride often effective; pyloric surgery sometimes required.

C.46**

Foot care: need to avoid barefoot walking and self-pedicure, especially once feet are 'at risk' (neuropathy and/or peripheral vascular disease). Correct cutting of nails to avoid injury. Correct footwear and dangers of tight shoes. Avoidance of over-the-counter corn and callus cures. Hazards of incorrect footwear. Prompt notification of doctor, nurse, or clinic if any weeping foot lesion or discoloration noted. Importance of daily washing, drying, and careful examination of feet. (Ulceration and gangrene represents the single biggest personal and cost factor in diabetics.)

Avoidance/cessation of smoking: its relation to development of vascular disease in cerebral, coronary, and peripheral arterial systems. The benefits of ceasing smoking, even after decades. The consequences of occlusive disease in the three main arterial territories.

Diet and nutrition: avoidance of obesity, by maintaining appropriate food intake and highest attainable levels of exercise. Concepts of reducing fat intake (vascular and obesity risk) and the problem of 'hidden fats'. Limited allowance of refined carbohydrate (when mixed with other nutrients). The importance of fibre. Advantages of regular meals and the appropriate use of snacks. Avoidance of commercial 'diabetic foods' (on basis of expense and undesirability). Timing of meals in relation to hypoglycaemic drugs. Salt and alcohol limits.

Self-monitoring of glycaemic control: need for daily-alternate daily assessments. Blood monitoring more informative than urine (indeed essential in IDDM). Recording of results and the reasons for 'abnormal' readings as a form of biofeedback. The importance of negative urinalysis/optimal blood glucose levels ('diabetic control') in the context of avoiding/reducing complications. The need to consult nurse or doctor in the event of loss of control (as defined). Back-up confirmation of control by doctor's/clinic's assessment of HbA1c or fructosamine.

Blood pressure: the importance of maintaining normal blood pressure, and the potential consequences of not doing so. The need for checks ideally at 6-monthly intervals: more frequent if on hypotensive drugs.

How to avoid ketoacidosis/major loss of control: sick day rules: (a) need to continue hypoglycaemic medication, even if not eating; (b) continue calorie intake, in liquid if solids not tolerated; (c) more frequent self-monitoring when ill; (d) notify doctor/nurse if consistent high readings or polyuric/polydipsic; (d) in IDDM, test for ketones if urine blood glucose high, and notify doctor/nurse if positive; (e) the significance of vomiting and need to notify.

How to avoid/treat hypoglycaemia: recognizing hypoglycaemia. Risks of hypoglycaemia, acute and cumulative. The role of exercise and food omission as the major causes. Food supplement/dose reductions of hypoglycaemic drugs with increase of exercise. Anticipating the problem. Need to carry sugar/Dextrosol at all times. The role of snacks (especially bedtime) in IDDM patients.

Long-term complications and how to avoid them: the major impact on eyes, kidneys, and nerves. The importance of blood sugar, blood pressure, blood lipids, and smoking. The need for the annual review.

Annual review: The patient's responsibility for ensuring that it actually happens. What needs to be done for self-assurance [checks on BP, eyes (retinae/visual acuity), feet, glycaemic control—HbA1/fructosamine and what they mean, blood lipids, and diet.]

Pregnancy and its problems: optimal contraception. The need for good glycaemic control at conception. Possible complications of diabetic pregnancy. Relevant genetics of diabetes.

Driving (if applicable): potential dangers of delayed meals/hypoglycaemia, specific avoidance and actions to be taken (stop!). DVLA notification. Carry ID, in the context of accidents.

Identification: need to carry ID, preferably bracelet/pendant so that easily seen in event of accident. Reasons for this strategy, especially in IDDM.

C.47**

Overall increase of rate of infection due to poor humoral and cellular responses to infection in diabetes in general, and when uncontrolled in particular.

Staphylococcal infections: as related to poor diabetic control. Boils/furuncles and styes as frequent initially presenting clinical features.

Fungus/yeast skin infections: also related to poor control, especially in perineal and fingernail areas.

Necrobiosis lipoidica: unknown aetiology, but significant microvascular component: ulceration, paper-thin scarring, and serious disfigurement.

Xanthomas: eruptive (back, limbs, and buttocks) and tendon (hands, elbows, and knees): indicative of underlying dyslipidaemia, sometimes secondary to poor glycaemic control.

Xanthelasmata: location on upper and lower eyelids: not necessarily indicative of underlying dyslipidaemia (if so, usually type 2a).

Acanthosis nigricans: ridged, pigmented, hyperkeratotic lesions in axillae, groins, and neck folds. Its relation to *hyper*androgenism and to *i*nsulin *r*esistance (HAIR-AN syndrome).

Fournier's gangrene: necrotic perineal infection with ischaemic component.

References

Physiology

Topic: Hypertension and insulin resistance (metabolic abnormalities).

Livingstone, C. *et al.* (1995). *Clinical Science*, **89**, 109–16.

Topic: Insulin receptor substrate proteins and intracellular signalling.

Myers, M.G. *et al.* (1995). *Trends in Endocrinology and Metabolism*, **6**, 209–13.

Topic: Regulation of gene expression by insulin.

O'Brien, R.M. *et al.* (1996). *Physiological Reviews*, **76**, 1106–61.

Clinical

Topic: Diabetic microalbuminuria.

Alzaid, A. (1996). *Diabetes care*, **19**, 79–89.

Topic: Pathogenesis of insulin-dependent diabetes.

Atkinson, M.A. *et al.* (1994). *New England Journal of Medicine*, **331**, 1428–36.

Topic: The diabetic foot (symposium).

Bakker, K. *et al.* (1996). *Diabetic Medicine*, **13**, S5–S61.

Topic: Diabetes in pregnancy.

Hadden, D. (1996). *Postgraduate Medical Journal*, **72**, 525–31.

Topic: Impaired glucose tolerance (IGT) and undiagnosed diabetes.

Heine, R. *et al.* (1996). *Postgraduate Medical Journal*, **72**, 67–71.

Topic: Insulin resistance.

Krentz, A. (1996). *British Medical Journal*, **313**, 1385–95.

Topic: Diabetic ketoacidosis.

Lebowitz, H.E. (1995). *Lancet*, **345**, 767–72.

Topic: Long-term complications of diabetes. Nathan, D. (1993*a*). *New England Journal of Medicine*, **328**, 1076–85.

Topic: Diabetes control and complications trial (DCCT).

Nathan, D. *et al.* (1993*b*). *New England Journal of Medicine*, **329**, 977–86.

Topic: Therapy of type 2 diabetes.

Wolfenbuttel, B. *et al.* (1996). *Postgraduate Medical Journal*, **72**, 657–62.

Topic: Pathogenesis of non-insulin dependent diabetes.

Yki-Jarvinen, H. (1995). *Diabetologia*, **38**, 1378–88.

11 Hypoglycaemia and pancreatic tumours (Clinical)

Multiple Choice Questions

C.1

In regard to spontaneous hypoglycaemia (i.e. not related to antidiabetic hypoglycaemic drugs), which of the following is/are true?

a The usual threshold for development of symptoms is a blood glucose of 3.6–4.0 mmol/litre (65–72 mg/100 ml)
b Some insulin must be present in the circulation for neuroglycopaenic symptoms to occur
c Recovery from hypoglycaemia is mainly mediated by the action of glucagon
d Cortisol and growth hormone deficiency result in low blood glucose levels, but recovery from hypoglycaemia is not impaired
e The glucose threshold for triggering the release of each of the four major counter-regulatory hormones is identical

C.2

Which of the following drugs may alone cause hypoglycaemia (in the absence of other contributory factors)?

a Metformin
b Alcohol
c Beta-adrenergic blocking drugs
d Galactose
e Oral sulphonylureas

C.3

Which of the following may produce symptoms suggestive of, but not due to hypoglycaemia?

a Postural hypotension
b Hyperventilation syndrome
c Temporal lobe epilepsy (TLE)
d Transient (cerebral) ischaemic attacks (TIA)
e Phaeochromocytoma

C.4

A 45-year-old woman presents with a 6-month history of episodes of faintness, preceded by sweating and tremor. They appear to be aborted by eating sweets. You suspect hypoglycarmia, and a blood glucose level taken early next morning (pre-prandial) with various other blood tests reveals a value of 3.0 mmol/litre (55 mg/100 ml). Which of the following strategies would be appropriate as a next step?

a Self-testing of blood glucose by the patient on the occasion of the next episode
b Repeat blood glucose level after a 12-hour fast, with simultaneous measurement of serum insulin
c Hospitalization for a prolonged 72-hour fast
d A prolonged 5-hour glucose tolerance test
e Insulin suppression test

C.5

In the same patient hypoglycaemia with typical symptoms occurs after 14 hours of inpatient supervised fasting. Blood glucose is 1.5 mmol/litre (27 mg/100 ml), and the symptoms are rapidly absorbed with 50 g oral dextrose. Three days later, the laboratory reports serum insulin of 35 mU/litre (normally less than 6 mU/litre in presence of hypoglycaemia) Serum C peptide is also raised to 5 times the upper limit of normal. Which of the following diagnoses would fit this constellation of findings?

a Surreptitious administration of insulin
b Surreptitious administration of glibenclamide (sulphonylurea)
c Insulinoma
d Autoimmune hypoglycaemia
e Tumour-associated hypoglycaemia

C.6

In the above patient, sulphonylurea assay by HPLC is negative. She is now having frequent hypoglycaemic attacks which are difficult to control with oral glucose. Which of the following are appropriate next steps?

a Commence treatment with diazoxide to control her blood glucose levels
b Arrange MRI scan to image her (presumed) tumour
c Check serum calcium and prolactin levels
d Maintain a high level of physical activity pending treatment
e Avoid alcoholic drinks

C.7

A 65-year-old man presents with persistent dyspepsia. Gastrectomy and selective vagotomy were performed 5 years previously for a bleeding duodenal ulcer. He has been on a proton-pump inhibitor drug ever since, and dyspepsia recurs whenever this is ceased. Which of the following approaches may be of value in clarifying his problem?

a Check current drug-taking profile
b Take a detailed social history
c Refer for consideration of further gastric surgery
d Check serum calcium
e Check serum gastrin

MCQ Answers

C.1 a **False.** Blood glucose must fall below 3.0 mmol/litre (55 mg/100 ml) before symptoms occur. The concept that a rapidly falling blood glucose may cause symptoms at higher levels has been largely disproven.

b **False.** Glucose entry into neural tissue is entirely independent of insulin.

c **True.** Glucagon is the primary defence against hypoglycaemia, and without it full recovery does not occur: adrenaline is only important for glucose counter-regulation if glucagon is absent. Primary deficiencies of either do not cause hypoglycaemia, but if both are absent fasting hypoglycaemia will occur.

d **True.** These deficiencies both result in low fasting blood glucose levels, and a tendency to induction of hypoglycaemia by other factors. However, recovery from a hypoglycaemic episode is unimpaired (due to adrenaline and glucagon release).

e **False.** For adrenaline, glucagon, and growth hormone, the threshold for response is close to 3.7 mmol/litre (66 mg/100 ml). For cortisol, the levels is significantly lower at approximately 2.8 mmol/litre (50 mg/100 ml). There are further inter-individual variations.

C.2 a **False.** This drug increases glucose uptake by muscle cells by enhancing (insulin-independent) anaerobic glycolysis. However, suppression of insulin levels occurs as blood glucose levels fall, preventing hypoglycaemia. Accordingly, metformin only produces hypoglycaemia in the presence of insulin (either administered or stimulated by oral sulphonylurea drugs).

b **False.** Alcohol blocks glycogenolysis, but this is usually only clinically significant if glycogen stores are already depleted (prolonged illness or emaciation of any cause), or in acute or prolonged fasting. Alcohol also potentiates the hypoglycaemia produced by any other mechanism, since the normal (glucagon and adrenaline) corrective response to hypoglycaemia is dependent on glycogenolysis.

c **False.** They block the important adrenergic response to hypoglycaemia, but do not themselves cause hypoglycaemia, unless it has been induced by another drug (e.g. sulphonylureas or particularly insulin).

d **False.** Galactose only causes hypoglycaemia in the presence of the rare

(1:30 000) hereditary deficiency of galactose-1-phosphate uridyl transferase (due to a variety of mutations), which results in deficient glucose-1-phosphate and hence hypoglycaemia.

e **True.** Sulphonylureas are a major cause of hypoglycaemia, either in diabetics or more subtly taken 'factitiously', where the condition masquerades as an insulinoma.

C.3 a **True.** Sweating, faint feelings, and loss of consciousness are all part of this syndrome. In autonomic neuropathy, the symptoms are more marked in the presence of low blood glucose levels (especially if insulin-induced, although even then the symptoms are not due to hypoglycaemia itself.

b **True.** The hypocapnia and alkalosis secondary to this psychological response to stress/anxiety induces feelings of faintness, sometimes hunger and occasional loss of consciousness. Even 'simple' panic attacks simulate hypoglycaemia by inducing adrenergic discharge: dominantly sweating and tremor.

c **True.** The vegetative symptoms of TLE are highly variable, including sensations of hunger and faintness, sometimes culminating in abnormal behaviour and loss of consciousness.

d **True.** Although the age group is usually much higher than in the preceding disorders, faintness due to TIA may dominate. Of greater importance is the atypical presentation of hypoglycaemia in patients with coexisting cerebrovascular disease. Anatomically selective neuroglycopaenia occurs in those areas of the brain already compromised by borderline cerebral perfusion.

e **True.** The intermittent adrenergic discharge stimulates hypoglycaemia. In fact, during such episodes, blood glucose may actually be raised, due to catecholamine-induced gluconeogenesis from fat and glycogen.

C.4 a **False.** This is not an ideal approach. During hypoglycaemia, cerebral function may be impaired, and the test therefore may be unreliably performed and interpreted. However, it may be reasonable for a third party to do the test.

b **True.** This is all that is necessary in many cases and is the optimal first-line approach. A blood glucose less than 2.2 mmol/litre (40 mg/100 ml) coupled to a serum insulin of 10 mU/litre or more is highly suggestive. Nevertheless, the sensitivity of the test is well below 90%: further investigation is needed even if negative.

c **True.** This remains the definitive test. Failure to lower blood glucose to 2.2 mmol/litre (40 mg/100 ml) after 72 hours of fasting excludes insulinoma. The fast must be very closely supervised (for safety and for compliance!). It provides the opportunity of demonstrating Whipples triad: fasting-induced symptoms, verified (laboratory) hypoglycaemia at the time of the symptom(s), and a clinical response to correction with administered dextrose. At the time of the symptom(s) the sample is also split for insulin, C peptide, and proinsulin. Assay for sylphonylurea content is also essential (factitious hypoglycaemia).

d **False.** This is not very useful. Reactive lypoglycaemia (blood glucose falling to less than 3.0 mmol/litre (55 mg/100 ml) is found in 20% of normal subjects: only rarely is there a correlation between such 'hypoglycaemia' and symptoms. The condition is overdiagnosed and only occurs with significant frequency after gastric surgery (due to abnormally rapid glucose absorption) or in the early stages of diabetes mellitus (where there is delay in insulin release in response to the glucose challenge).

e **True.** Autonomously raised insulin secretion (as in insulinoma) can be identified either by giving IV insulin and demonstrating failed suppression of C peptide concentrations in response to the induced hypoglycaemia, or giving biologically active (but non-immuno-assayable) insulin (e.g. fish insulin), and demonstrating failed suppression of immuno-reactive insulin.

C.5 a **False.** Covert administration of insulin may even be achieved in a well-supervised hospital ward. However, exogenous insulin would reduce glucose which would in turn suppress C peptide secretion.

b **True.** Sulphonylureas produce roughly equimolar increases in endogenous insulin and C peptide. Serum assay for sulphonylurea compounds (by high pressure liquid chromatography: HPLC) forms a routine approach with this constellation of findings. (Accidental sulphonylurea administration in hospitalized patients is not rare, due to confusion with names of other drugs.)

c **True.** The findings are typical for insulinoma. However, it remains essential to differentiate the all-important covert administration of sulphonylureas (see b above) *in all cases*. Serum proinsulin is raised in insulinoma, but may also be elevated with sulponylureas.

d **False.** In this rare condition, islet-stimulating antibodies with intrinsic insulin-like action (analagous to stimulating thyrotrophin-like TSH receptor antibodies in Graves' disease) can induce hypoglycaemia. Depending on how these antibodies react in the insulin assay they register either high or low insulin levels, but C peptide concentrations are invariably reduced. Although islet cell-stimulating antibodies have also been proposed as a cause of hypoglycaemia, the condition is very rare. Theoretically, the constellation of findings would be similar to those of insulinoma and covert sulphonylurea administration.

e **False.** A variety of non-endocrine tumours particularly of mesenchymal origin produce IGF-II which has intrinsic insulin-like effects. Particularly large tumours also of mesenchymal origin appear to 'consume' glucose. By either mechanism, serum insulin and C peptide would be suppressed.

C.6 a **True.** As with all thiazide diuretics (but with greater potency and 'paradoxical' fluid retention), diazoxide suppresses insulin secretion and increases insulin resistance. It is capable of controlling blood glucose for many weeks or months. Verapamil, octreotide, and propranolol have also been used with some success.

b **True.** A number of imaging techniques could be undertaken. None is ideal. CT scanning, ultrasound (transoesophageal), and octreotide scanning can all be used and may display the tumour. Either coeliac axis angiography or (transhepatic) portal venous sampling are marginally better, while intraoperative ultrasound is often useful if preoperative localization is unsuccessful.

c **True.** Approximately 10% of insulinomas form part of a multiple endocrine adenoma syndrome (MEN-1). These tests form a suitable screening approach unless there are other significant clinical markers or a family history (where more detailed studies would be indicated).

d **False.** Physical exercise lowers blood glucose, more particularly in the presence of hyperinsulinism. It is to be avoided in this situation. Some patients with insulinoma first notice their hypoglycaemic symptoms during mild to moderate exercise.

e **True.** Alcohol potentiates hypoglycaemia however it is caused, by inhibiting glycogenolysis. This too should be avoided.

C.7 a **True.** Aspirin, non-steroidal anti-inflammatory drugs and therapeutic corticosteroids all produce recurrent dyspepsia and ulceration.

b **True.** Stress remains a potent cause of hyperchlorhydria and other functional disturbances of the upper gastrointestinal tract.

c **False.** This may prove to be necessary, but blocking drugs are often capable of maintaining such patients symptom-free indefinitely.

d **True.** Hyperparathyroidism (acting via hypercalcaemia) stimulates gastric acid secretion and accounts for part of the 'abdominal groans' symptom profile. In addition hyperparathyroidism forms part of the MEN-1 syndrome in which gastrinomas also figure prominently (see Chapter 14).

e **True.** Only measurement of serum gastrin will lead to a diagnosis of the rare gastrinoma. False elevation of serum gastrin is found in patients on H2 receptor blocking and proton-pump inhibiting drugs, so that these need to be discontinued for several days prior to sampling.

References

Clinical

Topic: Somatostatin analogue treatment of neuroendocrine tumours.
de Herder, W.W. *et al.* (1996). *Postgraduate Medical Journal*, 72, 403–8.
Topic: Gastrinoma.
Ellison, E.C. (1995). *Annals of Surgery*, 222, 511–21.

Topic: Localization of pancreatic tumours.
Hammond, P.J. *et al.* (1994). *Clinical Endocrinology*, 40, 3–14.
Topic: Investigation of hypoglycaemia.
Marks, V. *et al.* (1996). *Clinical Endocrinology*, 44, 133–6.
Topic: Functioning islet-cell tumours.
Perry, R.R. *et al.* (1995). *Journal of Clinical Endocrinology and Metabolism*, 80, 2273–8.
Topic: Drug-induced hypoglycaemia.
Selzer, H.S. (1989). *Endocrine and Metabolic Clinics of North America*, 18, 163–84.
Topic: Insulinoma.
Service, F.J. *et al.* (1991). *Mayo Clinic Proceedings*, 66, 711–19.

12 Growth and development (Physiology)

Multiple Choice Questions

See also (Chapter 3 (Qs 5, 12–14, 35): Chapter 8 (Q 6); and Chapter 10 (Q 7)

P.1 Fetal growth
a occurs at the fastest rate just before birth
b is influenced by maternal nutrition
c is independent of sex
d is stimulated by fetal insulin production
e is generally reduced in mothers who drink more than 40 g alcohol daily

P.2 The pubertal growth spurt
a generally occurs earlier in boys than in girls
b is preceded by increased adrenal androgen production in both sexes
c is associated with an increase in somatotrophin production
d begins after sexual maturation has occurred
e is associated with increased bone density

P.3 In girls
a the first menstrual cycle usually occurs between the ages of 8 and 10 years
b the age of onset of puberty is earlier now than it was 150 years ago
c breast development is associated with increased oestrogen production
d the pubertal growth spurt is often associated with greater fat deposition than in boys
e puberty is delayed if blind from birth

P.4 In boys
a penile development is the first indicator of the pubertal growth spurt
b puberty is delayed or absent when adrenal corticosteroid production is increased
c peaks of increased gonadotrophin secretion first occur at night
d the gonadotrophin response to an exogenous bolus of gonadotrophin releasing hormone (GnRH) decreases after puberty
e the prepubertal plasma sex hormone binding globulin concentration is greater than in girls

P.5 *Tissue growth and development in adults*
  a occurs at an increased rate with age
  b is regulated mainly by adrenal androgens
  c is generally impaired in hypopituitarism
  d is influenced by thyroidal iodothyronines
  e normally is dependent on an adequate nutrition

P.6 *The growth and maintenance of tissues*
  a is generally influenced by locally produced factors
  b can be stimulated by oncogene products
  c such as blood vessels may be stimulated as a consequence of reduced blood flow
  d such as muscle is stimulated by excess circulating glucocorticoid concentrations
  e can be generally stimulated by increasing the daily food intake above the normal daily requirement

Short Answer Questions

P.7
Name *two* hormones which influence fetal growth and *briefly* indicate what effect an increased production of each of these hormones might have on it.

P.8
List *two* environmental and *two* fetal factors which might influence fetal growth, *briefly* explaining how the birth size/weight could be affected by each of them.

P.9
Briefly explain how the age of onset of puberty has altered over the last 150 years. Identify two possible reasons which could account for this phenomenon and *briefly* give one item of supportive evidence in favour of your considered most likely explanation.

P.10
Identify three hormones which influence growth and development of tissues in the adult, *briefly* explaining how any one of your three chosen hormones influences the growth process.

MCQ Answers

P.1 a **False.** The peak growth rate, estimated at approximately 30 mm/day, occurs at around the week 20 *in utero*. At no other time throughout life is there such rapid growth rate.

b **True.** Maternal nutrition is very important in determining fetal growth, as determined by direct measurement (e.g. using ultrasound) or from birth weight. A restricted food intake, for whatever reason, is associated with a reduced birth weight for example, even after taking account of other commonly linked economic and social factors. In addition to quantity, however, the nature of the food intake can also influence fetal growth. Thus, if the maternal diet contains more than average protein content, the baby at birth tends to have an increased linear growth, while if the intake contains more fat than the baby will also tend to be fatter at birth.

c **False.** On average, baby boys are bigger than baby girls at birth, and this is exemplified particularly in studies on twins. The reason is that male fetuses produce greater amounts of anabolic androgens than females, and they consequently have greater growth *in utero*.

d **True.** One demonstration of the growth-promoting effect of insulin *in utero* is seen in babies born of mothers who develop diabetes during pregnancy. These babies tend to be larger than average, and the explanation is that the raised blood glucose level in the mother stimulates the fetal β cells of the developing islets of Langerhans which consequently produce more insulin. The insulin controls the fetal blood glucose level but in addition it promotes protein synthesis.

e **True.** Various drugs, including nicotine and alcohol, have a detrimental effect on fetal growth even after taking account of other influencing factors which may be present, such as reduced diet. Consequently, birth weight is usually reduced and there is an increased rate of premature births (which is associated with decreased survival). Some surveys have indicated that impaired physical and mental growth and development is still apparent in children at the age of 11.

P.2 a **False.** The pubertal growth spurt begins approximately 2 years earlier, on average, in girls than in boys. In general girls begin their growth spurt between the ages of 10–14 years while boys usually reach this stage between 12–16 years.

b **True.** The first endocrine manifestation of impending pubertal growth spurt is the increased production of androgens from the adrenal cortex, in both sexes. This event is called adrenarche, and it occurs approximately 2 years before the more obvious manifestations of puberty. The role of the adrenal androgens is still unclear although one effect is to stimulate the growth of axillary and pubic hair.

c **True.** An increased amplitude of pulses of somatotrophin, coinciding with increased gonadal steroid production, acting together are likely to be the principal stimulators of the pubertal growth spurt and the development and maturation of the gonads, the reproductive tracts, and the secondary sex characteristics.

d **False.** The pubertal growth spurt begins before sexual maturation has occurred. However, by the time the pubertal growth spurt has ended, sexual maturity will have been reached in both sexes.

e **True.** Most tissues undergo growth and development at this stage, and this includes bone which does indeed develop an increased bone density, probably under the influence of the androgens and oestrogens.

P.3 a **False.** The occurrence of the first menstrual cycle is called menarche, and it usually occurs between the ages of 11 and 15, the average being of the order of 13 years. If any sign of sexual maturation occurs earlier than at 8 years of age it is considered to be indicative of precocious puberty.

b **True.** Records from many Western industralized countries have shown that the age of onset of puberty has declined steadily during the last 150 years, although latest studies show that the decline has halted (and indeed may even be reversing!).

c **True.** An early manifestation of the pubertal growth spurt is the development of the breasts. This is under ovarian oestrogen control, and five stages can be clearly identified. Stage 1 is the preadolescent phase, with only the papilla raised; stage 2 is the early breast bud stage; stage 3 is the further enlargement of the breast and the areola, the two still following the same contour; stage 4 is when the areola and papilla form a secondary mound above the general breast contour; finally, stage 5 is the adult breast when the enlarged areola has recessed back into the general breast contour, with only the papilla projecting out.

d **True.** Body composition in the two sexes at adulthood tend to differ, and the difference begins at puberty. Boys develop a greater lean body mass during adolescence (the period during which pubertal changes take place) than girls, who in contrast have approximately twice as much body fat by the end of the growth spurt.

e **False.** One of the possible explanations for the earlier onset of puberty since the Industrial Revolution some 150 years ago is our increased exposure to light. Certainly other animals are clearly influenced (e.g. sexually, cf. rutting in deer) by the seasonal changes in daylight, so it is a possibility. However, at least one study of the age of onset of puberty in girls who were blind from birth suggests that it is unlikely that exposure to light is a key factor. (See also Chapter 12, P.9.)

P.4 a **False.** In males genital development takes place under testicular androgen influence in clearly defined stages which compare with the stages of breast development in girls. Stage 1 is the preadolescent stage; stage 2 is the early growth of the testes in their scrotal sac (this certainly being an early indicator of pubertal growth), the texture of the scrotal skin becoming coarser and wrinkled; stage 3 is associated with further growth of the testes and scrotum but there is now an enlargement (in length and breadth) of the penis; stage 4 involves the further enlargement of the penis (the glans in particular) while the scrotal skin becomes darker; the final stage 5 is reached when adult proportions for the penis and testes have been reached.

b **False.** An increase in adrenal corticosteroids, particularly the adrenal androgens, will not have any inhibitory effect on the pubertal growth spurt although excessive glucocorticoids (e.g. cortisol) can inhibit linear growth. The onset of puberty is probably controlled by the hypothalamo–adenohypophysial axis, and involves the maturation of those neurones which release pulses of gonadotrophin releasing hormone (GnRH) into the hypothalamo–hypophysial portal system. The consequent increase in gonadotrophin production then stimulates gonadal steroid hormone synthesis and release, these being important determinants of pubertal growth.

c **True.** The gonadotrophins luteinizing hormone (PH) and follicle-stimulating hormone (FSH) are released in larger pulses during sleep, and this increased production will stimulate the development of the male genitalia. The first manifestation of sexual maturation in adolescent boys, comparable to menarche in girls, is probably erection of the penis (and spontaneous ejaculation) occurring at night.

d **False.** There is an increased release of gonadotrophins in response to an exogenous single bolus of GnRH in pubertal boys and girls which is similar to that seen in adults. This does not occur *before* puberty, when the response is greatly attenuated.

e **False.** Before puberty, the concentrations of sex hormone binding globulin (SHBG) in boys and girls are similar. At puberty there is a decrease in circulating SHBG concentration in both sexes but the decrease is greater in adolescent boys than girls.

P.5 a **False.** The processes of tissue growth and development (e.g. repair and replacement) tend to *decrease* with age.

b **False.** There will be many hormonal influences on tissue growth and development throughout adult life, one of which might well be by adrenal androgens. However, any effects of these hormones will be minimal, other hormones such as somatotrophin, and thyroidal iodothyronines, and insulin being examples.

c **True.** Hypopituitarism is associated with a decrease in circulating somatotrophin concentrations in addition to deficiencies in other adenohypophysial hormones. One important role of somatotrophin is to stimulate somatomedin production in the liver and other tissues, the somatomedins (insulin-like growth factors, IGF-I and IGF-II) acting as potent growth promoters. Thus, low levels of circulating somatotrophin and the somatomedins may result in attenuated cell proliferation and differentiation.

d **True.** The iodothyronines stimulate growth and the maintenance of tissues, and impaired repair and replacement of tissues is a common feature of hypothyroidism. At least part of the explanation at local tissue level may be the greatly reduced concentrations of IGF-I in the thyroid hormone deficiency state.

e **True.** In nutrition-deficient states tissue growth and development processes are impaired. Again, part of the effect is probably the decrease in circulating IGF-I concentration associated with reduced availability of protein and other energy substrates, even when somatotrophin concentrations may be within normal limits.

P.6 a **True.** Locally produced factors are probably the ultimate regulators of cell proliferation (mitosis) and growth (hypertrophy). They include many molecules, generally polypeptides, which may be ubiquitous such as IGF-I and IGF-II, or more tissue-specific such as nerve growth factors. The more ubiquitous molecules can be considered to belong to growth factor superfamilies such as the somatomedins, epidermal growth factors, fibroblast growth factors, platelet-derived growth factors, and the transforming growth factors. The more tissue-specific growth factors are also numerous and include the nerve growth factors, the cytokines (which include the interleukins) and the haematopoietic growth factors.

b **True.** Oncogenes are portions of viral genome which can induce neoplasia (tumorous growth) in host tissues. Some oncogenes contain the DNA code for normal cell products such as growth factors, while others encode for intracellular transcription factors or membrane protein kinases such as tyrosine kinase.

c **True.** One example is the serious complication of diabetes mellitus called proliferative retinopathy. This is believed to be a proliferation of new blood vessels into an area of the retina, brought about by local ischaemia of the tissue. The causes of the ischaemia are probably multiple and will be a consequence of the loss of insulin and its regulatory role on metabolism, particularly that of glucose. The thickening of basement membranes, the loss of endothelial cells, and the focal occlusion of capillaries will combine with other local pathogenic events to produce the retinal ischaemia which is associated with the promotion of new blood vessel growth.

d **False.** The opposite is more likely, in the presence of excess circulating glucocorticoid concentrations since cortisol stimulates protein catabolism. Indeed, the increased protein catabolism in Cushing's syndrome (due to excessive circulating glucocorticoids, e.g. cortisol) is associated with thin arms and legs, and a thin layer of skin over susceptible blood vessels which results in easy bruising.

e **False.** Providing that the level of nutrition is adequate, any further increase in daily food intake is unlikely to increase the growth and maintenance of tissues (other than adipose) generally.

SAQ Answers

P.7

The main hormones which influence fetal growth are insulin and the androgens, iodothyronines and oestrogens also having an effect. Somatotrophin and the somatomedins may have minor influences as may other hormones such as prolactin.

Insulin and the gonadal steroids stimulate protein synthesis promoting growth. Thus babies born of untreated diabetic mothers tend to be larger than average because the raised maternal blood glucose concentration stimulates fetal insulin production which results in increased protein synthesis. Likewise, male babies tend on average to be bigger than otherwise similar female babies because of the protein anabolic effects of androgens.

Oestrogens are milder protein anabolic agents which also increase fat deposition. Iodothyronines stimulate metabolism generally, and are important regulators of physical and mental growth and development after birth. However, thyroid deficiency *in utero* is not necessarily associated with a lower birth weight so the physiological importance of the iodothyronines on fetal growth is questionable. The adenohypophysial hormone, somatotrophin, is very important as a growth promoter after birth, but again its physiological relevance on fetal growth is in doubt. For example, anencephalopic fetuses (lacking hypothalamus) are not necessarily associated with a lower birth weight once the lacking tissue has been taken into account.

P.8

Various environmental and fetal factors determine fetal growth, any suitable combination of which would provide a correct answer. Many environmental factors may be directly linked to the mother, for instance, nutritional status, drug intake (e.g. alcohol, nicotine, etc.), diet, maternal age, and maternal weight, all of which may be related to socioeconomic status. Others may be indirectly linked to the mother, and these would include pollutants in the air (e.g. lead) or in the food (e.g. pesticides), or again nutritional status (e.g. famine and starvation). Many of these environmental factors which directly or indirectly linked to the mother, are associated with reduced birth weight and increased prematurity, the latter being associated with increased child mortality. Thus reduced nutritional intake, poor diet (e.g. low vegetable content resulting in reduced vitamin intake), drug abuse (alcohol, smoking, and other narcotics), youth and low maternal weight, and various pollutants in the environment have all been associated with a lower than normal birth weight and an increased prematurity rate.

P.9

Over the last 150 years, coinciding with the time elapsed since the beginning of the Industrial Revolution, the time of onset of puberty has decreased from an average age of 16 years to an age of approximately 13 years, as indicated by the age at menarche (AM). Over the last two decades there is evidence that the decrease has halted, and that the AM has stabilized, or even been reversed. Two possible explanations for the gradual decrease over the last century are: (a) the improvement in nutrition and health and (b) the increased exposure to light.

Various items of evidence, either supportive or dismissive, are available. Examples are the following:

(i) coincidence of social and economic improvements in conjunction with the development of technology and medicine, for instance regarding preventative medicine (e.g. realization of the importance of hygiene, purity of drinking water, sewage disposal, etc.);

(ii) that nutrition may be a key factor in determining sexual maturation (attainment of a target body weight correlates with age at menarche); and

(iii) that other animals have a sexual development that is determined at least party by the length of exposure to daylight; this may be related to pineal gland function. Normal sighted girls and girls born blind have a similar age at menarche (indicating that in humans, at least, exposure to light is not a key factor).

P.10

Various hormones influence the growth and development of tissues in the adult. These include somatotrophin, the somatomedins, insulin, androgens such as testosterone, oestrogens such as 17β-oestradiol, and the iodothyronines. In addition to the principal hormones stimulating metabolic processes, there are many local factors which are either specific or non-specific to particular cell types which stimulate growth and development at the local level, i.e. via paracine (cell to cell) or autocrine (cell on itself) effects.

The principal metabolic feature of tissue growth and development is protein synthesis, and somatotrophin (at least partly via the somatomedins), androgens, oestrogens (to a limited extent), and iodothyronines all stimulate protein synthesis. This metabolic process can be stimulated either directly by a genomic effect (e.g. by somatotrophin, somatomedins, androgens, insulin, etc.), or indirectly by stimulating amino acid movement into cells (e.g. somatotrophin, insulin, iodothyronines). Protein synthesis results from the formation of peptide bonds linking amino acids in a particular sequence, usually determined by the translation of the necessary information from mRNA synthesized in the nucleus following initial transcription from the DNA code present in the chromosomal genes.

Growth and development (Clinical)

Multiple Choice Questions

See also Chapter 4 (Qs 5, 6); Chapter 7 (Q10); Chapter 8 (Q14); Chapter 9 (Q4d, e)

C.1

In the documentation and interpretation of child and adolescent growth, which of the following statements is/are true?

a Growth velocity increases gradually from the time of birth until the immediate pre-pubertal period

b A 50% increase of growth velocity is usual at the time of puberty

c Three-monthly longitudinal/height measurement is necessary to establish a growth pattern

d Height-age represents the horizontal intercept on the 50th centile curve plotted from current height

e The mid parental height (MPH) is the mean of the heights of the parents

C.2

In deciding the need for further investigation of apparent 'growth failure', which of the following statements is/are true?

a A one-year prepubertal growth velocity above 6 cm per annum is unlikely to represent a significant growth problem

b In a short child, delayed bone age compared with height age is predictive of poor outcome of height at maturity, and an unlikely response to intervention

c The mid parental height (MPH) is a valid indicator of expected mature height (EMH) of the child under investigation

d An assessment of weight–age is unlikely to contribute important diagnostic information

e In pubertal or postpubertal short stature, knee epiphyseal maturity established by radiology provides a reliable indication of remaining growth potential

C.3

Which of the following conditions may be associated with prepubertal growth failure?

a Primary hypothyroidism

b Congenital adrenal hyperplasia (21-hydroxylase-deficient)

c Diabetes mellitus
d Klinefelter's syndrome
e Cranial irradiation

C.4**

In which of the following situations is short stature due to resistance to growth hormone action?

a Prolonged therapeutic corticosteroid therapy
b Malnutrition
c Cancer chemotherapy
d Hereditary GH receptor defects
e Turner's syndrome (gonadal dysgenesis)

C.5

In the syndrome of delayed puberty (small-delay syndrome: constitutional delay in growth and adolescence, CGDA) which of the following observations is/are true?

a The condition is more common in females
b A positive parental history of CDGA is common
c Bone age is markedly reduced compared to height age
d Serum gonadal and gonadotrophic hormone concentrations are usually diagnostic
e Intervention is required to avoid low final mature height

C.6**

Low birth weight and length (intrauterine growth retardation: IUGR) may have implications for subsequent development. In regard to this group of disorders, which of the following statements is/are true?

a Potentially preventable maternal factors are often present
b In the majority of cases, therapeutic interventions will not benefit final mature height
c Catch-up growth occurs in most cases
d Growth hormone deficiency is an important cause
e Low birth weight in an otherwise healthy infant is relevant to the development of disease syndromes in the adult

C.7

Which of the following conditions may be associated with excessively rapid growth velocity and tall stature during adolescence?

a Marfan's syndrome
b Klinefelter's syndrome
c Growth hormone producing pituitary tumour
d Congenital adrenal hyperplasia
e Hyperthyroidism

C.8

Most tallness is due to polygenic factors reflecting parental tallness. In this context, which of the following statements is/are true?

a Mature height can be estimated by doubling the child's height at age $1\frac{1}{2}$ years (girls) and 2 years (boys).
b Mid-parental height is a reliable method of predicting mature height
c Bone age is a critical variable influencing height predictions
d Early induction of puberty by gonadal hormone administration is a potential method of reducing final mature height
e Familial 'idiopathic' tallness is not mediated by endocrine mechanisms

C.9

In relation to the entity of *true precocious puberty*, which of the following statements is/are true?

a Most cases can be shown to have an underlying structural hypothalamic/ pituitary lesion
b Male patients are more likely to have an 'idiopathic' form of the disorder
c Serum LH and FSH concentrations are normal for the clinical stage of puberty
d GnRH stimulation fails to induce a rise in LH and FSH
e Treatment directed towards delaying pubertal progression is mostly necessary

C.10

In relation to the entity of *pseudo-precocious puberty*, which of the following statements is/are true?

a Hyperfunctioning gonadal tumours are a common cause of isosexual precocity
b Congenital adrenal hyperplasia is the commonest cause of contrasexual precocity
c Café-au-lait skin patches identify a specific adrenal cause
d Hyperthyroidism may present as precocious puberty
e Gonadotrophin agonists are not effective in treating pseudo-precocity

MCQ Answers

C.1 a **False.** Growth rate progressively declines from about 12–16 cm per annum in the first year to between 4 and 7 cm per annum immediately before puberty. Growth failure is evaluated either as relative shortness compared with centile distribution at the current age, and/or as reduced growth velocity. The usual criterion for concern is a measurement below 3rd centile. Both centile height as well as centile growth velocity charts are necessary for interpretation.

b **True.** Puberty growth spurt occurs about 2 years earlier in females than males, due to earlier maturation of the hypothalamic–pituitary–gonadal axis in girls. Gonadal hormones potentiate other growth factors, including growth hormone. It is often because of absence of the (expected) growth spurt that parents (and the child him or herself) is first aware of a problem in growth.

c **True.** Given the inaccuracy and observer variation in growth measurements, even if a quality stadiometer is used, 3-monthly measurement is essential to plot a reliable growth curve. Unless current height is well below the 3rd centile, growth velocity in the first observational year is an important parameter both for diagnosis, as well as for interpretation of response to any treatment provided.

d **True.** Height–age is an important extrapolation of current height. It is used as a point of comparison with simultaneous bone–age estimates, using reference hand X-ray norms based on Greulich and Pyle or Tanner–Whitehouse standards.

e **False.** Mid parental height (MPH) is the mean of: (a) the actual height of the isosexual parent and (b) the centile position of the heterosexual parent's height, transferred from the heterosexual to the isosexual growth chart.

C.2 a **True.** A growth velocity of 6 cm per annum represents the approximate 50th centile measurement for boys and girls in the three to four pre-pubertal years. Even if current height is 'suboptimal', growth velocities above 6 cm per annum are unlikely to identify signify a remediable cause.

b **False.** Bone age closely approximates neuroendocrine maturation, and correlates with pubertal rather than chronological age. It is inversely proportional to the potential for epiphyseal cartilaginous growth. In general, the more delayed bone–age compared with height–age, the greater the potential for growth and for response to endocrine or other interventions.

c **False.** The MPH is a useful indicator of ultimate height of the offspring (plus or minus 4–5 cm), but only assuming that no organic lesion is present. It represents physiological expectations, and is of greatest value in reassuring parents of children who are short due to the common paraphysiological entity of delayed puberty.

d **False.** Nutritional causes of short stature are common, particularly in developing countries. A weight–age less than height–age is generally found where there is a primary or secondary nutritional component to the short stature under investigation.

e **True.** Complete or near-complete fusion of knee epiphyses signifies that little if any further growth is possible, irrespective of cause, and provides guidance on the intensity with which further investigations should be pursued.

C.3 a **True.** In juvenile hypothroidism, growth failure may be the dominant or sole clinical presenting feature. Thyroid hormone is essential for the triple processes of pituitary growth hormone release, hepatic IGF-I production as well as response of growing epiphyseal cartilage. Bone–age is often lower than height–age (see also 8C14)

b **False.** This common form of congenital adrenal hyperplasia results in excess androgen production in both females and males (see also Chapter 5, C.9, 10). This is associated with growth stimulation prepubertally: children have above average height *initially*, but if either unrecognized (which may occur in less severe cases) or incompletely treated, they subsequently suffer premature epiphyseal fusion with a low *final* mature height.

c **True.** Poorly controlled juvenile diabetes (IDDM) results in poor growth rate as well as delay in puberty: good glycaemic control prevents this phenomenon. The mechanism may involve deficient IGF-I production secondary to insulin deficiency (which impairs GH binding protein and hence receptor function). In its extreme form (Mauriac syndrome), there is hepatomegaly coupled to extreme growth retardation. Short stature is also seen in rare syndromes manifesting peripheral tissue insulin resistance (leprechaunism and Rabson–Mendenhall syndromes).

d **False.** Klinefelter's syndrome is associated with hypergonadotrophic hypogonadism. Since almost all cases have some residual Leydig cell function, there is sufficient circulating testosterone to provide adjuvant growth activity for growth hormone action. Affected males are therefore of normal height during the prepubertal phase of growth. There is no pubertal growth spurt however, and androgen deficiency delays epiphyseal fusion, so that final mature height is on average above normal.

e **True.** This treatment is used for meningeal leukaemia and brain tumours in children, and in the past was also used to 'ablate' the thymus. Cranial doses upwards of 18 Gy increase the risk of pituitary damage, of which growth hormone secretion is the most sensitive indicator. Hypothalamic damage may be more important than involvement of the pituitary itself, since the hypothalamus is more radiosensitive.

C.4** a **True.** Glucocorticoids exert profound effects on growth. Even inhaled corticosteroids share this adverse reaction. Although high-dose cortisol and its analogues blunt hGH release in high dosage, and may temporarily reduce serum IGF-I, the major effects are on inhibiting the action of growth hormone and IGF-I on cartilage, suppressing chondrocyte mitosis and collagen synthesis. As expected, concurrent growth hormone therapy only partially reverses these processes.

b **True.** The effects of malnutrition are only partly mediated by a lack of nutritional substrate. IGF-I production is reduced secondary to malnutrition, and circulating hGH levels rise substantially, with increased hGH pulse frequency and amplitude.

c **False.** Cancer chemotherapy of different types induce gonadal damage but this is not likely to be a factor. It compounds the central (hypothalamic–pituitary) hGH effects of radiotherapy when used in treatment of leukaemia. Hypothalamic hypothyroidism also result from cranial irradiation. Only the malnutrition of the underlying disorder (see C.4b above) is likely to represent a contribution of growth hormone resistance.

d **True.** The so-called Laron dwarf represents a mutation in the hGH receptor gene; a complete absence of GHBP which is the extracellular domain of the growth hormone receptor. Growth response to administered IGF-I has been documented. Pygmies and other ethnically small races such as the Loja of Ecuador and the mountain Ok of New Guinea have variable resistance to hGH, due to reduced levels of GHBP.

e **True.** The short stature of Turner's syndrome is due to defective receptors in bone for both growth hormone and somatomedin (IGF-I). The defect is, however, only partial, and high doses of both hGH and IGF-I are individually capable of modestly increasing growth velocity and final mature height.

C.5 a **False.** Males are more commonly affected, for reasons which are not clear. CDGA is a diagnosis which should only be made in females after the most careful exclusion of other pathology.

b **True.** The age of hypothalamic 'maturation', characterized by the acquisition of LH and FSH pulsatility, is partly inherited. 'Immature' patterns of growth hormone release may also occur in CGDA: suboptimal growth hormone responses to provocative stimuli (e.g. exercise, arginine, hypoglycaemia) which are correctable by testosterone or oestrogen priming. The absence of a parental history increases the likelihood of an diagnosis other than CGDA.

c **False.** The stated combination is more consistent with primary hypothyroidism. In delayed puberty, bone–age and height–age are usually similar. In contrast, in growth hormone deficiency, height–age is usually disproportionately reduced compared to bone–age.

d **False.** The low serum gonadal and gonadotrophic hormone concentrations which are found in CGDA may also be encountered in hypopituitarism, malabsorption syndrome, and many other causes: only in gonadal dysgenesis is there a characteristic pattern of low gonadal and high gonadotrophic hormone concentrations. Both exercise and pharmacologically induced growth hormone responses may be confusingly low in CGDA, but be returned to normal by gonadal hormone and other forms of hypothalamic 'priming'.

e **False.** CGDA represents one extreme of a physiological range. A late growth spurt occurs with delayed epiphyseal fusion ensuring that final mature height is unaffected. Short-term testosterone or gonadotrophin therapy will trigger pubertal development, but not affect ultimate height. Such 'triggering therapy' may become preferred therapy if reduced bone density is confirmed in the follow-up of CGDA.

C.6** a **True.** Maternal undernutrition, alcohol excess, addictive drugs, and smoking are preventable factors. Nicotine reduces placental blood flow and affects placental structure. Evidence supports nutritional protein as contributing to linear growth, while fats contribute to fetal weight.

b **True.** Chromosomal anomalies (e.g. Turner's syndrome), osteochondro-dysplasias, and a variety of eponymous disorders of unknown aetiology (Seckel, Russell–Silver, Noonan, and Smith–Lemli–Opitz syndromes) account for a high proportion of cases. Gene mutations are probably responsible, and render the prospect of intervention remote. High-dose growth hormone therapy has been successful in some cases while epiphyses remain open.

c **False.** Catch-up growth is unpredictable, but the estimated mature height (based on mid parental height) is unlikely to be achieved in more than 50% of cases. It is more likely where maternal factors were responsible.

d **False.** Intrauterine growth is independent of growth hormone and its related somatomedin (IGF-I). A variety of other growth factors, particularly insulin, are highly relevant. In fetal life, insulin effects on intermediary metabolism are subdued, while growth-promoting effects dominate (see also Chapter 10, C.37d).

e **True.** Low birth-weight has been linked to a substantially higher preval-ence of obesity, diabetes, atherosclerosis, and hypertension in later life. The mechanism of this phenomenon is currently unknown, but it relates to babies who although small are otherwise normal, rather than suffering from any of the more defined causes of intrauterine growth retardation.

C.7 a **True.** This is due to a mutation in the epidermal growth factor region within the fibrillin gene (on chromosome 15). This defect subsequently affects a variety of tissues including the suspensory ligament of the lens (causing dislocation) and aorta (causing dilatation and aneurysm). The precise link with tall stature and long fingers (arachnodactyly) is still unclear. Homocystinuria and Sipple's syndrome (MEN-2) may produce a marfanoid appearance.

b **False.** Adolescent growth is normal, or even slightly delayed due to deficiency of androgens which are cofactors for both the release and action of growth hormone. However, androgen deficiency delays epiphyseal fusion so that the growth period is extended and average final mature height is approximately 5 cm above what would be expected on the basis of mid parental height.

c **True.** Growth hormone producing tumours are rare in adolescence, but do produce gigantism. Cerebral gigantism (Sotos' syndrome) confers acromegaloid features without growth hormone excess. A dilated ventricular system and mental retardation are common. The neuroendocrine mechanism of this disorder is unknown.

d **True.** In males and females with CAH, androgen excess leads to enhanced growth velocity in childhood. Accordingly, in untreated or suboptimally controlled cases, height in (early) adolescence is above normal. However, androgen-induced premature epiphyseal fusion in later adolescence risks ultimate below-normal stature.

e **True.** Thyroid hormones, acting via the thyroid hormone T_3 receptor complex directly increase the expression of the hGH gene and hence growth hormone release. Thyroid hormones also act directly via thyroid receptor β-isoforms found on osteoblasts and osteoclasts. The corollary is dwarfism seen in hypothyroidism and peripheral thyroid hormone resistance (see Chapter 8, C.14).

C.8 a **False.** This is an unreliable method, and the estimate only broadly valid for population means rather than assessment of individuals.

b **True.** Providing that accurate assessments of height are available for both parents, this method provides an EMH with an accuracy within plus or minus 4–5 cm. The method is described in C.1e. As mentioned in C.2c, it holds true only where no growth-limiting or -accelerating disorder coexists.

c **True.** Any disorder which delays or accelerates bone–age may invalidate the method referred to in C.8b above. Tables (Bayley and Pinneau) have been designed to assist prediction in this situation, taking into account the variables of current height, bone–age and the interval between bone and chronological age. Accuracy is again within plus or minus 5 cm.

d **True.** In principle, oestrogen administration to girls with enhanced 'normal' growth should accelerate epiphyseal fusion. In practice, such patients are often referred too late (beyond age 11) for benefit to be conferred. Furthermore, there are often psychological consequences of rapid and early induction of puberty. Treatment is even less successful in boys.

e **False.** Although non-endocrine genetic factors almost certainly predominate, tall stature may result from a familial trend to growth hormone hypersecretion and elevated IGF-I levels. Paradoxical hGH responses to both TRH and glucose (as seen in acromegaly) have been reported in some tall families (see Chapter 4, C.3). Conversely, parental heights of children with 'idiopathic' growth hormone deficiency have been reported as below average in some studies, here too suggesting familial growth hormone dysfunction.

C.9 a **False.** No identifiable lesion can be identified in more than 75% of cases. The disorder then represents an extreme end of the physiological range. As is the case in delayed puberty, it may be familial. However, an MRI scan is essential in all cases with pubertal onset under age 10 to exclude benign and malignant tumours such as hamartomas and gliomas, and benign lesions such as arachnoid cysts.

b **False.** Males are far more likely to have an identifiable organic, structural cause: 'idiopathic' cases are very uncommon. The reverse is true for females.

c **True.** In contrast to pseudo-precocious puberty (where LH and FSH serum levels are suppressed), serum LH, FSH, and gonadal hormone levels correspond to those expected for the pubertal stage. Females menstruate early, and both female and male patients are usually fertile.

d **False.** In keeping with pubertal stage, a positive response to GnRH identifies true precocious puberty, in contrast to pseudo-precocious puberty where this response is absent. It is this response, coupled to the biochemical characteristics noted in c above which in effect characterize true precocity.

e **True.** Untreated, the consequences consist of psychological disturbance (embarrassment and risk of sexual abuse in females) and short stature resulting from premature epiphyseal fusion. High-dose GnRH agonists down-regulate pituitary GnRH receptors and put puberty 'on hold'. They are frequently indicated, even where a structural lesion is identified and independently treated.

C.10 a **False.** Although testosterone producing interstitial cell tumours of the testis and granulosa cell tumours of the ovary do occur, they are uncommon. Similarly rare disorders include familial Leydig cell hyperfunction (testotoxicosis) due to a putative LH-like stimulator, and hCG producing teratomas and hepatomas.

b **True.** In females, late-presenting (non-salt-losing) 21-hydroxylase-deficient congenital adrenal hyperplasia is a common cause of contrasexual precocity. The same lesion in males produces isosexual pseudo-precocity.

c **False.** In the McCune–Albright syndrome, polyostotic fibrous dysplasia of bone coexist with patches, together with enlarged, sometimes cystic ovaries which are responsible for the hyper-oestrogenaemia these (the adrenals are normal). The precise genetic defect is unknown.

d **True.** Rarely, hyperthyroidism can occur as part of the (above) McCune–Albright syndrome. However, primary *hypothyroidism* is much more often responsible for precocious puberty (Van Wyk–Grumbach syndrome), in this instance paradoxically associated with short stature due to impaired growth hormone release and receptor function (see also C.3a). The precocity may be due to the effect of the excess α-subunit which is common to TSH, LH, and FSH.

e **True.** LH secretion is almost invariably suppressed. The only effect of GnRH agonists is to reduce pituitary LH release, so that this treatment is ineffective in psuedo-precocity. Where the underlying disorder cannot be directly corrected or reversed, antiandrogens such as cyproterone or the imidazole compound, ketoconazole (which inhibits conversion of 17-hydroxyprogesterone to androstenedione) can be used. In girls, tamoxifen may be effective.

References

Physiology

Topic: Review of growth hormone, insulin-like growth factors, their receptors and binding proteins.

Feld, S. *et al.* (1996). *Endocrine Reviews*, 17, 423–80.

Topic: Physiological effects of insulin-like growth factors.

Stewart, C.E.H. *et al.* (1996). *Physiological Reviews*, 76, 1005–26.

Topic: Growth hormone and ageing.

Xu, X. *et al.* (1996). *Trends in Endocrinology and Metabolism*, 7, 145–50.

Clinical

Topic: Precocious puberty.

Brook, C.D.G. (1995). *Clinical Endocrinology*, 42, 647–50.

Topic: Pseudo-hypopituitary syndromes.

Heinze, E. *et al.* (1992). In *Clinical Endocrinology and metabolism*,Vol. 6, pp. 557–71. Baillière Tindall, London.

Topic: Investigation of short stature.

Hindmarsh, P. *et al.* (1995). *Clinial Endocrinology*, 43, 133–42.

Topic: Delayed puberty.

Kulin, H. (1996). *Journal of Clinical Endocrinology and Metabolism*, 81, 3460–4.

Topic: Growth hormone insensitivity syndromes.

Savage, M.O. *et al.* (1995). *Acta Paediatrica*, 411(**Suppl.**), 1465–71.

13 Obesity, lipid metabolism and its disorders (Physiology)

Multiple Choice Questions

See also Chapters 4 (Q 14); Chapter 7 (Q 13)

P.1 Dietary lipids
   a are mainly digested in the stomach
   b such as the triglycerides are converted to cholesterol in the gut lumen
   c form micelles with the bile salts
   d are absorbed mainly along the duodenum
   e are absorbed by a carrier-mediated transport process involving sodium ions

P.2 Lipid digestion products
   a are normally over 95% absorbed on a moderate fat diet
   b reach the general circulation via lacteal vessels of the lymphatic system
   c are generally transported in the blood in association with lipoproteins
   d are removed from lipoproteins by the action of endothelial lipoprotein lipase
   e if present in excessive quantities in the circulation are usually associated with obesity

P.3 Plasma lipid regulation
   a is influenced by the iodothyronines from the thyroid gland
   b is abnormal in chronic insulin deficiency
   c is dependent on availability of apolipoproteins in the blood
   d is associated with glucocorticoid activity
   e is not related to adipose tissue mass

P.4 The body's metabolic requirements
   a are normally provided solely by the adipose tissue
   b depend on its energy expenditure
   c are regulated at least partly by the hypothalamus
   d are related to the maintenance of the basal body temperature
   e influence adaptive behaviours

P.5 Adipose tissue

a is composed of lipid-filled adipocytes
b normally comprises over 50% of the body mass
c takes up glucose when stimulated by insulin
d is a source of oestrogens
e is normally present in greater amounts in men than in women

P.6 Appetite

a is stimulated by leptin
b is controlled by the hypothalamus
c is depressed by exercise
d varies inversely with body weight
e increases whenever the satiety centre in the brain is stimulated

P.7 Food intake

a is normally under the control of the hypothalamus
b is increased when the external temperature rises above 22 °C
c decreases in diabetes mellitus
d is purely under endocrine control
e is partly genetically determined

MCQ Answers

P.1 a **False.** Very little lipid is digested in the stomach, the main gastric secretions (acid and proteolytic enzymes) favouring the breakdown of proteins. However, a small amount of gastric lipase is produced and this, together with the churning motions of the stomach do begin the fat digestion process and assist the breaking down of large globules to smaller ones.

b **False.** Dietary lipids are mainly triglycerides, phospholipids, and cholesterol. The triglycerides are digested down to fatty acids, diglycerides, and glycerol, while cholesterol enters the gastrointestinal tract mainly as a dietary component usually as a cholesterol ester.

c **True.** Once the lipids have entered the duodenum, they are emulsified by the intestinal contractions in the presence of bile salts which act as stabilizers. Micelles are then formed, these being aggregations of lipids in a central core surrounded by bile salt molecules such that their hydrophobic ends face inwards with the hydrophilic ends outwards. Pancreatic lipase enzyme molecules break down the large triglycerides to smaller molecules (fatty acids, glycerol, and 2-monoglycerides) by acting at the water–lipid interface. Cholesterol esters are hydrolysed by esterase enzymes released into the duodenum.

d **True.** Most of the lipids are absorbed in the duodenum and jejunum although some is absorbed in the ileum. Fatty acids, monoglycerides, and cholesterol reach the intestinal mucosal cells in the micelles.

e **False.** The small fatty acids (less than 10 carbon atoms) enter the mucosal cells by passive diffusion and pass into the portal blood directly. Larger fatty acids are converted back into triglycerides in the mucosal cells and, together with cholesterol and phospholipids, become coated by proteins to form chylomicrons which then enter the lymphatics by exocytosis. A lot of the cholesterol is probably absorbed in the distal parts of the small intestine.

P.2 a **True.** In adults, faecal fat represents approximately 3% of the stools, although the percentage can increase if the diet contain greater than normal quantities of fat. In new-born babies a greater proportion of fat is excreted in the stools (approximately 10% or more) because the absorptive process is not yet fully functional.

b **True.** Most of the absorbed lipids, (i.e. the phospholipids and cholesterol together with reformed triglyceride molecules), together with their lipoprotein 'coat' are transported as chylomicrons in the lacteal vessels. The lymphatic system eventually feeds the chylomicrons into the general circulation in the vena cava. Only the small fatty acids can be transported to the liver directly, unesterified (i.e. free), in the portal blood or bound to albumin.

c **True.** There are various lipid–lipoprotein fractions in the blood. The largest complexes are the chylomicrons formed in the intestinal mucosa (see above), and the smaller chylomicron remnants. Smaller lipoprotein complexes contain differing proportions of triglyceride, cholesterol, protein, and phospholipid. As the proportions of triglyceride and cholesterol decrease, so the proportions of protein and phospholipid increase. In order of decreasing triglyceride and cholesterol, the various complexes are: (a) the very low density lipoproteins (VLDL), (b) the intermediate density lipoproteins (IDL), (c) the low density lipoproteins (LDL), and (d) the high density lipoproteins (HDL).

d **True.** Endothelial lipoprotein lipase in the capillaries removes the chylomicrons and the VLDL complexes from the circulation by catalysing the breakdown of triglyceride to fatty acids and glycerol which can then enter cells (e.g. adipocytes). The smaller complexes which remain (i.e. the chylomicron remnants and the IDL) reach the liver where they are internalized. The LDL and HDL are formed in the liver, the LDL transporting lipids to the cells while the HDL clear the lipids, primarily cholesterol, from the blood by transporting them back to the liver.

e **True.** If the diet is rich in fats, there will be increased circulating lipids in the form of lipoprotein complexes, as well as free fatty acids and cholesterol. In the chronic state, this will usually be associated with the increased deposition of fat in adipose tissue.

P.3   a   **True.** The iodothyromines increase lipid metabolism by increasing lipolysis in adipose tissue which can be associated with an increase in plasma non-esterified free fatty acid concentrations in the blood. However, the iodothyronines also increase fatty acid oxidation in tissue and this effect is more prominent, so that in the presence of excess circulating iodothyronines (i.e. hyperthyroidism) there is usually a weight loss and decreased circulating concentrations of fatty acids as well as triglycerides, phospholipids, and cholesterol. Part of the effect of the iodothyronines on circulating lipids is by its action on the lipoproteins in the blood. For example, iodothyronines increase LDL receptor synthesis which results in an increased removal of lipoprotein and associated lipids by the cells.

   b   **True.** Insulin deficiency (i.e. diabetes mellitus) is associated with raised circulating triglyceride, cholesterol, and LDL concentrations and at the same time reduced HDL concentrations. Re-establishment of normo-glycaemia following appropriate treatment with insulin is accompanied by a restoration of normal lipid metabolism. The alteration in circulating lipid concentrations in the absence of insulin is at least partly due to the lack of control over glucose metabolism, which results in cells being 'starved' of principal energy substrate and consequently increasing their utilization of lipids. This probably accounts for the increased incidence of atherosclerosis in diabetic patients. Furthermore, long-term complications of diabetes are associated with altered lipid metabolism.

   c   **True.** Regulation of the various apolipoproteins (proteins prior to binding lipid components) which are associated with the transport of lipids such as cholesterol, fatty acids, and phospholipids, is necessary otherwise abnormal quantities of lipids circulating in the blood get deposited in the blood vessels (atherosclerosis) and in other tissues (e.g. the kidneys) resulting in clinical disease. Catecholamines stimulate apolipoprotein synthesis and thus influence lipid metabolism indirectly; thus chronic administration of catecholamines prevent the increase in circulating lipids (despite stimulating lipolysis) because of the simultaneous rise in apolipoprotein synthesis. Other factors, including other hormones, also influence the regulation of apolipoprotein synthesis.

   d   **False.** Glucocorticoids certainly stimulate protein catabolism but changes in circulating lipoprotein concentrations are not associated with clinical conditions associated with hypo- or hyper-secretion of glucocorticoids into the blood.

e **False.** Normally, lipid metabolism is directly associated with circulating plasma lipid concentrations via the production of molecules such as leptin from adipose tissue. Leptin inhibits food intake as one part of the regulatory process. This results in decreased storage of fat in adipose tissue.

P.4 a **False.** The body's immediate requirements are normally provided by carbohydrates, particularly blood glucose and tissue glycogen. Longer-term energy requirements are provided by the triglycerides stored in adipose tissue which produce 9 calories/gram compared with the 4 calories/gram produced by the metabolism of glucose.

b **True.** The body's requirement for energy substrates will indeed be determined by the amount of energy being expended, including the energy expended by the various activities we perform in addition to the basal metabolism of cells.

c **True.** While many aspects of metabolic control are unclear it is evidence that the brain, in particular the hypothalamus, has various regulatory influences. For example, through the hypothalamic production of thyrotrophin releasing hormone the adenohypophysial influence on the thyroid gland is largely maintained. The thyroidal iodothyronines have an important influence on metabolic rate (e.g. basal metabolism can increase by 100% or more in the presence of excessive amounts of circulating hormone). The hypothalamus also contains a thermoregulatory centre as well as nuclei which are concerned with regulation of hunger and satiety.

d **True.** The basal body temperature is maintained as a consequence of basal metabolism. If the basal metabolic rate, and consequently basal body temperature, increases this will be associated with an increase in the body's metabolic requirements. The iodothyronines have an important role in regulating basal metabolism and body temperature.

e **True.** Various adaptive behaviours will be influenced by the body's metabolic requirements. For example, if these requirements should increase appetite will be stimulated resulting in food-seeking behaviour. Furthermore, if the requirement has increased because of the need to maintain the basal body temperature then seeking shelter and donning warm clothing would be suitable adaptive responses.

P.5 a **True.** Adipocytes are the cellular constituents of adipose tissue. Large amounts of triglycerides are stored within these cells.

b **False.** Skeletal muscle provides approximately 60% of the total body mass so the adipose tissue normally provides *less* than 50% of the total body mass.

c **True.** Adipocytes, like muscle cells, contain insulin-sensitive glucose transporter molecules (GLUT 4) in their plasma cell membranes. Consequently, glucose enters these cells rapidly down their concentration gradients by means of this specialized transporter system in the presence of insulin.

d **True.** Certain androgens are aromatized to weak oestrogens in adipose tissue. Androstenedione, a weak androgen derived from ovarian and adrenal sources, is aromatized mainly to oestrone. This extra-ovarian source of oestrogen becomes increasingly important after the menopause. Indeed, it has been estimated that the total oestrogen production in very obese women can be greater than the normal production of oestrogens in premenopausal women because of the contribution by the large amounts of adipose tissue. Presumably the oestrogen production in similarly obese men is also considerably raised in comparison with men of normal size.

e **False.** Oestrogens increase fat deposition, so that from puberty women normally have a greater contribution to their body weight from adipose tissue compared with men of a similar body weight (men having a relatively greater muscle mass instead).

P.6 a **False.** Leptin is a protein produced by adipose tissue which seems to act as a hormonal negative feedback signal to the hypothalamus (particularly the paraventricular nucleus). It inhibits feeding, thereby reducing fat cell size. Thus, a mutation of the leptin gene in obese ob/ob mice results in a lack of gene expression and a decrease in the protein product; consequently, food intake is increased and obesity ensues. Another molecule, glucagon-like peptide-1, also inhibits feeding but probably acts at least partly by blocking the central action of the very powerful appetite stimulant neuropeptide-Y.

b **True.** The hypothalamus plays a key role in regulating food intake, via the drive to eat (the hunger, or 'appetite' centre) and opposing feeling of 'fullness' (via a satiety centre). Key areas of the hypothalamus associated with eating are the paraventricular nucleus and the ventromedial hypothalamus. Lesions in the latter area produce an overeating disorder in rats which consequently become immensely obese.

c **True.** Exercise is certainly to be recommended for decreasing stores of adipose tissue by increasing energy consumption. While it might be expected that appetite be stimulated because of the increased utilization of energy substrates, it is in fact decreased in prolonged moderate–severe exercise.

d **False.** If appetite decreased as body weight increased, there would be a built-in negative feedback loop which would prevent the development of obesity. Since obese people eat as much (or more) than others, it would seem that such a feedback system is either non-existent or is easily overridden by other stimuli.

e **False.** In general appetite is *depressed* whenever the satiety centre is stimulated. Glugacon-like peptide-1 is believed to stimulate the hypothalamic satiety centre, reducing food intake. Thus, a specific inhibitor of this polypeptide, when administered intracerebro-ventricularly, blocks its inhibitory effect on food intake in satiated rats, more than doubling food intake.

P.7 a **True.** Food intake is regulated by the hypothalamic appetite and satiety centres. The appetite (or hunger) centre is located in the anterior hypo-thalamus while the satiety centre is located in the ventromedial hypothalamus. Both of these centres receive neural input from other parts of the hypothalamus (and brain) and are also influenced by hormones which cross the blood–brain barrier. Metabolites such as glucose may also have an effect on these centres.

b **False.** Appetite usually increases when the external temperature falls, therefore in cold weather we tend to eat more in order to provide the extra energy required to maintain the basal body temperature.

c **False.** In diabetes mellitus appetite is not usually affected, although a craving for sweet foods may occur. Interestingly, if the blood glucose concentration decreases markedly, there may be an increase in appetite, but this is likely to be a pathological effect.

d **False.** While various hormones probably influence appetite (see above, and also the iodothyronines and other hormones), they are not the only determinants. Neural influences from other parts of the brain (e.g. from within the hypothalamus, even) and possible influences from metabolite concentrations in the cerebrospinal fluid also have effects on appetite and food intake.

e **True.** There is likely to be a genetic influence on appetite (and on food intake). Studies on twins certainly support the view that genetic factors need to be considered. However, the genetic influence is no more than that, since it is clear that other factors (e.g. hormonal and neural) also affect food intake.

Obesity, lipid metabolism, and its disorders (Clinical)

Multiple Choice Questions

C.1

With regard to the effects of coexistent obesity on the prevalence and behaviour of other disorders, which of the following statements is/are correct?

a Obesity plays only a small part in the variation of diabetes prevalence between different ethnic groups

b Body weight is a major determinant of blood pressure level

c The pattern of fat distribution within the body relates to morbidity and mortality from macrovascular occlusive events

d Postoperative complications are no more frequent in the obese than in people of normal weight

e Once obese, the mortality risk is not reversible by weight reduction

C.2

In regard to appetite and food intake, and their relationship to obesity, which of the following statements is/are correct?

a Blood glucose is a minor determinant of appetite

b There is evidence for a direct effect of adipose tissue mass on appetite regulation

c Abnormalities within critical hypothalamic centres are common determinants of obesity

d Psychological factors are common determinants of appetite and body weight

e Inter-individual variation in afferent neural and humoral signals from the gastrointestinal tract determine body weight.

C.3

In regard to energy storage in adipose tissue, which of the following statements is/are true?

a Reduced dietary-induced thermogenesis is a relevant phenomenon in the genesis of human obesity

b Relative adipocyte hyperplasia represents a genetic contribution to the cause of obesity

c Adipocyte hypertrophy in response to prolonged overeating is a reversible phenomenon

d A defect in lipolysis is fundamental to the aetiology of human obesity e Endocrine factors in obesity operate mainly by affecting energy storage in adipose tissue

C.4

A 35-year-old woman presents with moderate and increasing obesity (BMI 30 kg/m²), together with mild hirsutism and infrequent, irregular periods. Over the last 5 years she has been in new employment largely involving desk work and higher-level responsibility for 15 other staff in an open plan office based in a new multi-storey city development. During this period alone, she has steadily gained 14 kg (31 lb). Apart from mild hypertension (BP 155/90), some hair growth on chin, upper lip and sideburn areas, and largely abdominal obesity, clinical examination is normal. Which of the following statements would you endorse in the context of this patient's problems?

a Acquisition of a positive energy balance is most unlikely to explain all the above clinical features

b An acquired adrenal lesion is likely to underlie her weight and other changes

c Ovarian abnormalities may explain her clinical presentation

d Comprehensive investigation of her hypertension is an important element of your diagnostic work-up

e Sociopsychological factors are worth pursuing in clarifying her problem

C.5

In the same patient, further discussion does disclose some concern about her 'image' in front of working colleagues. She also admits to considerable stress-related binge eating and snacking. Investigations show a normally suppressible serum cortisol in the overnight dexamethasone suppression test. Thyroid function is normal, but SHBG is reduced and free androgen index (testosterone/SHBG ratio) is 8.2 (N < 4.5). At the follow-up visit, her blood pressure has fallen to 150/80. What principles would you then follow in her management?

a Advise a psychological assessment or a change in employment

b Provide guidelines on healthier snacking and eating

c Negotiate methods of increasing her exercise-related energy expenditure

d Prescribe an appetite-suppressant drug to give her an initial boost

e Further investigate her recently identified androgen excess

C.6

One year later she has gained a further 10 kg (22 lb) and is severely depressed. Her blood pressure is 180/105 (even with a broad cuff and after resting). Her periods have ceased, loss of her job is imminent, and she admits to continued snacking and bingeing. Which of the following approaches is/are indicated?

a Refer for a psychiatric opinion

b Hospitalize and institute strict caloric restriction

c Refer to a surgeon for consideration of gastroplasty

d Commence on beta-adrenergic blocking drugs for treatment of her hypertension

e Restore her menstrual pattern by prescribing some for of oral contraceptive

C.7

The process of atherogenesis is fundamental to the common critical life events of stroke and myocardial infarction. In relation to this important phenomenon, which of the following statements is/are true?

a The postmenopausal state in women represents a higher coronary risk period than in age-matched men, when all other risk factors are held constant

b Hypercholesterolaemia of 7 mmol/litre is a greater risk for coronary heart disease (CHD) than smoking 20 cigarettes per day, when other risk factors are held constant

c Diabetes increases the risk of CHD by 50%, all other risk factors being held constant

d The deleterious effects of hypertension on coronary and stroke risk are not related to any direct effect on prevalence of atherosclerosis

e The familial component of coronary heart disease is based entirely on hereditary disorders of lipid metabolism

C.8

In relation to serum lipids and coronary artery disease, which of the following statements is/are true?

a There is a cut-off point of serum total and LDL cholesterol below which epidemiological studies show no further reduction in coronary risk

b In non-diabetics, serum triglyceride is a minor factor in determining coronary risk, compared with total and LDL–cholesterol

c Abnormality in the intravascular coagulation process is an effect of hyperlipidaemia, additional to its deleterious effects on the arterial wall

d Low serum HDL represents an independent risk factor for CHD

e Lipoprotein (a) is a major determinant of risk in coronary artery disease

C.9

Hyperlipidaemia is based on both hereditary/genetic as well as environmental/acquired factors. Considering the latter causes, which of the following statements is/are true?

a A total serum cholesterol of 10.2 mmol/litre is unlikely to be due solely to dietary factors

b Hypercholesterolaemia may be secondary to hypothyroidism

c Raised serum triglyceride is the dominant feature of alcohol excess

d The lipid disturbance of chronic glomerular failure is dominantly hypercholesterolaemia e The oestrogenic component of the combined contraceptive pill conveys deleterious effects on the serum lipid profile

C.10

In relation to the non-atherosclerotic clinical features of hyperlipidaemia, which of the following statements is/are true?

a Xanthelasmata are virtually pathognomonic of hypercholesterolaemia
b Eruptive xanthomas are almost always a manifestation of hypertriglyceridaemia
c Tendon xanthomas are a feature of combined (cholesterol and triglyceride) hyperlipidaemia
d Pancreatitis may be a manifestation of hypertriglyceridaemia
e Haemolysis is a rare complication of hypertriglyceridaemia

C.11

A 65-year-old man with a BMI of 28 kg/m^2 sustains a myocardial infarct. He is a non-smoker. A serum cholesterol taken on admission reveals a total serum cholesterol of 8.8 mmol/litre. LDL–cholesterol is 6.9 mmol/litre (N < 4.8), and HDL–cholesterol 0.9 mmol/litre (NR 1.1–1.8). Serum triglyceride is 2.2 mmol/litre (NR 0.9–1.8). His father (also a non-smoker) died of a myocardial infarct age 55. Although he will proceed to exercise testing and probably coronary angiography, which of the following additional steps directed towards his lipid profile would be appropriate?

a Take no action at the present time
b Refer to a dietitian for dietary review and advice
c Commence lipid-lowering drug therapy
d Check his children and siblings for hypercholesterolaemia
e Check thyroid function tests

C.12

A premenopausal woman age 50 of normal weight (BMI 21 kg/m^2) has an 'executive screen', in which a serum cholesterol of 5.8 mmol/litre and triglyceride of 4.4 mmol/litre (NR 0.7–1.9) are identified. Serum LDL–cholesterol is 3.7 mmol/litre (NR 0.5–4.9) and HDL–cholesterol is 0.7 mmol/litre (NR 1.1–1.9). She is not diabetic, has no family history CHD, is not hypertensive and is a non-smoker. She consumes 12 units of alcohol weekly. Which of the following statements is appropriate?

a Her cardiovascular risk is no greater than someone with a normal lipid profile
b Diet and exercise advice should be provided
c One should attempt to correct her abnormal lipid profile, with drugs if necessary
d Since she is perimenopausal, oestrogen replacement (HRT) should be seriously considered
e Family studies should be undertaken

C.13

In relation to the use of lipid lowering drugs, which of the following statements is/are true?

a Statins represent optimal therapy for hypercholesterolaemia unresponsive to diet, and justifying treatment on other grounds
b A combination of statins and fibrates is safe and appropriate for initial therapy of combined (cholesterol and triglyceride) hyperlipidaemia
c Nicotinic acid derivatives correct both high LDL– as well as low HDL–cholesterol
d Bile acid sequestrants are potentially dangerous because of their systemic side-effects
e Probucol is of no proven value in reducing atherosclerotic risk

Short Answer Question

C.14

'Coronary artery disease is a major cause of morbidity and mortality. Reducing serum cholesterol is a worthwhile public health target in the process of reducing cardiovascular risk.' Write *short* notes contrasting the strategies of: (a) population cholesterol screening and selective therapy with (b) a population-based coronary risk education programme.

MCQ Answers

C.1 a **False.** Both within and between ethnic and racial groups, body weight is the largest determinant of diabetes incidence and prevalence. In one study, prevalence was 50% greater with weight 10% above average, and 300% greater with weight 20% above average. It achieves this influence by increasing insulin resistance, although the precise link is not known.

b **True.** The most important contribution to this relationship is the false hypertension resulting from use of a standard width blood pressure cuff in (obese) patients with increased upper arm circumference. Use of a wide (thigh) cuff reduces (but does not eliminate) the relationship between body weight and blood pressure. The mechanism of hypertension in obesity is unknown, but weight reduction mostly lowers pressure.

c **True.** The pattern of fat distribution with weight gain varies greatly. Intra-abdominal obesity (a high waist/hip ratio) defines a greater risk of hyperlipidaemia and cardio- and cerebrovascular disease than those who are obese and have a normal waist/hip ratio. These characteristics ('apple' and 'pear' body fat distribution respectively) are thought to be genetic rather than being related to environmental factors such as exercise or food type.

d **False.** Obesity causes a higher incidence of poor wound healing and infection (unrelated to diabetes) and deep vein thrombosis and thromboembolism. Reduced chest wall compliance and hypoventilation causes stasis of secretions within airways and consequent superinfection. This gives rise to the high incidence of postoperative pneumonia.

e **False.** Even reversal of very longstanding obesity is followed by improvement in mortality. This may relate to correction of hyperlipidaemia and hypertension as well as to other subtle factors affecting respiratory and neurological function.

C.2 a **True.** A pathological fall of blood glucose represents an appetite trigger. Hyperglycaemia (as in diabetes) does not have the inverse effect. Other nutrients such as amino acids and fatty acids as well as humoral factors including circulating catecholamines and serotonin are probably of greater importance in appetite regulation and eating behaviour.

b **True.** Circulating levels of the recently identified peptide, leptin, correlate with adipose tissue mass. In turn, leptin suppresses appetite in experimental animals. Variation in leptin receptor activity may represent a theoretical basis for comparative stability or 'tracking' of weight in individuals.

c **False.** Hypothalamic tumours affecting the ventromedial and lateral nucleus certainly cause appetite disturbance, and this can be mimicked by experimental destructive lesions in animals. However, only in rare congenital syndromes such as those of Laurence–Moon–Biedl and Prader–Willi is it likely that a hypothalamic lesion is responsible for the (often gross) obesity. Even here, low physical activity related to mental subnormality may be contributory.

d **True.** Approximately one-third of the population respond to stress by eating more, and another one-third by eating less. Although not all psychologically disturbed patients are obese, there is a higher prevalence of stress-triggered eating within an obese population. The adverse reciprocal effects of 'being obese' on well-being should not be forgotten.

e **False.** There are afferent signals from different levels of the gastrointestinal tract mediated by adrenergic and cholinergic neurotransmitters, and by humoral factors such as cholecystokinin. However, there is no evidence that variation in the activity of any element of this hypothalamic feedback system is responsible for obesity. These pathways may nevertheless explain the differing satiety effects of 'snacking' when compared with standard meals.

C.3 a **False.** The mechanisms underlying the adaptive thermogenesis seen with overeating are still unknown. Thyroid hormones play a part in ATP economy via sodium-dependent ATPase pump activity. Increased levels of (biologically inactive) reverse T_3 are also seen in the opposite state of fasting. However, obesity is not associated with clearcut differences in either basal metabolic rate or exercise- or diet-induced thermogenesis.

b **False.** Adipocyte hyperplasia is an acquired reaction to positive energy balance, almost uniquely confined to growth periods in human development. This phenomenon almost certainly underlies the comparative resistance to diet in obese subjects who were overfed in childhood and teenage years, since this hyperplastic adipocyte mass is irreversible. There is no evidence that proneness to adipocyte hyperplasia is genetic.

c **True.** Adipocyte hypertrophy is the (potentially) reversible component of obesity, at any age. Changes in the volume of adipocytes are the reflection of the normal month to month weight variation seen in man.

d **False.** Although isolated reports of defective lipolysis in response to traditional stimuli (fasting and catecholamines) have been reported in rare cases of familial obesity, there is no evidence that such defects underlie common forms of obesity.

e **True.** Classical endocrine syndromes often include mild obesity. Thus patients with phaeochromocytoma are often slim (catecholamine-mediated lipolysis), hypothyroidism causes mild obesity (reduced thermogenesis), and acromegaly is associated with markedly reduced subcutaneous tissue (growth-hormone dependent lipolysis). Corticosteroid therapy and Cushing's syndrome is associated with mild to moderate obesity due to enhanced lipogenesis (but also substantially increased appetite).

C.4 a **False.** Acquisition of weight at the rate of 3 kg (6.5 lb) per year is consistent with 'simple obesity'. Obesity also carries with it a number of secondary changes, including hypertension and a reduction in sex-hormone binding globulin (SHBG). See also 7C4b.

b **False.** The statistical likelihood of a causative adrenal lesion (e.g. Cushings disease) is extremely small. However, no one could be reproached for doing an overnight dexamethason suppression test or 24-hour urinary cortisol estimation!

c **True.** Polycystic ovary syndrome or one of its variants is present in 10% or more of the female population. The androgen excess state which it produces may not be apparent until weight gain induces a typical reduction of SHBG, and a proportionate increase in free testosterone. The hyperinsulinaemia characteristic of obesity is also thought to induce synthesis of androgens.

d **False.** The likelihood is that she is just a little tense at her visit to your surgery or clinic. 'White coat' hypertension is a more likely cause . . . or did you forget to use a wide cuff for its measurement? Check her blood pressure again on her subsequent visit.

e **True.** In every obese patient, this is an important strategy. Embarrassment and self-consciousness about her weight and hirsutism may be the real reason for her wanting to see you. Conversely, stress levels and associated hyperphagia may be at the root of her weight gain problem.

C.5 a **False.** Despite knowledge of the dynamics on overeating in response to stress, psychological intervention rarely achieves anything but short-term weight loss. Even behavioural modification techniques rarely achieve significant long-term weight control. This approach can be deferred for the time being. Although she must be made aware of the risks of obesity, she probably is aware of at least some, and fear is an emotion which must be avoided.

b **True.** This is always worth a try, although most people do know what they are 'doing wrong'. A dietitian would, however, provide advice on lower calorie snacks, more regular 'sit-down' meals and advise a calorie counter (most obese patients will not lose weight on anything less than 1500 kcal daily). The dietitian may also provide some behavioural guidelines, including the avoidance of visual and olfactory cues to eating.

c **True.** This is an important step. Using the stairs rather than the elevator: walking rather than driving; getting off the bus or train one or more stops earlier (and then walking); taking up regular sport, and a general increase in incidental exercise all help. An extra hour of brisk continuous walking each day will alone result in weight loss of 1 kg (2 lb) per month.

d **False.** Most appetite-suppressants act by providing catecholaminergic suppression of the appetite centre(s). Tachyphylaxis (progressively larger dose requirement due to loss of effect) and habituation are common. Since they are only licensed for short-term use, they do not represent a long-term solution. Leptin and glucagon-related peptide (GLP-1) are newly identified peptides which provide negative (inhibitory) feedback to appetite centres. These compounds or their analogues may prove useful in the future. Similarly, antagonists of peptides that stimulate appetite may achieve similar effects.

e **False.** Although you have probably identified associated polycystic ovary syndrome, weight loss itself is likely to normalize her periods, and possible reduce pathological hair growth, all mediated by elevating her SHBG levels. This is the time to make further investigations (ovarian ultrasound) and treat (using supplemental oestrogen) if weight reduction fails: indeed explanation of these dynamics may provide her with useful motivation.

C.6 a **True.** Her phychological state now probably has two components: that which is causing her hyperphagia and obesity, and that which results from the feelings of inadequacy and poor body image consequent on her obesity. 'Talking treatment' (psychotherapy) either with a psychologist or a psychiatrist may help her (although not necessarily her weight!). One of the serotonin re-uptake receptor inhibitors (SSRI) group of drugs such as fluoxetine may be helpful at this stage, since they are antidepressants and have direct hypothalamic effects. Tricyclic antidepressants might actually cause her to gain weight.

b **False.** No doubt she would lose some weight on a regimen of enforced 600–800 calorie intake coupled to an intense exercise programme. However, this is expensive short-term strategy, and follow-up indicates poor long-term results.

c **False.** She is not really heavy enough, nor is her obesity sufficiently 'complicated' to justify the risks of such major surgery, which essentially creates a small gastric pouch in lieu of the normal stomach. Nevertheless, at a later stage, this may be worth considering. Jaw-wiring (only temporary benefit) and jejuno-ileal bypass (side-effects from the resulting malabsorption) have been largely superseded by gastric surgery, as above.

d **False.** Although hypertension should be treated at this level, beta-adrenergic blocking drugs inhibit weight loss by blocking catechol-amine-mediated lipolysis. They also increase serum triglyceride levels and may enhance the risk of atherosclerosis with long-term use. ACE inhibitors, alpha-adrenergic and calcium channel blocking drugs are free of lipid effects.

e **False.** She is unlikely to be very concerned about her amenorrhoea, and any oestrogen administered may make the process of weight loss more difficult.

C.7 a **True.** Until the menopause, the protective effect of oestrogen limits coronary risk to between 30% and 50% of age-matched men. By age 65, coronary risk in women already exceeds that of age-matched men, all other variables being taken into consideration. Current data support a 30–50% reduction in coronary events as a result of ongoing menopausal oestrogen replacement, which corrects the raised LDL and reduced HDL levels often found in the oestrogen-deficient state.

b **False.** Smoking remains the biggest risk factor for atherosclerosis and it has vaso-occlusive consequences. Smoking induces increased levels of oxidized LDL which are more atherogenic, together with a fall in HDL cholesterol. However, these changes are insufficient to explain the substantial effects on atherogenesis and represent factors of minor significance.

c **False.** The relative risk of coronary events is 300% in male and 600% in female diabetics compared with non-diabetics. The additional presence of proteinuria (nephropathy) multiples this risk a further 4–10 times!

One of the main mediators of the increased risk in diabetes is the combination of raised serum triglyceride and reduced HDL–cholesterol: raised LDL and hypercholesterolaemia is no more common in *well-controlled* diabetics than in an age-matched population. When present, hypercholesterolaemia compounds the cardiovascular risk.

d **False.** The effects of atherosclerosis and hypertension are reciprocal. Reduced compliance of atherosclerotic vessels increases (particularly) systolic blood pressure. Conversely, studies on atherogenesis confirm a role of hypertension in arterial wall lipid accumulation.

e **False.** Genetic factors are certainly known to be relevant for both familial hypercholesterolaemia and familial combined hyperlipidaemia. Serum fibrinogen concentrations are partly genetically determined, as is the insulin resistance syndrome which constitutes an independent risk factor. Familial trends in eating patterns are relevant, as are familial obesity trends. There remain factors which should be clarified by future research. Genetic variation in the geography of the coronary 'tree' may also prove to be relevant.

C.8 a **False.** There is a continuum of risk for coronary morbidity and mortality from the highest to the lowest serum total cholesterol. Within this relationship, a serum cholesterol reduction of 0.6 mmol/litre (i.e. approximately 10%) has been estimated to reduce incidence of coronary occlusive events in the UK population by approximately 50% at age 40, 40% at age 50, and 20% at age 70. Even in a country like China with low CHD rates and low fat intakes, CHD event prevalence relates to serum cholesterol within that population's range of 2.4–4.2 mmol/litre. However, in most populations, no further reduction in coronary events is seen with LDL levels below 2.5 mmol/litre.

b **True.** The role of triglyceride in atherogenesis remains unclear, but is undoubtedly far less important than total or LDL–cholesterol, even in diabetics. In a Norwegian study, triglyceride levels were predictive of coronary events. Levels of serum triglyceride above 1.5 mmol/litre are associated with small, dense LDL particle size, in turn thought to be more atherogenic by virtue of being more prone to oxidation. Triglyceride levels are also correlated with serum factor VII concentrations.

c **True.** Platelet activity and survival are adversely affected in the presence of elevated LDL levels. Within the coagulation cascade, oxidized LDL has been shown to increase the expression of tissue thromboplastin, and increases the level of plasminogen activator inhibitor (PAI-1), which in turn inhibits fibrinolysis. Antioxidants may prove useful in inhibiting this (and other) critical reactions leading to intravascular thrombosis as well as arterial wall changes.

d **True.** The 'protective' effect of HDL identified in cross-sectional studies probably reflects its role in reverse cholesterol transport from peripheral tissues back to the liver. Because of the closely related metabolism of HDL–cholesterol and triglyceride, the inverse relation between HDL–cholesterol and coronary risk may be responsible for part of the apparent role of triglyceride as a coronary risk factor.

e   **True.** Although lipoprotein (a) (Lp(a)) correlates with CHD events, and is undoubtedly a subsidiary coronary risk factor, a temporary rise of Lp(a) may also be secondary to ischaemic damage. A raised serum Lp(a) appears to carry a similar atherogenic risk to raised serum fibrinogen levels.

C.9   a   **True.** Dietary cholesterol varies greatly, and at most 40% is absorbed. A high saturated to polyunsaturated ratio of fat intake also causes down-regulation of LDL receptors, causing additional increases in cholesterol-rich LDL particles. The extent of this process is broadly proportional to the number of double bonds in the saturated fat. At the level of serum cholesterol in this patient, however, it is unlikely that dietary fat and cholesterol are (solely) responsible.

b   **True.** Between 5% and 10% of patients with serum cholesterol above 7.0 mmol/litre have unrecognized biochemical or overt hypothroidism: low thyroid hormones reduce both lipoprotein lipase as well as LDL receptor activity. Hypothyroidism is recognized as predisposing to atherosclerosis. Thyroid function tests should be checked in every hyper-cholesterolaemic patient, since both the abnormalities and coronary-proneness are reversible by correction of the hypothyroidism.

c   **True.** Alcohol increases hepatic synthesis of triglyceride, which is incorporated into VLDL. Serum HDL–cholesterol is normal and often raised, while Lp(a) is also reduced in advanced alcoholic liver disease. These combined features may explain why moderate consumption of alcohol is associated with lower prevalence of atherosclerosis. However, heavy alcohol intake is often associated with very marked hyper-triglyceridaemia.

d   **False.** *The nephrotic syndrome*, however caused, results in raised VLDL and associated hypertriglyceridaemia, but also raised LDL and cholesterol levels: the mechanism for the latter is thought to be the hypo-albuminaemia which is invariably present in severe forms, and which non-specifically stimulates hepatic protein synthesis, including Lp(a). In *chronic glomerular failure*, hypertriglyceridaemia is more prominent, due to reduced hepatic lipase and postheparin lipolytic activity. The hyperlipidaemia may itself accelerate deterioration of renal function, and may also be responsible for the markedly raised risk of stroke and myocardial infarction which occurs in diabetics when renal failure supervenes.

e   **False.** The oestrogenic component of the combined pill reduced LDL and raises HDL–cholesterol levels, a profile which also reflects the cardiovascular benefit of oestrogen in the postmenopausal state. Pregnane-derived progestogens are virtually devoid of lipoprotein effects, although they are now less frequently used because of the higher prevalence of venous thromboembolism (the mechanism of which is still unclear). More frequently used 19-nortestosterone-derived progestogens partially reverse the advantageous effects of oestrogen, by decreasing HDL-2 and increasing LDL–cholesterol. These adverse factors may represent the cause of the marginally increased risk of myocardial infarction seen with use of the combined pill, although additional prothrombotic effects may be operative.

C.10 a **False.** Xanthelasmata do occur in hypercholesterolaemia (particularly with levels above 8 mmol/l and in the familial form: Fredricksen type 2a). They are also occasionally seen with isolated reductions of HDL–cholesterol. However, more frequently they are unassociated with any lipid disturbance. As with the broadly related corneal arcus, they are due to lipid deposition, but the pathogenesis in patients with normal lipid levels is unknown.

b **True.** These lesions are most commonly seen with the grossly raised serum triglycerides found in alcohol abuse or in severely uncontrolled diabetes mellitus. More rarely, familial hypertriglyceridaemia may also cause this skin eruption.

c **False.** Tendon xanthomas occur almost exclusively in severe forms of hypercholesterolaemia (homozygous or heterozygous familial) and in the rare condition of familial dysbetalipoproteinaemia (Fredricksen type 3).

d **True.** When hypertriglyceridaemia is particularly severe (as is the case with heavy alcohol excess), incorporation of triglyceride into chylomicrons is accelerated, giving rise to opalescent serum. In extreme forms of chylomicronaemia, abdominal pain occurs due to pancreatitis (possibly due to fatty acid release from chylomicrons 'trapped' in pancreatic capillaries). Deposition of chylomicrons in reticuloendothelial tissue of the liver and spleen give rise to coexistent hepatosplenomegaly. Lipaemia retinalis is often also present. The same constellation of findings is also seen in familial lipoprotein lipase deficiency.

e **True.** Particularly in poorly nourished alcoholics the occurrence of lipid-rich erythrocytes leads to sufficient red cell deformity so that haemolysis and (haemolytic) jaundice occur, referred to as Zieve's syndrome, usually in association with the clinical features mentioned in d above.

C.11 a **False.** Current data from many studies reveal an approximate 30% reduction in mortality and re-infarction rate in patients treated with the statin group of drugs (achieving a 25% and 35% reduction in total and LDL–cholesterol levels, respectively). There is also an approximate 35% reduction in the need for either angioplasty or coronary artery bypass surgery. Furthermore, there is increasing data on actual regression of atherosclerotic lesions as a result of lipid-lowering therapy, with statins, fibrates, nicotinic acid derivatives, or with cholestyramine. Targets of total cholesterol below 4.5 and LDL–cholesterol below 2.6 mmol/litre have been recommended by several advisory bodies. There are also data to show that even lowering serum cholesterol within the normal range reduces coronary risk.

b **True.** Weight reduction improves the cardiac prognosis: he is certainly overweight. Advice on lipid-lowering diet is the first step in such a patient, although the height of serum cholesterol suggests that diet alone may not be enough.

c **False.** There is no urgency: it is better to wait until serum cholesterol and weight reach a low plateau, perhaps after 3–6 months, so that it will be possible to assess more precisely the effects of added lipid-lowering drugs. Motivation to diet will also be better if the 'crutch' of hypo-lipidaemic agents is not applied too soon.

d **True.** The family history and height of serum cholesterol in the absence of cutaneous manifestations certainly suggest familial or polygenic hypercholesterolaemia. Both hypercholesterolaemic siblings and children are likely to be of an age where institution of therapy (if appropriate) would be valuable, acceptable, and rational. Data are now available to show that coronary risk is reduced by cholesterol-lowering statins even without a preceding myocardial infarction (i.e. primary prevention is effective).

e **True.** As mentioned above, with isolated hypercholesterolaemia he has a 5–10% chance of being hypothyroid: it would be a shame to miss a readily correctable cause.

C.12 a **False.** Epidemiological studies show raised serum triglyceride to represent a CHD risk, but to a lesser degree than raised cholesterol. the mechanism is likely to be the generation of small, dense (and more atherogenic) LDL particles which occurs with serum trigyceride levels above 1.6 mmol/litre. The combination with low HDL constitutes a somewhat higher risk.

b **True.** Diet and exercise have been shown to have some benefit on serum triglyceride, but HDL is not likely to be responsive.

c **False.** At the present time, there is inadequate evidence to indicate that correction of this profile reduces cardiovascular risk However the fibrate group of drugs is capable of correcting this abnormal lipid pattern, and in a secondary prevention trial coronary benefit appeared to relate to changes in HDL. More data are required. In diabetics, it may be justified to treat this profile.

d **True.** In this lady, the menopause will almost certainly result in lower HDL levels. Supplemental oestrogen will reverse/prevent this biochemical change. The evidence of current (non-prospective) studies suggest that oestrogen has benefits over and above effects on serum lipids. Unless there are contra-indications, HRT would be advisable. However, oral oestrogen increases serum triglyceride, while transdermal oestrogen does not: the latter may be preferable.

e **False.** Familial occurrence of this profile is rare.

C.13 a **True.** *Statins* are HMG-CoA reductase inhibitors which inhibit cholesterol synthesis. They also increase the number and affinity of LDL receptors, so reducing LDL–cholesterol. Less than 1% of patients have disturbance of liver function tests, which are usually minor and do not contra-indicate continued use. They are currently the most effective, best-tolerated drug for lowering serum cholesterol. Target levels are listed in C.11a, although controversial.

b **False.** *Fibrates* act mainly by activating lipoprotein lipase, so reducing serum triglycerides. The combination with statins is certainly often effective. However, statins alone have beneficial effects on mild to moderate hypertriglyceridaemia; conversely fibrates also lower serum cholesterol. Individual drugs should be tried before giving them jointly. The combination of these drugs risks myopathy (rhabdomyolysis) and liver dysfunction of sufficient severity to discontinue therapy.

c **True.** *Nicotinic acid* derivatives reduce hepatic VLDL synthesis and all other lipoproteins (including LDL) in the metabolic 'cascade'. There is no convincing mechanism for the HDL rise of 10–30% recorded in most studies. They also lower Lp(a) which may be advantageous.

d **False.** *Bile acid sequestrants* are not absorbed from the gastrointestinal tract, so that serious side-effects are therefore rare. Nausea, bloating, and constipation do occur and limit compliance. They act by interrupting the enterohepatic circulation of cholesterol, depleting hepatic cholesterol content, up-regulating LDL receptor affinity, and thereby lowering total and LDL–cholesterol. Serum triglyceride levels, however, do increase, although the mechanism of this is not clear.

e **True.** *Probucol* increases LDL catabolism, and as an antioxidant decreases oxidized LDL particles thought to be most atherogenic. However it decreases serum HDL, and apart from animal studies has not been shown conclusively to carry any benefits in clinical arterial disease. This is in contrast to fibrates, statins, bile acid sequestrants, and nicotinic acid derivatives, all of which have been demonstrated to cause either regression of atheromatous lesions or a reduction in vascular occlusive events.

SAQ Answer

C.14

Population screening

In favour: restricts diet and drug treatment to those at major risk; motivation may be enhanced in those screening positive, in terms of undertaking associated diet, smoking, and exercise modification; interim benefits visible (serum cholesterol lowering).

Against: costly (£136 000 per life year saved without known CHD: £32 000 per life year saved with CHD); drug therapy may act as crutch, rather than attacking coexistent risk factors; unless performed as a 'organized' public service, regional and district differences likely; process will take up doctors' time.

Population education

In favour: multifactorial aetiologies of CHD (i.e. exercise, smoking, diet) can be simultaneously addressed; allows application already in schools, setting patterns for life; potential benefits of genuine primary prevention as compared with secondary prevention (i.e. targeting those with raised serum cholesterol levels).

Against: little evidence that the public will be responsive, except with substantial 'political' backing; an idealistic ineffective programme may turn out to be more expensive (in cost/benefit terms) than screening; nihilists may be just as negative with education as they would be with their response to screening.

References

Physiology

Topic: Nutritional regulation of fatty acids.

Hillgartner, F.B. *et al.* (1995). *Physiological Reviews*, 75, 47–76.

Topic: Leptin and feeding behaviour (Editorial).

Steiner, R.A. (1996). *Endocrinology*, 137, 4533–5.

Topic: Glucagon-like peptide-1 and central regulation of food intake.

Turton, M.D. *et al.* (1996). *Nature*, 379, 69–72.

Clinical

Topic: Aetiology of obesity.

Beales, P.L. *et al.* (1996). *Clinical Endocrinology*, 45, 373–8.

Topic: Overweight: prevalence and risks.

Bray, G. (1987). *Annals of the New York Academy of Sciences*, 499, 14–28.

Topic: Lipoprotein (a).

Durrington, P. (1995). In *Clinics in endocrinology and metabolism*, Vol. 9, pp. 773–96. Baillière Tindall; London.

Topic: Benefits and risks of cholesterol-lowering strategies.

Gaziano, J. (1996). *Annals of Internal Medicine*, 124, 914–18.

Topic: Lipid lowering in coronary artery disease prevention.

Haq, I.W. *et al*. (1996). *Clinical Science*, 91, 399–413.

Topic: Lipid profiles in prediction of CAD.

Kannel, W.B. *et al*. (1992). *American Heart Journal*, 124, 768–74.

Topic: Investigation of obesity.

Kopelman, P. (1994). *Clinical Endocrinology*, 41, 703–8.

Topic: Treatment of hyperlipidaemia (diet).

Neil, H.A.W. *et al*. (1995). *British Medical Journal*, 310, 569–73.

14 Ectopic and familial polyglandular syndromes (Clinical)

Multiple Choice Questions

C.1

In regard to ectopic hormone syndromes (the production of hormones from non-endocrine tumour tissue), which of the following is/are true?

a The incidence and spectrum of hormone excess is similar whatever primary tumour is considered

b The syndromes most commonly result from tumour synthesis and release of simple peptides resembling those of normal hypothalamic origin

c Hormone secretion is an epiphenomenon of advanced tumour status, and is normally of minor clinical significance.

d Ectopic secretion is a reflection of the pluripotential genetic endowment of all body cells.

e Not all peptides released are biologically active

C.2

In the ectopic ACTH syndrome

a The features of mineralocorticoid excess usually predominate over those reflecting glucocorticoid excess

b The syndrome is biochemically indistinguishable from that of pituitary-dependent Cushing's syndrome

c Osteoporosis and pathological fracture are significant consequences

d In addition to small cell bronchogenic carcinoma, C cell tumours are a common cause

e Treatment by bilateral adrenalectomy is the usual therapeutic approach

C.3

In the hypercalcaemia of malignancy

a Serum levels of PTH measured by immunoradiometric assay are usually raised

b Tumour production of a parathormone-related peptide is the major cause

c Muscular weakness is often the first and major symptom

d Rehydration is an important principle of emergency treatment e Corticosteroid therapy represents appropriate medium and long-term treatment in most cases

C.4

Hyponatraemia is often encountered in patients with malignant disease, particularly in advanced cases. In relation to this finding, which of the following statements is/are true?

a Hyponatraemia may represent a consequence of the 'sick-cell syndrome'
b The tumour may be actively secreting antidiuretic hormone (ADH, AVP)
c Metastatic involvement of the adrenal needs to be considered
d Cancer chemotherapy drugs may be responsible
e The hyponatraemia of ectopic ADH/AVP syndromes is not amenable to therapy other than that directed against the tumour itself

C.5 **

Which of the following hormones has/have been shown to be released ectopically?

a Insulin
b Gonadotrophins
c Thyrotrophin
d Somatotrophin (hGH)
e Erythropoeitin

C.6 **

A 35-year-old woman has been diagnosed as having autoimmune hypothyroidism. Which of the following statements is/are true?

a The prevalence of autoimmune thyroid dysfunction in her first degree family members is approximately 20%
b A concordance rate of 50% would be expected in her identical twin
c The likelihood of her developing a second organ-specific autoimmune disorder is approximately 10%
d A predisposition to familial and pluriglandular autoimmune endocrine dysfunction can be identified by characteristic genetic markers
e If occurring as part of a polyglandular deficiency syndrome the clinical features of her hypothyroidism would be different from those of monoglandular cases

C.7

In which of the following non-endocrine disorders is there an increased incidence of endocrine autoimmunity?

a Turner's syndrome (gonadal dysgenesis)
b Pernicious anaemia
c Systematic lupus erythematosus

d Mucocutaneous candidiasis
e Vitiligo

C.8

Which of the following endocrine tumours may occur in the multiple endocrine neoplasia (MEN-1) syndrome?

a Growth hormone producing pituitary adenoma (acromegaly)
b Gastrinoma
c Phaeochromocytoma
d Testicular teratoma
e Parathyroid adenoma

C.9

Which of the following features may be present as part of the multiple endocrine neoplasia (MEN-2) syndrome?

a Phaeochromocytoma
b Papillary thyroid carcinoma
c Parathyroid adenoma
d Lipoma
e Carcinoid tumour

C.10**

In screening for MEN syndromes, which of the following statements is/are correct?

a Patients with (apparently) sporadic pituitary or parathyroid adenomas and their relatives should be screened for MEN-1 related endocrine disorders
b Following identification of a proband with MEN-1 syndrome, all first and second degree relatives require periodic biochemical screening
c Histological characteristics of excised thyroid tissue in (apparently) sporadic medullary thyroid carcinoma (MTC) reliably identify individuals, whose relatives should be screened for familial MTC and MEN-2 syndromes
d In screening relatives for familial MTC, a normal basal serum calcitonin value suffices to exclude MTC
e In a patient with a phaeochromocytoma, characteristic mucocutaneous lesions and a family history of MEN-2B, thyroidectomy is mandatory

C.11**

In the management of MEN syndromes, which of the following statements is/are correct?

a Total parathyroidectomy is the treatment of choice in hyperparathyroid patients with MEN-1 syndrome
b Pituitary tumours require more radical therapy if within the MEN-1 syndrome than in sporadic forms

c Medical therapy of gastrinomas is often necessary

d In MEN-2 related phaeochromocytoma, bilateral adrenalectomy is appropriate, even in the presence of anatomically confirmed unilateral tumour

e Malignant tumours within the MEN syndromes are often sensitive to cytotoxic chemotherapy drugs

MCQ Answers

C.1 a **False.** Not all tumour cell types behave the same when they undergo malignant change. Small-cell bronchial carcinoma is particularly prone to acquire hormone secretory status. APUD (amine-precursor-uptake and decarboxylation) cells, which are widespread in different organs and normally synthesize cell-specific hormones, are uniquely prone to acquire additional abnormal secretory potential. However, ectopic hormone production has been recorded from almost every organ cell-type.

b **False.** Although some tumours synthesize biologically active hypo-thalamic-like peptides (particularly CRH and hGH-RH), the majority of syndromes result from secretion of non-hypothalamic and indeed sometimes non-pituitary peptides.

c **False.** Although in some cases the syndrome resulting from hormone excess is clinically inapparent, in many cases the symptoms are super-imposed on those of the underlying tumour and contribute significantly to ill-health. Furthermore, in some instances ectopic syndromes antedate the clinical appearance and recognition of the primary tumour, and simulate the corresponding 'natural' hormone excess syndromes.

d **True.** Current research favours a process of random de-repression of sections of the genome present in pluripotential body cells, and which therefore become available for transcription. Steroid hormones are not ectopically produced. It is reasoned that the complex and multiple enzymatic pathways which would be necessary for steroid synthesis are unlikely to be facilitated by the random derepression process which constitutes malignant change.

e **True.** Typical exceptions are carcinoembryonic antigen (CEA) and alpha-fetoprotein (AFP), both of which however are useful tumour markers. In addition, biologically inactive variants of peptides have been reported. Conversely, almost certainly some tumours produce peptides which are currently unidentified and yet are responsible for some clinical features of advanced malignancy.

C.2 a **True.** Physiologically, mineralocorticoid production and release are negligibly influenced by ACTH. However, the very high plasma ACTH levels found in ectopic ACTH syndromes do induce aldosterone and desoxycorticosterone excess. Weakness due to hypokalaemic alkalosis is often the dominant symptom. The speed of development of the syndrome often results in insufficient time to manifest glucocorticoid-dependent features: cushingoid facies and habitus are uncommon.

b **False.** High serum ACTH and varying degrees of dexamethasone non-suppressibility of a raised cortisol concentration occur in both conditions. ACTH (and cortisol) levels are mostly, but not invariably much higher than in 'natural' Cushing's syndrome. In addition, the de-repression process results in tumour secretion of POMC and other ACTH precursors which can be assayed. Above all, non-response of ACTH to CRH stimulation contrasts with the hyper-response usually seen in more than 90% of patients with pituitary-dependent Cushing's syndrome (see also 5C1, 2). In contrast, CRH itself has been reported as the ectopic hormone in a small number of cases: in these, CRH responsiveness has been retained.

c **False.** Bone effects are uncommon because of the comparatively short periods of cortisol hypersecretion leading up to the time of diagnosis.

d **True.** The characteristic tumour is medullary carcinoma of the thyroid, whose C cells are of neural crest origin. Bronchial, thymic, and pancreatic carcinoid tumours as well as phaeochromocytoma are of similar cellular derivation, and share a particular potential for ectopic ACTH secretion.

e **False.** Although adrenalectomy may be necessary, adrenal blocking drugs such as metyrapone and aminoglutethimide are often adequate to block excess cortisol production. Blocking renal tubular mineralo-corticoid receptors with spironolactone is also useful. Correction of the syndrome by excision of the primary tumour is only occasionally successful because of early metastatic spread in many cases.

C.3 a **False.** 'Native' PTH (immunometrically assayed as intact (i) PTH) is never the cause of hypercalcaemia of malignancy: levels are always suppressed by hypercalcaemia, which has its origins in other patho-physiological mechanisms. However, primary hyperparathyroidism is a common disorder, and therefore may be coincidentally identified by the combination of hypercalcaemia and a raised serum iPTH.

b **False.** PTHrP (which has homology with PTH in residues 2—13) may be secreted from breast, pancreatic, and renal carcinoma, as well as from lymphoma and squamous cell tumours. It can be independently assayed. However, hypercalcaemia may also be caused by excess $1,25(OH)_2$ vitamin D activity in some lymphomas. In addition, prostaglandins, transforming growth factor (TGFα), and other cytokines have osteoclastic potential. Some bone metastases release osteoclastic cytokines locally: metastases are the commonest cause of malignant hypercalcaemia.

c **True.** Some degree of hypercalcaemic myopathy is usually present with serum calcium levels above 3.5 mmol/litre (NR 2.1–2.5). The weakness may be compounded by hypomagnesaemia and hypokalaemia, both of which are mainly consequences of hypercalcaemia-induced renal tubular toxicity and may require independent correction.

d **True.** ADH resistance occurs with consequent nephrogenic diabetes insipidus. This is based on largely reversible hypercalcaemic renal tubular (and glomerular) nephropathy. Dehydration reduces renal calcium clearance and potentiates hypercalcaemia. Rehydration reverses these events, improves renal function and provides time to institute more specific therapy.

e **False.** Steroids down-regulate PTH (i.e. PTHrP) receptors and inhibit cytokine action, but are probably most effective when excess vitamin D-like activity is responsible (i.e. in myelo- or lympho-proliferative disorders). Side-effects even in medium-term therapy, and a comparatively narrow band of effectiveness make this group of drugs a subsidiary option. Since increased osteoclastic activity is the mechanism of almost all causes of malignant hypercalcaemia, bisphosphonates are effective in treatment, with a low side-effect profile. Calcitonin is also sometimes useful.

C.4 a **True.** In a wide variety of nutritional, cardiac and infective disorders, but particularly in advanced malignancy there is disturbed Na^+/K^+-ATPase activity. This failure of the sodium pump causes intracellular sodium and extracellular potassium shifts. Specific correction is not possible.

b **True.** Bronchial small-cell carcinoma (but also a wide variety of other tumours) have been shown to secrete ADH: as high as 40% in some studies. Water 'intoxication' with confusion, vomiting, drowsiness, and coma are typical symptoms. In some patients, absence of tumour AVP content suggests an alternative mechanism involving reset of the hypothalamic osmostat: a true SIADH syndrome.

c **True.** Both carcinoma as well as lymphoma commonly metastasize to the adrenals, causing adrenocortical insufficiency with hyponatraemia and often hyperkalaemia.

d **True.** Vincristine, vinblastine, and cyclophoshamide may cause it (as may phenothiazines and tricyclic antidepressant drugs which may be used in cases with advanced malignancy). The mechanism of action is unknown, although cytotoxic drugs may induce a type of sick-cell syndrome referred in a above.

e **False.** Fluid restriction is the single most important therapeutic step. Drugs which induce nephrogenic diabetes insipidus, such as demeclocycline are also useful in more refractory cases.

C.5** a **False.** Large mesenchymal tumours do produce hypoglycaemia. However, insulin is not the mediator, and incompletely processed pro-insulin-like ('big') IGF-II peptides have been isolated in a number of cases. These peptides induce hypoglycaemia and sometimes acromegaloid features. Some cases are responsive to corticosteroid therapy.

b **True.** Hepatoma and bronchial oat cell carcinoma are particularly associated with this syndrome, manifest by gynaecomastia and caused by the synthesis of a peptide resembling human chorionic gonadotrophin (hCG). Teratomas may also be responsible. CG is present in many tissues, and the glycosylation which occurs in tumours is thought to enhance CG bioactivity.

c **True.** Since TSH shares its α subunit with hCG, clinical and biochemical hyperthyroidism frequently occurs 'ectopically' in choriocarcinoma in which hCG is grossly hypersecreted. Bronchial and ovarian carcinoma may also cause hyperthyroidism, due to TSH synthesis and release.

d **True.** Bronchial carcinoid and small-cell tumours may cause acromegaly, in some cases by production of hGH-RH rather than hGH itself. As mentioned in a above, acromegaly may also be a consequence of tumour-associated somatomedin synthesis and release.

e **False.** Erythropoietin is normally synthesized in the kidney. Polycythaemia seen in 5–10% of renal tumours is probably due to regional hypoxia (the stimulus for enhanced erythropoietin synthesis), in turn caused by the anatomical encroachment on normal renal tissue by the tumour. The same mechanism may apply to the polycythaemia of massive uterine fibromyomata. Cerebellar haemangiomata and hepatomas are associated with polycythaemia, but have not been proven to synthesize erythropoietin.

C.6** a **True.** Approximately 20% of first degree relatives of patients with any autoimmune thyroid disorder, when screened cross-sectionally will prove to have (often subclinical) thyroid dysfunction (hyperthyroidism or hypothyroidism) or non-toxic goitre, and a high prevalence of thyroid peroxidase antibodies.

b **True.** Her identical twin is significantly more likely than even an HLA-identical sibling to 'share' this disorder. This highlights the existence and relevance of as yet uncharacterized genes outside the HLA region. Increasing age and acquired factors also play a role in triggering overt disease. Iodine and viral infection (retroviruses in particular) have been implicated.

c **True.** Every endocrine organ can be involved in this process: insulin-dependent diabetes, Addison's disease (eponymously termed Schmidt's syndrome when associated with autoimmune hypothyroidism), hypoparathyroidism, hypopituitarism, and premature ovarian failure (in descending order of likelihood). Again, these disorders would be expected with increased frequency in her first-degree relatives. The term 'type II polyglandular disorder' is applied to this complex.

d **False.** All individual organ-specific immune disorders (listed in c above) have an increased association with HLA-DR3 and DR4 and certain DQ haplotypes. There is no specific genetic marker profile for the combination of disorders within the type II polyglandular syndrome.

e **False.** There is no difference, either in age of onset or other clinical characteristic between familial and sporadic cases.

C.7 a **True.** In addition, there is a higher incidence in patients with Klinefelter's syndrome (XXY). In Down's syndrome (trisomy 21), the prevalence of TPO positivity and thyroid dysfunction is about 4 times higher than in a control population. The reason for these chromosome-related variations in prevalence is obscure, since the major gene (MHC) determinant of organ-specific autoimmune disease lies on (unrelated) chromosome 6.

b **True.** Pernicious anaemia is in fact more frequently associated with autoimmune thyroid disorders than any of the other endocrine disorders mentioned in C.6. Intrinsic factor antibody (and to a lesser extent parietal cell antibody) positivity are the serological 'hallmarks'. Idiopathic thrombocytopaenic purpura (ITP) is also associated.

c **True.** Both systemic lupus erythematosus and rheumatoid arthritis are specifically associated with autoimmune thyroid disease. In Sjögren's (sicca) syndrome, the prevalence of TPO positivity has been as high as 40% in some series. Coeliac disease (gluten-sensitive enteropathy) also forms part of this complex.

d **True.** This condition is linked to impaired cell-mediated immunity, and has a specifically high association with Addison's disease and hypoparathyroidism. The complex has been referred to as type I polyglandular syndrome, occurs at an earlier age than type II, does not have associated HLA linkage, despite occasional co-incidence of autoimmune thyroid, and other endocrine deficiency syndromes.

e **True.** Vitiligo is present in approximately 20% of patients with Addison's disease and 10% of patients with autoimmune thyroid disease, and may precede these conditions by more than 10 years. Antimelanocyte antibodies are detectable in most instances, directed towards the 69 kDa protein tyrosinase, which has a key role in melanin synthesis.

C.8 a **True.** Any pituitary adenoma may occur within the MEN-1 (Wermer) syndrome, either non-functioning (50% of cases) or functioning tumours such as prolactinoma, Cushing's disease (ACTH-producing adenoma), and prolactinoma. By age 20 apparently non-functioning tumours of considerable size may be present, only later in life acquiring secretory potential.

b **True.** Either gastrinoma or insulinoma is the presenting tumour in almost 70% of cases. In contrast to sporadic cases, they are often multifocal. Diarrhoea may figure strongly in the symptom complex of gastrinoma as part of the Zollinger–Ellison syndrome. Insulinoma is less likely to be malignant than in its sporadic form, gastrinoma is more likely to be malignant and metastatic by the time it is diagnosed. Somatostatinoma and pancreatic or intestinal carcinoid may also rarely occur in this syndrome.

c **False.** Adrenal medullary tumours are not part of he MEN-1 syndrome. However, non-functioning and also occasionally functioning adrenal cortical (cortisol or aldosterone-producing) adenomas are found in some cases.

d **False.** Although teratomas are often functioning tumours (secreting LH or hCG), they are of germ cell origin and sporadic.

e **True.** Hyperparathyroidism is eventually present in 90% of cases of MEN-1, and may be asymptomatic for many years. In contrast to sporadic cases, hypercalcaemia may suddenly escalate with typical clinical consequences. Multifocal adenomas are usual, superimposed on an underlying hyperplastic process.

C.9 a **True.** This is present in approximately 50% of MEN-2 cases (also known as Sipple's syndrome), with bilateral pathological hyperplasis as the underlying process ultimately leading to formation of tumours, 70% of which are eventually bilateral, but only occasionally malignant. Not all cases are hypertensive.

b **False.** Differentiated (papillary or follicular) carcinoma is a rare component only of the *MEN-1* syndrome. *Medullary* thyroid carcinoma (MTC), based on underlying neural crest-derived C cell hyperplasia is often already metastatic at diagnosis. It may occur without other endocrine abnormality in a familial form (FMTC), which has a more benign course. More commonly it is the principal association with phaeochromocytoma in both the MEN-2A and MEN-2B 'sub' syndromes. Severe diarrhoea is often present, presumably mediated by a peptide cosecreted with calcitonin, although calcitonin itself increases terminal ileal secretions and may contribute in some cases. Ectopic ACTH is common.

c **True.** Compared with MEN-1, it is less frequently present and less progressive. It is even more uncommon in the MEN-2B variant.

d **False.** Lipomas are the only (uncommon) cutaneous components of the *MEN-1* syndrome. However, nodular neuromas of the eyelids, tongue, and gastrointestinal mucosa identify the MEN-2B syndrome, often accompanied by marfanoid features (tallness, arched palate, arachnodactyly). MEN-2B is also known MEN-3 syndrome.

e **False.** These are usually sporadic, but may occur as an uncommon feature of *MEN-1*, either in the bronchus, thymus, pancreas, stomach, or small bowel. Typical flushing, diarrhoea, and metastatic potential is present in all sites, together with a proneness to ectopic ACTH production.

*C.10*** a **False.** The likelihood of identifying other MEN-1 pathology related to these two tumours is sufficiently low that screening is not justified. The hypercalcaemia of hyperparathyroidism is sometimes associated with elevated serum gastrin levels. Although these may normalize after parathyroidectomy, there is a high incidence of later development of gastrinoma. However, with an (apparently) sporadic islet cell tumour, the 15% likelihood of MEN-2 probably does justify the patient having periodic serum calcium checks and one-off MRI pituitary imaging.

  b **True.** There is currently no genetic marker for MEN-1. However, RFLP analysis of DNA in two affected members of an MEN-1 kindred allows more than 95% identification or exclusion of MEN-1 in other members, thereby identifying the 50% 'at risk' population. In the absence of such selectivity, annual clinical evaluation together with measurements of serum calcium and prolactin together with a gut hormone profile currently represents an appropriate screening protocol.

  c **True.** In the absence of C cell hyperplasia, familial MTC or MEN-2 is most unlikely. However, the recent ability to detect mutations activating a specific (RET) proto-oncogene now permits identification of this genotype, and allows more effective screening and treatment. Abnormalities of RET are found in less than 5% of patients with apparently sporadic MTC.

  d **False.** Elevation of basal serum calcitonin is expected with larger tumours. However, it is important to identify relatives with C cell hyperplasia, a number of whom will also harbour single, or quite often multi-focal microscopic tumours. To this end, the pentagastrin stimulation is an appropriate test, providing diagnostic rises of calcitonin in 95% of such patients. However, availability of (RET) pro-oncogene screening should allow simpler and totally confident identification of all affected relatives.

  e **True.** In an MEN-2B kindred, of which this patient must be a member, all affected individuals have C cell hyperplasia and more than 80% have or will develop MTC: early total thyroidectomy is therefore the treatment of choice. Additional assessment is required to establish whether MTC is already metastatic. The behaviour of MTC in MEN-2B is more aggressive than in MEN-2A.

C.11 a **True.** Diffuse parathyroid hyperplasia and the incidence of multiple adenomas makes this approach essential, followed either by re-implanting some excised parathyroid tissue into an accessible subcutaneous site, or treating with calcium and vitamin D replacement. In MEN-2, this radical approach is not necessary. Large and obvious parathyroid tumours are removed at the time of thyroidectomy. Hypercalcaemia may revert following thyroidectomy, and rarely evolves subsequently, suggesting either accidental parathyroid damage or removal of a parathyroid-stimulating factor (? calcitonin).

b **False.** Pituitary tumours do not behave more aggressively in MEN-1 kindreds than in the sporadic forms. However, the likelihood of functioning tumours is higher. The indications for surgery and medical therapy are identical.

c **True.** Gastrinomas are frequently multifocal and malignant at diagnosis. Once metastatic, surgical removal of imaged tumour masses has not been shown to improve prognosis. Many patients require H2 receptor antagonist or proton-pump inhibitor therapy for control of both the hyperacidity (dyspepsia) and the resulting diarrhoea.

d **False.** The underlying pathology in MEN-2 related adrenal disease is indeed bilateral diffuse or nodular adrenal medullary hyperplasia. However, if bilateral tumours are not anatomically confirmed, only 30% of patients will eventually require removal of the second adrenal: bearing in mind the low risk of malignancy, the remaining 70% can be spared the risks of steroid dependancy and simply screened regularly.

e **False.** There has been little progress with developing effective drugs for malignant MEN tumours. Fortunately, although they may metastasize early, progression of tumours and their metastases is comparatively slow. Furthermore, octreotide and its longer-acting analogues are effective in reducing hypersecretion from pancreatic tumours (including somatostatinomas and glucagonomas), as a supplement to the acid-inhibiting drugs. Diazoxide is available for inhibiting insulin secretion in the rare malignant insulinoma. Indeed, pharmacological approaches are available for all hypersecretory syndromes, although they are all only palliative.

References

Topic: Multiple endocrine neoplasia syndromes
(Detailed multi-author reviews). (1995). *Journal of Internal Medicine*, **238**, No. 10 (October).
Topic: Paraneoplastic (ectopic hormone) syndromes.
Agarwala, S.S. (1996). *Medical Clinics of North America*, **80**, 173–84.
Topic: MEN 2 syndromes.
Eng, C. (1996). *New England Journal of Medicine*, **335**, 943–51.
Topic: The MEN 1 syndrome.
Teh, B.T. *et al.* (1995). *Australian and New Zealand Journal of Surgery*, **65**, 708–13.
Topic: Autoimmunity in familial polyendocrine syndromes.
Weetman, A.P. (1995). *Clinical Endocrinology and Metabolism*, **9**, 157–76.

The entries in **bold** *refer to pages on which* **questions** *are devoted mainly to the topic indexed.*